ART THERAPY AND HEALTH CARE

ART THERAPY
and HEALTH CARE

EDITED BY

Cathy A. Malchiodi

THE GUILFORD PRESS
New York   London

© 2013 The Guilford Press
A Division of Guilford Publications, Inc.
72 Spring Street, New York, NY 10012
www.guilford.com

Printed in the United States of America

This book is printed on acid-free paper.

Last digit is print number: 9   8   7   6   5   4   3   2   1

The authors have checked with sources believed to be reliable in their efforts to provide
information that is complete and generally in accord with the standards of practice that
are accepted at the time of publication. However, in view of the possibility of human
error or changes in medical sciences, neither the authors, nor the editor and publisher,
nor any other party who has been involved in the preparation or publication of this work
warrants that the information contained herein is in every respect accurate or complete,
and they are not responsible for any errors or omissions or the results obtained from the
use of such information. Readers are encouraged to confirm the information contained
in this book with other sources.

Library of Congress Cataloging-in-Publication Data

Art therapy and health care / edited by Cathy A. Malchiodi.
    p. cm.
  Includes bibliographical references and index.
  ISBN 978-1-4625-0716-0 (hardcover: alk. paper)
  1. Art therapy.   I. Malchiodi, Cathy A.
  RC489.A7A7675 2013
  616.89′1656—dc23

                                      2012029733

About the Editor

Cathy A. Malchiodi, PhD, ATR-BC, LPAT, LPCC, is an art therapist, expressive arts therapist, and clinical mental health counselor, as well as a recognized authority on art therapy with children, adults, and families. She is on the faculty of Lesley University and is a visiting professor to universities in the United States and internationally. She is also founder of the Trauma-Informed Practices Institute and President of Art Therapy Without Borders. The first person to have received all three of the American Art Therapy Association's highest honors—the Distinguished Service Award, Clinician Award, and Honorary Life Member Award—Dr. Malchiodi has also received honors from the Kennedy Center and Very Special Arts in Washington, DC. She has published numerous books, articles, and chapters, and has given more than 350 presentations on art therapy.

Contributors

Anya Beebe, MA, LPC, Whole HeART Therapy, LLC, Denver, Colorado

Margaret Carpenter Arnett, BSN, ATR, University of Washington Medical Center, and Childhaven, Seattle, Washington; Yakima Valley Memorial Hospital, Yakima, Washington

Susana Catarino, MA, clinical psychologist and art therapist/art psychotherapist; Portuguese Society of Art Therapy; and Saint House of Mercy, Lisbon, Portugal

Fiona Chang, REAT, RSW, MSocSc, Department of Social Work and Social Administration, University of Hong Kong, and Art in Hospital, Hong Kong, China

Catherine Donovan, BSN (retired), Neonatal Intensive Care Unit, University of California, Davis, Children's Hospital, Sacramento, California

Angel C. Duncan, MA, MFT, ATR, Cognitive Connections, a national art therapy program of the Cognitive Dynamics Foundation, Tuscaloosa, Alabama

Luis Formaiano, MA, BSc, private practice; art therapy with HIV-positive/AIDS patients, Centro Cultural Literario; and Art Therapy Program for Psychiatric Patients, Clínica Las Heras, Buenos Aires, Argentina

Ellen Goldring, ATR-BC, CCLS, LPC, Child Life/Creative Arts Therapy, Joseph M. Sanzari Children's Hospital, Hackensack University Medical Center, Hackensack, New Jersey

Janice Havlena, MA, ATR-BC, Art Therapy Program, Edgewood College, Madison, Wisconsin

Hannah K. Hunter, MFA, Child Life and Creative Arts Therapy Department, University of California, Davis, Children's Hospital, Sacramento, California

Ephrat Huss, PhD, Department of Social Work, Ben Gurion University of the Negev, Beer Sheva, Israel

Emily R. Johnson, MA, ATR, LPCC, Norton Cancer Institute at Kosair Children's Hospital, Louisville, Kentucky

Deborah Koff-Chapin, BFA, Expressive Art Therapy Program, California Institute of Integral Studies, San Francisco, California; Center for Touch Drawing, Langley, Washington

Donald Lewis, LCSW, Hospice Program, University of California, Davis, Health System, Sacramento, California

John Lorance, MS, ATR, LPCA, LMFTA, private practice; Integrative Art Psychotherapy and Counseling, Charlotte, North Carolina

Cathy A. Malchiodi, PhD, ATR-BC, LPAT, LPCC, Division of Expressive Therapies, Lesley University, Cambridge, Massachusetts; Trauma-Informed Practices Institute, Louisville, Kentucky

Elizabeth Sanders Martin, LPCC, LPAT, CCLS, Kosair Children's Hospital, Louisville, Kentucky

Margaret M. McGuinness, MA, MEd, ATR-BC, independent practitioner; Center for Therapeutic Learning and Communication, Clinton Township, Michigan; The Epilepsy Foundation of Michigan, Studio E: the Epilepsy Art Therapy Program, Detroit, Michigan

Jill V. McNutt, MS, ATR-BC, Division of Expressive Therapies, Lesley University, Cambridge, Massachusetts; Department of Art Therapy, Mount Mary College, and Art Therapy, Aurora Healthcare, Milwaukee, Wisconsin

Rebekah Near, CAGS, LCAT, The Art 2 Heart Project, Albany, New York; Community Expressive Arts Project, a division of the Trustee Leader Scholar Program, Bard College, Annandale-on-Hudson, New York

Shari L. Racut, MA, ATR-BC, PCC, Family and Child Life Services Department, Rainbow Babies and Children's Hospital, Cleveland, Ohio

Laury Rappaport, PhD, ATR-BC, REAT, LMFT, LMHC, Focusing and Expressive Arts Institute, Santa Rosa, California; Five Branches Mind–Body Center, Five Branches University, Santa Cruz, California; Division of Expressive Therapies, Lesley University, Cambridge, Massachusetts

Orly Sarid, PhD, Department of Social Work, Ben Gurion University of the Negev, Beer Sheva, Israel

Kathy J. Schnur, RN, Med, ATR-BC, private practice; Willows Creek Counseling and Art Center, Lake Orion, Michigan

Rachel C. Schreibman, MA, Fairfax County Public Schools, Fairfax, Virginia; Art Therapy Dialysis Program, Renal Support Network, Glendale, California

Carl E. Stafstrom, MD, PhD, Pediatric Neurology Section, Department of Neurology, University of Wisconsin–Madison, Madison, Wisconsin

Marta Tagarro, MA, clinical psychologist and art therapist/art psychotherapist; Portuguese Society of Art Therapy, Lisbon, Portugal; Department of Education and Curriculum, Superior School of Education of Santarém, Santarém, Portugal

Pamela Ullmann, MS, ATR-BC, LCAT, CCLS, Colors of Play, LLC, Healing Arts Family Connection, Bergen County, New Jersey; Heartsong, Westchester, New York

Elizabeth Warson, PhD, ATR-BC, LPC, NCC, Graduate Art Therapy Program, The George Washington University, Alexandria, Virginia

Marcia Weisbrot, MA, MFA, ATR-BC, professional artist and art therapy consultant, San Francisco, California

Contents

Introduction to Art Therapy in Health Care Settings

Cathy A. Malchiodi

In working on this book, I recalled many children and adults living with serious or chronic illnesses or physical challenges who I have been privileged to encounter in art therapy sessions over the last two decades. Many have had cancer. Others have struggled with autoimmune illnesses like rheumatoid arthritis. Some have had to adjust to traumatic brain injury, paraplegia, or chronic pain due to accidents, disasters, or war. While each has had a lasting impact on me, one individual's story comes to mind in particular because it eloquently summarizes how art therapy makes a difference in the lives of people confronted with a medical illness or physical disability.

At the age of 43, Michaela was diagnosed with ovarian cancer. For most of her adult life she had been a triathlete and a self-proclaimed "health nut" who was careful about her diet and health. She was also nurse who worked in the adult oncology unit and assisted in surgery at a university hospital. Because of her medical background as a nurse, Michaela knew in great detail what a diagnosis of ovarian cancer meant and the challenges that were ahead of her, including treatment that would be physically exhausting and often toxic in order to rid her body of cancer. When I met her for our first few art therapy sessions, Michaela explained to me that she wanted to include art making and creative writing as part of her treatment. She jokingly referred to her illness as "cancer schmancer," maintaining a uniquely positive attitude during what were months of debilitating side effects of chemotherapy and fatigue resulting from radiation. From the outset, Michaela committed herself to do whatever possible to treat not only the disease, but also to explore the "psycho-social-spiritual" effects of the illness on mind and body with everything available, including art therapy.

Michaela had never considered herself a creative person, but she decided to risk expressing herself in art and writing as a way to cope with her diagnosis, medical interventions, medications, and changes in her life. In initial sessions, we focused on the

1

feelings she had about her cancer diagnosis through drawings and collage. One of the first images Michaela created (see Figure 1) was a drawing of her anger; for the first time in her life, she felt deeply angry, even questioning and blaming herself for her illness despite her own medical knowledge about ovarian cancer. While she felt uncomfortable expressing this anger to even her closest family members and friends, drawing and writing about her feelings provided ways to acknowledge feelings, put her emotions into perspective, and release some of the stress associated with the challenges of being a patient for the first time in her life. We also explored the growing depression (see Figure 2) she was experiencing and how well she hid it from family, friends, and colleagues at the hospital. When we discussed the content of this particular drawing, Michaela immediately recognized how well she disguised her depression, keeping it deep inside herself, and how the lines in this art expression mimicked those in her anger drawing. These early art expressions became the basis for a series of larger drawings and paintings that Michaela eventually exhibited at the local Gilda's Club, a support program for cancer survivors, where she also shared her creative writing about her experiences with other patients and families.

A year after surgery, chemotherapy, and radiation treatments, Michaela's cancer went into remission. She began long distance running again, took on more responsibilities at work, and became more hopeful about her prognosis because there was no evidence of cancer according to tests. The remission was short-lived and 9 months later her cancer returned in an inoperable Stage 4 form in her liver and lungs. Right after this recurrence, her husband of 13 years decided that he did not want to remain in a marriage to a terminally ill wife and filed for divorce. As Michaela recalled, "things really have hit rock bottom," and she subsequently experienced a month of severe grief reactions and depression due to the divorce and her prognosis. Fortunately, she had extensive

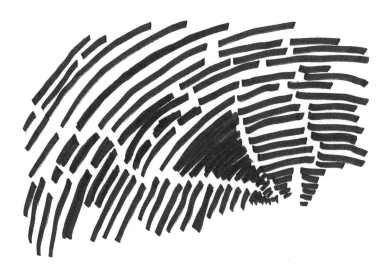

FIGURE 1. Michaela's "anger" drawing.

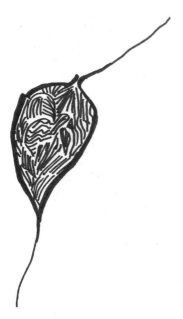

FIGURE 2. Michaela's depiction of "depression."

social support from family and friends who were available to help Michaela during the inevitable progression of the cancer and the loss of a primary relationship. In many art therapy sessions during this time she depicted what she called the "struggle between life and death," and we talked about the process of dying and if there was indeed an afterlife, soul, or spirit. Art making and writing strengthened Michaela's resolve to find peace from any lingering anger and sadness about simultaneously having cancer and enduring a divorce.

As Michaela became more physically debilitated, her visits to my office became too exhausting and I brought art materials to her apartment. In these final sessions before she became too ill to participate, I helped Michaela organize her writing journals and create colorful binders for them. She also continued to make art, working on what she called an "inner sense of compassion" for herself that she eventually symbolized in a small mixed media collage piece called "Buddha Blossom" (see Figure 3). Michaela created a hand-drawn image of a brilliant yellow, orange, and red rose blooming and placed it on a background that she said represented the cancer cells overtaking her body. In this artwork, she depicted her transformation into someone who was no longer a cancer patient. It had helped her to leave cancer behind and make peace with both the divorce and the process of dying.

Michaela's story is both compelling and inspiring to all those who confront mortality when living with a diagnosis of cancer or other condition. From working with Michaela, I learned much of what I now believe about the role of art expression as therapy for individuals and families with life-threatening or chronic illness. Michaela and I never discussed art therapy as a "cure" for her cancer, but we often talked about how her creative expression through art and writing were part of her "healing" in the

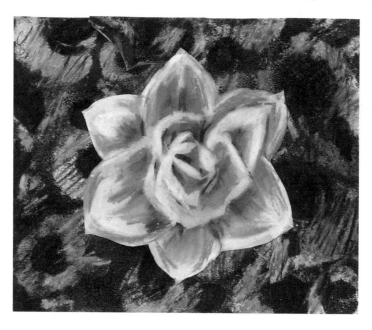

FIGURE 3. Michaela's mixed media collage: "Buddha Blossom."

sense of coming to terms with her illness, a divorce, and eventually the process of dying. After Michaela died peacefully at home with her family and hospice care at her bedside, I continued to work with her parents and her brother to help them through their grief. A large part of our family sessions were not only focused on commemorating Michaela's life through art expression, but also in collecting, reviewing, and framing many of the artworks she created during art therapy. Her writing journals became a treasured legacy and a record of a life well lived and well loved by family, friends, and colleagues.

In a growing number of hospitals and medical settings in the United States and internationally, many patients, not just those with cancer but also those of all ages with chronic or serious illnesses and physical challenges, are using art to express their experiences and reduce stress. Art therapy programs and services are finding their way into inpatient and outpatient treatment, complementary medicine, wellness programs, rehabilitation units, assisted care, and hospice/palliative care. These applications of art therapy are often defined as "medical art therapy," the clinical use of art expression and imagery with individuals who are physically ill, experiencing bodily trauma, or undergoing invasive or aggressive medical procedures such as surgery or chemotherapy (Long, Chapman, Appleton, Abrahms, & Palmer, 1989; Malchiodi, 1993, 1999a, 1999b, 2005, 2012a). Additionally, medical art therapy is part of the continuum of the "arts in healthcare," a wide-ranging international movement including art therapy and other creative arts therapies, that promotes the development and application of the arts, creativity, and imagination as agents of wellness. In a 2009 monograph, the Society for the Arts in Healthcare reported that hospitals and healthcare settings are increasingly applying the arts, including art therapy, as an important and integral part of health care.

GOALS OF ART THERAPY IN HEALTH CARE SETTINGS

This volume is rich in content and examples from practitioners on how art therapy is used with a variety of individuals and patient populations of all ages and in medical settings ranging from inpatient hospitals, outpatient clinics, hospice, assisted care, rehabilitation, open studios, and independent practice. Because of the diversity in settings and patient needs, art therapists often tailor treatment and intervention to meet individuals' unique needs and specific circumstances. However, there are also many goals that are part of most patients' art therapy in medical settings; these include, but are not limited to the following: (1) psychosocial care, (2) rehabilitation, (3) health benefits, and (4) reauthoring the dominant narrative of illness.

Psychosocial Care

In most inpatient hospital settings, the central goal of art therapy is to address and enhance the psychosocial care of patients. In brief, psychosocial care focuses on psychological and social aspects of cognitive and emotional growth and development. For example, art-based interventions may be used to support children's self-expression of perceptions and emotions about having cancer or a chronic illness, or social aspects such as the capacity to form attachments to caregivers, family, and peers and to maintain relationships during medical treatment and recovery. The overall goal of psychosocial care is to support and enhance patients' growth and recovery by addressing emotional, cognitive, and social needs. With children, developmental characteristics are central to successful psychosocial intervention (see Chapter 3, this volume, for more information on psychosocial care).

Supporting a sense of control (Councill, 2012; Malchiodi, 2012a) is central to the application of art therapy as a psychosocial intervention with patients who often find themselves losing control when hospitalized or incapacitated. For example, consider the child or adult who is told to "hold still" for a painful procedure or test and often one that they do not understand (Rollins & Riccio, 2003); patients often feel fearful, powerless, and confused about medical interventions despite health care professionals' best efforts to provide comfort and assurance. In reference to work with adult cancer patients like Michaela:

> Art expression is a way to convey painful, confusing, and contradictory experiences of illness that are difficult to communicate with words alone; in this sense, its central purpose is meaning-making. In addition, the very act of drawing, painting, or constructing can be a personally empowering experience in contrast to the loss of control that generally accompanies illness. For example, patients who are seriously ill often lose control of their time during their hospitalization because of the hospital's schedule and necessary medical treatments; they also may lose control of their bodies due to disease, medical intervention, surgery, or disability. In these circumstances art expression can help people regain some measure of control in their lives by providing an active process involving the freedom to

choose materials, style, and subject matter; to play freely with color, lines, forms, and textures; and to create what one wants to create. This element of choice can contribute to feelings of autonomy and dignity when other aspects of life seem out of control. (Malchiodi, 2012a, p. 399)

In the field of health psychology, self-efficacy (the internal perception of control) is a determining factor as to whether an individual is empowered to adopt and maintain a health behavior and feels positive about health outcomes. For example, Cohen's (2006) studies of creativity and aging provide evidence that the experience of self-efficacy through the arts provides older adults with a heightened sense of control and mastery and thus increased participation in healthy behaviors. Councill (2012), in work with pediatric patients, notes that successful art therapy provides a sense of mastery over troubling events inherent to medical intervention, particularly when ameliorating psychological trauma associated with loss of control.

Additionally, medical art therapists use approaches that provide patients with the opportunity for symbolic expression through visual arts in order to develop appropriate psychosocial interventions. They often use drawing, in particular, as a way to provide a subjective measure of how an individual is dealing with illness and recovery, as a developmental assessment with children, and as a form of communication about medical treatment (Councill, 2012; Malchiodi, 1998, 1999b). While there are few specific ways to evaluate patients through art alone, a great deal can be learned from the metaphors and narratives about their creative expressions (see Chapter 2, this volume, for more information). Art therapists working on pediatric units are well versed in evaluating the content of children's art expressions and how they may communicate perceptions and experiences with hospitalization, illness, and death and dying (Councill, 2012; Malchiodi, 1998; 1999b). Also, practitioners working with older adults who may have Alzheimer's disease, dementia, or cognitive challenges due to stroke also capitalize on art expression as a way to evaluate and understand how memory and cognition may be compromised or affected by these conditions (Levine-Madori, 2009; Malchiodi, 2012c; Wald, 1999).

Rehabilitation

For patients who have survived traumatic accidents involving brain injuries or other physical injuries, art therapy not only enhances psychosocial care, but also physical and cognitive recovery. As McGraw (1999) notes after several decades of work with individuals with physical disabilities and medical conditions, traditional verbal psychotherapy is often inappropriate or impossible. These individuals may have mobility impairments from paraplegia or quadriplegia, amputation or burns, traumatic brain injury, multiple sclerosis, or strokes. What becomes important in addition to self-efficacy and self-expression is addressing motor function, improving memory skills, and increasing cognitive and physical functioning.

Medical rehabilitation (also called medical rehab) is the process of helping people achieve their most functional levels of ability after a disabling illness or accident. Art

therapy that capitalizes on manipulation of materials and media focuses on both rehabilitative and developmental aspects that build skills and improve functioning. For example,
young patients who may need to learn and practice age-appropriate developmental tasks
might be encouraged to put together a gadget, build an object with clay, or learn how to
hold a syringe filled with paint and create an image on paper. Because of physical challenges, some patients may need adaptations that make possible artistic expression when
fine motor skills are compromised. In Chapter 1, this volume, Ulmann describes various
ways to make adaptations in art materials to enable physically disabled children to benefit from art and improve developmental skills. McGuninness and Schnur (Chapter 17,
this volume) and Weisbrot (Chapter 16, this volume) underscore the value of art therapy
as a component of rehabilitation for a variety of conditions, including traumatic brain
injury, stroke, tumors, burns, spinal cord injuries, and arthritis. In particular, McGuinness and Schnur cite the importance of art therapy as remediation for executive functioning lost due to brain injuries and cite improvement in attention and independence as
important outcomes of structured art therapy interventions. Overall, art therapy, when
used as a complement to rehabilitation, provides uniquely creative methods that assist
in patient recovery by enhancing functionality and increasing or maintaining cognitive
abilities, while providing an opportunity for personal expression about disability and
physical challenges.

Health Benefits

While psychosocial and rehabilitative art-based intervention can be defined as health
enhancing, the rapidly increasing knowledge about art expression and the brain is providing information on how art therapy actually may complement medical treatment
in producing positive health outcomes. For example, Lusebrink (2004, 2010) observes
that images are a bridge between body and mind that influences information processing
and physiological and emotional changes in the body. Guided imagery, an experiential
process in which an individual is directed through relaxation followed by suggestions
to imagine specific images, has been used to reduce symptoms, change mood, and harness the body's healing capacities. Van Kuiken's (2004) meta-analysis of guided imagery literature since 1996 reported that imagery has the potential to improve immunity
and psychological resilience. Four different categories of imagery include: (1) pleasant
imagery, (2) physiologically focused imagery, (3) mental rehearsing or reframing, and
(4) receptive imagery. As our understanding of how the brain processes and responds to
imagery increases, art therapists and other professionals have applied these principles of
mental and guided imagery with art therapy in their work with individuals in a variety
of settings (Malchiodi, 1999a, 2012b) (see Chapter 9, this volume, for further discussion).

Additionally, most agree that art therapy can be used to tap the body's relaxation
response. Drawing, for example, is hypothesized to facilitate children's verbal reports of
emotionally laden events in several ways: reduction of anxiety, helping the child feel
comfortable with the therapist, increasing memory retrieval, organizing narratives, and
prompting the child to tell more details than in a solely verbal interview (Gross &

Haynes, 1998; Lev-Weisel & Liraz, 2007). Benson (1975; Benson & Proctor, 2010) pioneered medicine's understanding of the "relaxation response," a phenomenon that is now being embraced within psychosocial treatment of people with serious illness. Newer approaches such as mindfulness-based cognitive therapy and mindfulness-based stress reduction (Kabat-Zinn, 2006) have been adapted and integrated with art therapy for various medical populations including adult oncology (Monti et al., 2006), underscoring that art making is one way to reduce stress and, for some people, to induce the "relaxation response." Nainis, Paice, and Ratner (2006), in work with cancer patients, were able to demonstrate that even brief applications of art therapy reduces pain perception, a response often connected to relaxation. Because art making is a sensory activity, one that involves tactile, visual, kinesthetic, and other senses, it is naturally self-soothing and involves repetitive activity that can induce relaxation and well-being similar to what Benson reported in his studies (Malchiodi, 2008).

The following research provides evidence of the health-giving benefits of participating in visual arts or art therapy activities:

1. Several studies demonstrate that art therapy enhances the psychosocial treatment of cancer, including decreased symptoms of distress, improved quality of life, and perceptions of body image, reduction of pain perception, and general physical and psychological health (Monti et al., 2006; Nainis et al., 2002b; Oster & Svensk, 2006; Svensk et al., 2009).

2. Studies indicate a reduction of depression and fatigue levels in cancer patients on chemotherapy (Bar-Sela, Atid, Danos, Gabay, & Epelbaum, 2007).

3. Individuals who participate in an art therapy/museum education program experience increased perceptions of support, psychological strength, and insights about their cancer experience (Deanne, Fitch, & Carman, 2000).

4. Art therapy strengthens positive feelings, alleviates distress, and helps individuals to clarify existential questions for adult bone marrow transplant patients (Gabriel, Bromberg, Vandenbovenkamp, Kornblith, & Luzzato, 2001).

5. Research with children with cancer indicates that engaging in drawing and painting is an effective method for dealing with pain and other disturbing symptoms of illness and treatment (Rollins, 2005).

6. Research on art therapy with children with asthma indicates that it reduces anxiety, improve feelings of quality of life, and strengthen self-concept (Beebe, Gelfand, & Bender, 2010; also see Chapter 5, this volume).

7. Evidence indicates that art therapy and other creative arts therapies stimulate cognitive function in older adults who have dementia or related disorders (Levine-Madori, 2009) and may reduce depression in those with Parkinson's disease (Elkis-Abuhoff, Goldblatt, Gaydos, & Coratto, 2008).

8. Art making may reduce anxiety and stress reactions as measured by cortisol (Walsh, Radcliffe, Castillo, Kumar, & Broschard, 2007; see also Chapter 25, this volume).

9. Visual arts also serve as a diagnostic tool; asthma symptoms may be revealed in children's illness drawings (Gabriels, Wamboldt, McCormick, Adams, & McTaggart, 2000).

Re-Authoring the Dominant Narrative of Illness

Finally, art therapy provides a creative experience that is not clearly categorized as psychosocial, rehabilitative, or health giving. In brief, it is art therapy's ability to provide patients with the chance to re-author the dominant narrative of their illness or physical disability and provide a way to explore what is referred to as "posttraumatic growth" (Joseph, 2011). Returning to Michaela's story as a person with cancer, art therapy ultimately not only became a way to find meaning and express the story of her experiences with a cancer diagnosis and treatment and the process of death and dying, but also provided a medium for reframing her cancer narrative. Art expression often becomes a pathway for transforming feelings and perceptions into a new life story and, as a result, creating a new sense of self (Malchiodi, 1999a). This "re-authoring" of one's life story may be different for each person, and it often includes one or more of the following aspects: development of new outlooks; discovery of answers to the unanswered questions (e.g., Why did God do this to me?); revisions in the way one lives life; creation of solutions or resolutions to personal struggles; creation of a new "post-illness" identity; or discovery of an explanation for why one's life has been altered by illness, disability, or physical trauma. It is a form of "meaning making" that can be ultimately helpful in an individual's adjustment and acceptance of serious or life-threatening conditions (Collie & Kante, 2011).

I also believe that art expression is particularly helpful to individuals with medical illnesses because people who are seriously ill often have two explanations for their condition, one verbal and one nonverbal (Malchiodi, 1999b, 2008). Their verbal explanation is often a detailed description of the illness and a rational recounting of their conditions based on medical knowledge. Art and expressive work facilitates a nonverbal explanation, one is a more personal and idiosyncratic, and often private, perception of illness. This personal explanation may or may not be conscious and may involve confusion, misunderstanding, fear, or anxiety, but it is more often expressed in a nonverbal modality such as art rather than initially communicated with words. Oliver Sacks (1990), the well-known British neurosurgeon, describes this in his conceptualization of awakening that he describes as " . . . a reversal. The patient ceases to feel the presence of illness and the absence of the world, and comes to feel the absence of his illness and the full presence of the world" (p. 53). Because people often shift away from the presence of illness in their lives while making art, momentarily forgetting that they are sick or disabled, they have the opportunity to become "awakened" to experiences other than their illness and, through art expression and the guidance of the therapist, are able to develop and express new perspectives and reframe the dominant story of illness into transformative and empowering narratives.

CONCLUSION

As you will learn throughout this book, art therapy is being applied to a wide array of health issues including cancer; chronic illnesses such as asthma, epilepsy, and renal disease; neurological disorders and traumatic brain injuries; physical disabilities; and Alzheimer's disease and dementia to improve individuals' wellness, symptoms, and quality of life. Each chapter explains and illustrates how art therapy helps children and adults address the psychosocial challenges of illness, regain a sense of empowerment and efficacy, improve functioning, and enhance health and well-being. Although these chapters have been written by expert art therapy professionals throughout the United States and internationally, and the world, this book is also intended as a guide for all health care practitioners who want to learn more about how art therapy complements medical intervention and supports patients' adjustment and recovery. As mentor physician Bernie Siegel once noted, "I wish all physicians would add a box of crayons to their diagnostic and therapeutic tools" (1990, p. 114). His observation highlights what art therapists who work in medical settings already know—that art has a powerful role in treatment and restoration of health in patients of all ages.

REFERENCES

Bar-Sela, G., Atid, L., Danos, S., Gabay, N., & Epelbaum, P. (2007). Art therapy improved depression and influenced fatigue levels in cancer patients on chemotherapy. *Psychoonocology, 16,* 980–984.

Beebe, A., Gelfand, W., & Bender, B. (2010). A randomized trial to test the effectiveness of art therapy for children with asthma. *Journal of Allergy and Clinical Immunology, 126*(2), 263–266.

Benson, H. (1975). *The relaxation response.* New York: William Morrow.

Benson, H., & Proctor, W. (2010). *The relaxation revolution.* New York: Scribner.

Cohen, G. (2006). *The creativity and aging study: The impact of professionally conducted cultural programs on older adults.* Retrieved December 17, 2011, from *www.nea.gov/resources/accessibility/CnA-Rep4-30-06.pdf.*

Collie, K., & Kante, A. (2011). Art groups for marginalized women with breast cancer. *Qualitative Health Research, 21*(5), 652–661.

Councill, T. (2012). Medical art therapy with children. In C. A. Malchiodi (Ed.), *Handbook of art therapy* (2nd ed., pp. 222–240). New York: Guilford Press.

Deanne, K., Fitch, M., & Carman, M. (2000). An innovative art therapy program for cancer patients. *Canadian Oncology Nursing Journal, 10,* 147–157.

Elkis-Abuhoff, D., Goldblatt, R., Gaydos, M., & Coratto, S. (2008). The effects of clay manipulation on somatic dysfunction and emotional distress in patients diagnosed with Parkinson's disease. *Art Therapy: Journal of the American Art Therapy Association, 25*(3), 122–128.

Gabriel, B., Bromberg, E., Vandenbovenkamp, J., Kornblith, A., & Luzzato, P. (2001). Art therapy with adult bone marrow transplant patients in isolation: A pilot study. *Psycho-Oncology, 10,* 114–123.

Gabriels, R., Wamboldt, M., McCormick, D., Adams, T., & McTaggart, S. (2000). Children's illness drawings and asthma symptom awareness. *Journal of Asthma, 37*(7), 565–574.

Gross, J., & Haynes, H. (1998). Drawing facilitates children's verbal reports of emotional laden events. *Journal of Experimental Psychology, 4,* 163–179.

Hundleby, M., Collie, K., & Carlson, L. (2010). Creative arts in oncology. In D. Kissane, B. Bultz, P. Butow, & I. Finlay (Eds.), *Handbook of communication in cancer and palliative care.* New York: Oxford University Press.

Joseph, S. (2011). *What does not kill us: The new psychology of posttraumatic growth.* New York: Basic Books.

Kabat-Zinn, J. (2006). *Coming to our senses: Healing ourselves and the world through mindfulness.* New: York: Hyperion.

Lev-Wiesel, R., & Liraz, R. (2007). Drawings versus narratives: Drawing as a tool to encourage verbalization in children whose fathers are drug abusers. *Clinical Child Psychology and Psychiatry, 12*(1), 65–75.

Levine-Madori, L. (2009). Uses of therapeutic thematic arts programming (TTAP Method) for enhanced cognitive and psychosocial functioning in the geriatric population. *American Journal of Recreation Therapy, 8*(1), 25–31.

Long, J., Chapman, L., Appleton, V., Abrahms, L., & Palmer, S. (1989). Innovations in medical art therapy. In *Proceedings of the 20th annual American Art Therapy Association Conference.* Mundelein, IL: American Art Therapy Association.

Lusebrink, V. B. (2004). Art therapy and the brain: An attempt to understand the underlying processes of art expression in therapy. *Art Therapy: Journal of the American Art Therapy Association, 21*(3), 121–125.

Lusebrink, V. (2010). Assessment and therapeutic application of the Expressive Therapies Continuum. *Art Therapy: Journal of the American Art Therapy Association, 27*(4), 166–170.

Malchiodi, C. A. (1993). Medical art therapy: Contributions to the field of arts medicine. *International Journal of Arts Medicine, 2*(2), 28–31.

Malchiodi, C. A. (1997). Invasive art: Art as empowerment for women with breast cancer. In S. Hogan (Ed.), *Feminist approaches to art therapy* (pp. 49–64). London: Routledge.

Malchiodi, C. A. (1998). *Understanding children's drawings.* New York: Guilford Press.

Malchiodi, C. A. (Ed.). (1999a). *Medical art therapy with adults.* London: Jessica Kingsley.

Malchiodi, C. A. (Ed.). (1999b). *Medical art therapy with children.* London: Jessica Kingsley.

Malchiodi, C. A. (Ed.). (2005). *Expressive therapies.* New York: Guilford Press.

Malchiodi, C. A. (2008). *Creative interventions with traumatized children.* New York: Guilford Press.

Malchiodi, C. A. (2012a). Using art therapy with medical support groups. In C. A. Malchiodi (Ed.), *Handbook of art therapy* (2nd ed., pp. 397–408). New York: Guilford Press.

Malchiodi, C. A. (2012b). Art therapy and the brain. In C. A. Malchiodi (Ed.), *Handbook of art therapy* (2nd ed., pp. 17–26). New York: Guilford Press.

Malchiodi, C. A. (2012c). Creativity and aging: An art therapy perspective. In C. A. Malchiodi (Ed.), *Handbook of art therapy* (2nd ed., pp. 275–287). New York: Guilford Press.

McGraw, M. (1999). Studio-based art therapy for medically ill and physically disabled persons. In C. A. Malchiodi (Ed.), *Medical art therapy with adults* (pp. 243–260). London: Jesssica Kingsley.

Monti, D. A., Peterson, C., Kunkel, E., Hauck, W., Pequignot, E., Rhodes, L., & Brainard, G.

(2006). A randomized, controlled trial of mindfulness-based art therapy (MBAT) for women with cancer. *Psycho-Oncology, 15*(5), 363–373.

Nainis, N., Paice, J., & Ratner, J. (2006) Relieving symptoms in cancer: Innovative use of art therapy. *Journal of Pain and Symptom Management, 31*(2),162–169.

Oster, I., & Svensk, A. (2006). Art therapy improves coping resources: a randomized, controlled study among women with breast cancer. *Palliative Support Care, 4*(1), 57–64.

Rollins, J. (2005). Tell me about it: Drawing as a communication tool for children with cancer. *Journal of Pediatric Oncology Nursing, 22*(4), 203–221.

Rollins, J., & Riccio, L. (2003). *Art with a heart: An arts-in-healthcare program for children and families in home and hospice care.* Washington, DC: WVSA Arts Connection.

Sacks, O. (1990) *Awakenings.* New York: Harper Perennial.

Siegel, B. (1990). *Love, medicine and miracles.* New York: William Morrow.

Society for the Arts in Healthcare. (2009). *State of the field report: Arts in healthcare: 2009.* Washington, DC: Society for the Arts in Healthcare.

Svensk, A., Oster, I., Thyme, K., Magnusson, E., Sjodin, M., Eisemann, et al. (2009). Art therapy improves experienced quality of life among women undergoing treatment for breast cancer: A randomized controlled study. *European Journal of Cancer Care, 18*(1), 69–77.

Van Kuiken, D. (2004). A meta-analysis of the effect of guided imagery practice on outcomes. *Journal of Holistic Nursing, 22*(2), 164–179.

Wald, J. (1999). The role of art therapy in post-stroke rehabilitation. In C. A. Malchiodi (Ed.), *Medical art therapy with adults* (pp. 25–41). London: Jessica Kingsley.

Walsh, S. M., Radcliffe, R. S., Castillo, L. C., Kumar, A. M., & Broschard, D. M. (2007). A pilot study to test the effects of art-making classes for family caregivers of patients with cancer. *Oncology Nursing Forum, 34*(1), E9–E16.

PART I

ART THERAPY WITH CHILD AND ADOLESCENT PATIENTS

INTRODUCTION

All health care professionals would agree that hospitalization and other experiences associated with medical illness and disabling conditions are emotionally and physically difficult for children. For some, encounters with health care are brief; for others who have chronic or recurrent illnesses, there may be long-term or lifetime interactions with medical settings. In all cases, patients' self-perception, sense of control, and quality of life may be altered. For example, Rollins (2008) observes that being touched can bring either comfort or feelings of discomfort and confusing, especially when pediatric patients are examined in areas of their bodies that they have been educated to not let strangers touch. Others note that children and adolescents are afraid of one or more aspects of being in the hospital, such as nursing interventions (Salmela, Salantera, & Aronen, 2009) and separation from parents and family (Coyne, 2006). Developmental level (Malchiodi & Goldring, Chapter 3), the nature of the illness or disability, and previous trauma, loss, or separation affect pediatric patients' responses. Even for the most resilient children or teenagers, loss of privacy and self-efficacy may increase negative perceptions of hospitalization or treatment.

According to Hart and Rollins (2011), helping professionals are increasingly acknowledging the necessity of addressing psychosocial issues in pediatric patients; this recognition has intensified the need for services for children and adolescents that apply the same high standards of care that medical interventions offer. For this reason formal art therapy programs for young patients are becoming more commonplace, particularly in children's hospitals and as part of comprehensive creative arts therapies, child life services, and arts in hospitals programming. Despite this recent recognition, art therapy in health care environments has a lengthy history documenting the use of art and play-based interventions with a variety of pediatric populations (Councill, 1993; Gabriels, 1988; Goodman, 1991; Levinson & Ousterhout, 1979; Malchiodi, 1999; Perkins,

1977). Allied health professionals including child life specialists, play therapists, artists in residence, psychiatric nurses, and activity therapists have also included art expression in their work with hospitalized children and adolescents (Hart & Rollins, 2011; Rode, 1995). In addition, hospital arts and "arts in health care" programs have also contributed to the proliferation of therapeutic art-based services for children (Palmer & Nash, 1991; Society for the Arts in Healthcare, 2009).

This part provides an overview of many of the accepted and emerging "best practices" in art therapy with children and adolescents coping with health issues. Art therapists use a variety of approaches within healthcare settings, including: (1) spontaneous and unstructured art and play-based techniques to meet developmental needs, support gross and fine motor skills, and provide distraction and relaxation; (2) therapeutic art and play-based techniques to enhance self-expression or support catharsis; and (3) medical art therapy and play-based therapy to specifically address patients' perceptions of medical procedures, experiences of hospitalization or illness, and psychosocial challenges for patients and families (Malchiodi, 1999). In hospital settings, this continuum of techniques often includes an emphasis on medical themes and inclusion of medical supplies as art materials to encourage direct expression about worries and concerns regarding medications and treatments. While not a specific focus of this part, work with pediatric patients in hospitals and outpatient clinics also often addresses young patients' traumatic memories and trauma reactions related to medical issues. For example, some children may have survived accidents, physical or sexual assault, burns, or natural disasters. In other cases, the nature of the medical event itself is upsetting, including surgery, diagnostic tests, or invasive medical procedures. Medical art therapy and play-based approaches are used to help children not only express and explore trauma narratives, but also to identify adaptive coping skills, strengths, and resilience; for some, art therapy may be a means to posttraumatic growth (Malchiodi, 2008).

Art therapists are making significant contributions to research on how art expression makes a measurable difference in health care and health outcomes. For example, Havlena and Stafstrom (Chapter 4) describe a research collaboration combining art therapy and neurology to study how art therapy can be applied in work with children and adolescents with epilepsy to enhance quality of life. Beebe (Chapter 5) presents a randomized clinical trial and art therapy protocol with pediatric asthma patients; this study underscores how art therapy may reduce anxiety and strengthen self-concept in children with chronic asthma. The work of these art therapists not only adds to the growing list of studies that suggest art therapy is an effective intervention with patients with chronic illnesses, but also clarifies the need for emotional regulation and psychoeducation in the psychosocial care of pediatric patients.

These contributions also illustrate how art therapy is a mind–body approach to treatment that complements medical intervention and enhances health care professionals' understanding of patients' perceptions of illness and symptoms. The term "body image" is frequently used to describe how an individual mentally represents or perceives his or her body. Art therapists recognize that a child's body image can be threatened by illness, pain and other symptoms, invasive procedures, disfigurement, or surgery. These perceptions and experiences may emerge in drawings and other art expressions. For example, 8-year-old Brandi survived an accidental burning in a house fire and sustained first and some second degree burns to her body. When she came back to the hospital for follow-up visits with doctors, she also spent time with me drawing what she remembered about the fire and how it affected her body. Although her physical healing was progressing accordingly, she emphasized the exact areas of her body that were burned months before, using orange and yellow felt markers to show the first degree (more minor) burns and black to depict the areas of her torso where she experienced second degree (deeper and more extensive) burns (see Figure I.1). Like other children her age she used "hot colors" (yellow and orange) to represent burns and the color black to indicate where the most painful and serious damage from the accident occurred to her body. Other young patients may use art expression in similar ways to reflect a variety of physical aspects of illness and medical treatment including organ transplants, pain, cancer, chemotherapy and radiation, blood draws, or catheters (Carpenter Arnett & Malchiodi, Chapter 2).

Art therapist Tracy Councill summarizes the value of art therapy with children and adolescents coping with illness or disability as follows: "A visit from the art therapist, who brings familiar materials and an invitation to create, instead of needles or pills to

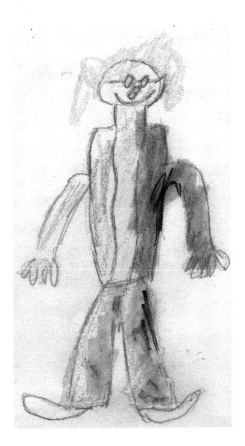

FIGURE I.1. Child's drawing of burns on her body.

swallow can be instantly comforting. Whether that first encounter leads to an expressive piece of artwork or just a few simple marks, it can establish a meaningful link to life outside the hospital and provide a concrete way to respond to the hospital experience" (2012, pp. 238–239). In sum, art therapy empowers young patients to regain a sense of control and mastery, preserve or improve functioning, and reconstruct and restore the self and in doing so, find the possibility for hope and emerge as emotionally whole.

REFERENCES

Councill, T. (1993). Art therapy with pediatric cancer patients: Helping normal children cope with abnormal circumstances. *Art Therapy: Journal of the American Art Therapy Association, 10*(2), 78–87.

Councill, T. (2012). Medical art therapy with children. In C. A. Malchiodi (Ed.), *Handbook of art therapy* (2nd ed., pp. 222–240). New York: Guilford Press.

Coyne, I. (2006). Children's experience of hospitalization. *Journal of Child Health Care, 10*(4), 326–336.

Gabriels, R. (1988). Art therapy assessment of coping styles of severe asthmatics. *Art Therapy: Journal of the American Art Therapy Association, 5*(2), 59–68.

Goodman, R. (1991). Diagnosis of childhood cancer: Case of Tim. In N. Webb (Ed.), *Play therapy with children in crisis*. New York: Guilford Press.

Hart, R., & Rollins, J. (2011). *Therapeutic activities for children and teens coping with health issues.* New York: Wiley.

Levinson, P., & Ousterhout, D. K. (1979). Art and play therapy with pediatric burn patients. *Journal of Burn Care and Rehabilitation, 1*, 42–46.

Malchiodi, C. A. (1999). *Medical art therapy with children.* London: Jessica Kingsley.

Malchiodi, C. A. (2008). *Creative interventions with traumatized children.* New York: Guilford Press.

Palmer. J., & Nash, F. (1991). *The hospital arts handbook.* Durham, NC: Duke University Press.

Perkins, C. F. (1977). The art of life-threatened children: A preliminary study. In R. H. Shoemaker & S. Gonick-Barris (Eds.), *Creativity and the art therapist's identity* (pp. 9–12). Baltimore: American Art Therapy Association.

Rode, D. (1995). Building bridges within the culture of pediatric medicine: The interface of art therapy and child life programming. *Art Therapy: Journal of the American Art Therapy Association, 12*(2), 104–110.

Rollins, J. (2008). The arts in children's health-care settings. In J. Rollins, R. Bolig, & C. Mahan (Eds.), *Meeting children's psychosocial needs across the health-care continuum* (pp. 119–174). Austin, TX: ProEd.

Samela, M., Salantera, S., & Aronen, E. (2009). Child-reported hospital fears in 4- to 6-year-old children. *Pediatric Nursing, 35*(5), 269–276.

Society for the Arts in Healthcare. (2009). *State of the field report: Arts in healthcare: 2009.* Washington, DC: Society for the Arts in Healthcare.

CHAPTER 1

Adaptive Art Therapy with Children Who Have Physical Challenges and Chronic Medical Issues

Pamela Ullmann

This chapter discusses how adaptive art therapy can be used to enhance children's abilities rather than focus on their disabilities and other medically related challenges. "Adaptive art therapy" is a term that describes the methods and techniques used to enable children with physical and medical challenges to experience successful opportunities in making art and engaging in creative expression. By providing opportunities for success, children can begin to feel a sense of pride and accomplishment, leading to more independence and self-mastery. Adaptive art therapy can provide children with physical challenges new modes of expression that, given their limitations, they may have not had the chance to experience. With newfound tools and skills in art making, these children can begin to explore the powerful and transforming world of creativity.

This chapter includes an overview of chronic medical conditions and the role of art therapy in the rehabilitation of children, emphasizing when and how to assist the child through modifications and adaptations, underscoring the use of the "third hand" (Kramer, 1986). My own adaptive art therapy program within a pediatric long-term care facility is described, and specific art therapy methods and materials are discussed.

CHRONIC MEDICAL ILLNESS AND CHILDREN

An "acute" disease or condition in childhood lasts for a short duration. For example, conditions such as tonsillitis or pneumonia may require limited hospitalization, but with family care and support a child generally recovers and goes on to a "normal" life. In contrast, a "chronic" medical condition or disability produces symptoms for a long period of time, perhaps even an entire lifetime. Chronic medical illnesses or conditions are generally defined as those that exist for a minimum of 3 months or longer. Children with ongoing medical issues may be sick or well at any point in time, but they are always living with their illness or condition. Chronic medical issues for children include but are not limited to conditions such as cancer and congenital heart defects, sickle cell anemia, AIDS, epilepsy, spina bifida, muscular dystrophy, cystic fibrosis, asthma, juvenile diabetes, cerebral palsy, allergies, and obesity; children may also have disabilities and challenges due to car accidents, fires or other events. Although these are very different conditions with diverse symptoms, children with chronic conditions have much in common. They often require numerous medical evaluations, long or repeated hospital stays, medical or adaptive equipment, and special accommodations at home and at school. They may perceive themselves as "different" than other children because of limitations, reduced activity levels, and changes in day-to-day life. Their parents, caretakers, siblings, and friends are also affected by the challenges of living or interacting with individuals with ongoing medical issues.

Chronic medical conditions affect children in a variety of ways depending on temperament, the illness or condition, family, culture, and other factors. A child's developmental stage also impacts how he or she responds to and copes with a chronic condition. For example, preschool children are beginning to develop a sense of autonomy. Because illness disrupts their growing independence, they may respond with a tantrum when parents try to administer medication. Being hospitalized may threaten their sense of control. They may also engage in magical thinking, believing that illness is a punishment for thinking "bad" thoughts, hitting a friend, or secretly wishing harm to someone else.

School-age children are mastering skills and their environment, and forming relationships with peers; a chronic medical condition may threaten self-worth and create a feeling of social isolation. In addition to their physical challenges, the pervasiveness of stigmatization toward them can create negative feelings with their peers, and this environment of unfavorable attitudes isolates children with disabilities and lessens their potential to develop a healthy sense of self (Barg, Armstrong, Hertz, & Latimer, 2010).

Chronic illnesses can have a profound impact on children's development and especially their education. Traditional transition plans that help children go from medical facilities back to school may no longer be effective, because the medical service delivery has been changed to reduce the length of hospital stays and has increased outpatient care instead. As a result, transitions from hospital to school emphasize more homebound strategies and flexible school days, and use of adaptive and differentiated instructional techniques to increase child autonomy and address affective issues (Shaw & McCabe, 2007).

SETTINGS FOR ADAPTIVE ART THERAPY

Children with ongoing medical issues may receive intervention while they are patients at a hospital. In this case, art therapy services may be part of an overall team treatment plan that includes nurses and allied health practitioners such as child life specialists, recreational therapists, occupational therapists, speech–language pathologists, and/or physical therapists (see Part I for more information on art therapy and team approaches). Children also may receive art therapy services for medically related disabilities as part of an individualized educational plan (also known as an IEP) through their school. These services may fall under "artistic/cultural therapies" that include the creative arts therapies (art, music, and dance therapy) required to assist children with disabilities or challenges that affect cognitive, behavioral, or physical performance in the classroom. In brief, art therapy may be used to assess functioning and enhance children's emotional, physical, and cognitive development impacted by chronic medical conditions. It may involve direct contact between the therapist and child at school or other facility, or the child's home. In this case, the therapist may also work to educate parents or caretakers and teachers about art-based strategies being employed. Additionally, a practitioner may provide indirect contact through consultation or supervision to help others (volunteers, paraprofessionals, and/or parents) provide appropriate adaptive activities to children in the classroom or at home.

WHAT IS ADAPTIVE ART THERAPY?

Adaptive art therapy, as used with children who are disabled or suffer from chronic medical conditions, is a specific methodology within the field of art therapy. Any form of adaptation is a modification of an organism or its parts that make it more fit for existence under the conditions of its environment. In the case of art therapy with children with disabilities, practitioners essentially modify the conditions by providing assistance when needed, develop techniques to aid in independence, and use tools that can help the children succeed. Keep in mind that there are so many levels of functionality within the scope of this population, depending on the diagnosis, available interventions, therapies, and other socioeconomic circumstances. Some of the severely physically challenged children possess otherwise healthy and normal intellects. Therefore, it is vital that practitioners provide opportunities for them to learn and grow in appropriate and normal environments (Henley, 1992). For the child with severe medical disabilities, it is important that the art therapist empathize with the child's predicament and also take proper steps to ensure safety and success (Henley, 1992, p. 67).

Historically, there are two ways to create positive environments for children requiring adaptive art therapy: ecological and normalization approaches (Anderson, 1992). The "ecological approach" views children in terms of their strengths and abilities, and how these correspond with their sociocultural background, environs, and primary relationships within the learning milieu. "Normalization" is enforced by the principle that emphasizes what the culture deems as "normative" in order to establish or maintain personal behaviors that are as culturally normative as possible (Anderson, 1992, p. 3). In terms of adaptive art making, "art experiences would occur in a context that is as near the age norm as possible" (p. 3). However, within the development of normalization experiences, the internal methods are adapted and formulated to enable the child to achieve mastery and independence.

Edith Kramer (1986) is credited with introducing another principle that is an important factor in exploring adaptive art therapy: the concept of the art therapist serving as the "third hand" for clients who need assistance for a variety of physical or neurological reasons. She defines the "third hand" as a metaphor to describe the art therapist's role and function to service others empathetically. In adaptive art therapy this concept is applied in a variety of ways. Whether assisting with their own hands, as in a method known as "hand over hand," or offering tools, the therapist's main objective is to ensure that clients are able to express what they need to, without attempting to influence their process or product. Kramer emphasizes that the third hand is "a hand that helps the creative process along without being intrusive, without distorting meaning or imposing pictorial ideas or preferences alien to the client" (p. 71).

When assisting children with physical disabilities, practitioners sometimes feel compelled to overassist out of their own need to rescue or to help. However, these actions often do not help the child at all; they should provide just enough assistance to help children achieve their own level of independence. The main goal in working with children who are physically challenged or medically impaired, as stated before, is to enable them to become more independent and to "normalize" their daily lives. In addition, many more goals and objectives that adaptive art therapy can support go beyond this first and fundamental one. Psychosocial functioning includes but is not limited to the following: (1) how a medical condition affects social and emotional well-being; (2) identification of a family support system that assists the child on a regular basis; and (3) what a child really understands about his or her chronic condition and how it affects self-perception (Childress, 2011). Art therapy is not only an adaptive means of building functionality, but it also can be used to tap into psychosocial issues throughout treatment. This is explored in a case study later in this chapter.

ADAPTIVE ART THERAPY AND REHABILITATION

The central goal of a child's stay in any hospital or rehabilitation facility is to heal and to focus first and foremost on his or her physical condition. To this end, rehabilitation therapists (physical therapists, occupational therapists, and speech–language therapists) work to improve overall physical, neurological, and cognitive functioning in children with medical conditions. Therefore, it is important that any adaptive art therapy complement rehabilitation therapists' goals and outcomes for children with chronic medical illnesses or conditions.

Physical therapists, sometimes referred to as PTs, are health care professionals who diagnose and treat individuals of all ages with medical problems or other health-related conditions, illnesses, or injuries that limit their abilities to move and perform functional activities as well as they would like in their daily lives. PTs who work with children either in private practice or in a facility with an interdisciplinary team examine each individual and develop a plan using treatment techniques that promote the ability to move, reduce pain, restore function, and prevent disability. In addition, PTs work with individuals to prevent the loss of mobility before it occurs by developing fitness- and wellness-oriented programs for healthier and more active lifestyles. Although PTs are not trained in mental health, those who work with children are often more sensitive and tuned into children's social and cognitive deficits. Consulting with a child's PT can be very helpful, because the therapist can learn about the child's limitations; the goals the child is working on; the current level of functioning; and most importantly, the behavioral challenges or resistance the PT may be experiencing during sessions with the child.

Occupational therapists, or OTs, help children who have physical, sensory, or cognitive disabilities carry out everyday activities such as brushing their teeth or putting on shoes and socks. An OT helps children with special needs be as independent as possible, whether in a hospital, school, or individual home-based setting. In terms of methods and techniques, most people think that OTs mainly build "fine motor" skills, but the emphasis overall is on how helping the child develop independence in daily life. OTs tend to be more concerned with the ways their work impacts the child's whole life and family experience. Some have a "family-centered" approach, because it is so important to have the family involved in the skills that are being built. In addition, an OT also uses evidence-based instruments that measure not only functionality but also psychosocial issues (Fingerhut, 2009). Since their focus is on functionality and fine motor skills, consultation with OTs is key to developing tools, strategies, and adaptive methods, and designing creative solutions to help children obtain independence through developmentally appropriate activities.

Speech–language pathologists, sometimes called speech therapists (STs), are professionals who assess, diagnose, treat, and help to prevent disorders related to speech, language, cognition, communication, voice, swallowing, and fluency. They work with individuals who either cannot produce sounds or cannot produce the sounds clearly, as well as with those who have speech rhythm and fluency problems, such as stuttering. STs working with disabled children often employ play therapy strategies with the scope of their work, using toys, books, and other "play" items to encourage communication and language skills. It is very helpful to work with STs, because they can provide the art therapist with information and insight about how the child communicates. They can tell us whether the child has receptive language skills (can understand us), expressive language skills (can relate ideas to others), and verbal speaking skills or challenges. This can help the art therapist work with the child more effectively, because children who are nonverbal or have very delayed skills in speech and language are trained in other forms of communication in lieu of or in addition to speaking. Art therapists can also learn and make use of these systems and devices when creating an adaptive program.

Child life specialists, although not considered rehabilitative professionals, are part of the allied health spectrum of services and work in many hospital pediatric departments. They are trained professionals with skill and knowledge in helping children and their families overcome challenging events due to health-related issues. Child life specialists have a strong background in child development and family systems, and promote effective psychosocial growth and coping through play, preparation, education, and self-expression activities. They provide emotional support for families and optimum development of children facing a variety of challenging experiences, particularly those related to health care and hospitalization. Child life specialists provide information, support, and guidance to parents, siblings, and other family members. They also play a vital role in educating caregivers, administrators, and the general public about the needs of children under stress. Many creative art therapists who work in hospital and health care settings choose dual-certification and get their child life credentials. This helps them provide a comprehensive array of clinical and therapeutic services for the children and their families.

Art therapists creating adaptive art therapy programs for children with physical and cognitive challenges in addition to chronic medical conditions need to seek out the professionals just described. By consulting with them, not only do therapists learn about successful adaptive methods and tools, but they also understand more accurately the child's overall response to treatment, resistances, and preferences. For example, the OT may be working to improve a child's grasping ability and fine motor skills; such a child may resist using small art tools or shy away from drawing directives and be more open to collage directives. By offering materials that are more conducive to children's functioning level, practitioners are able to increase chances of successes and mastery for them over time. A PT working with wheelchair-bound children may suggest optimal positioning for participation in activities and provide the physical supports or braces needed to enable children to have more control over their bodies.

ADAPTIVE ART THERAPY APPROACHES

In this section are descriptions of several adaptive art therapy techniques and methods that I developed or discovered while working with children at an inpatient long-term care facility in New York City from 2003 through 2008. In this particular facility there were 136 beds for children ranging from infancy to age 21 years. The diagnoses varied, ranging from mild to severe; they were mostly chronic conditions and occasionally some acute rehabilitation or "orthopedic" cases. Some children stayed several months, while others lived at the facility as their home. Most of the children's conditions comprised a variety of neurological and genetic disorders that impaired their ability to function; more than half were in wheelchairs and needed physical assistance with daily living skills.

Within this facility, children went to an onsite special education school in which the teachers and therapists were trained to create individualized programs. Because of their multiple medical needs, these children often had their nurses, aides, and other therapists come to the school to administer necessary medical treatments and interventions. Applying Kramer's third hand technique, as described earlier, there were opportunities to develop creative projects that supported this methodology. Art therapy interns, an important part of the program, were directed to adopt a "follow the lead of the child" approach, without pressuring the children to create an art product (Eddison, 2005). The concept of being impartial and assisting the children without directly influencing the artwork (Kramer, 1986) was also central.

As all professionals and interns became familiar with the treatment plans and limitations of each child, and consulted with each child's therapists, *adaptive art therapy* plans, projects, and approaches emerged. A typical adaptive art therapy treatment plan included several measurable goals that were recorded and documented quarterly in the child's "plan of care" under the therapeutic activities section in the medical chart. For example, a measurable goal might be "child will participate in a multisensory art making activity for 45 minutes, one time per week" or "child will use the paintbrush independently for 10 minutes during each session." Updates of the care plans were based on the progress of each child. In addition to the care plans, staff members would write progress notes in the mental health section that described child progress in a more narrative format including psychosocial gains.

The major components of adaptive art therapy I discovered while working in the facility included (1) *simple adjustments* to help the child participate; (2) *adaptive tools*, which "assist" the child's ability to make art; and (3) *becoming the art-making tool for the child*. With regard to the last component (becoming the art making tool), an adolescent boy needed help to participate in painting large murals. This young man had been an artist before his disease progressively made him totally unable to control his upper body and fine motor skills. He was cognitively aware and emotionally stable enough to create art. We became his art tools and paintbrushes by having him direct us to paint and tell us which colors and forms went where. We purchased a laser pointer with which he directed us to paint. He was able to get the results he wanted simply by telling us his vision. Although he did not physically paint the pieces, he was the artist and art director.

Additionally, with another child who had severe physical limitations with his arms, we incorporated "adaptive tools" by purchasing a commercially made "mouth stick," so the young patient was able to paint with his mouth. This made him feel so proud and enabled him to feel like the artist he wanted to be. We were fortunate to have an adaptive equipment department at this facility where staff were able to custom-make an easel to attach to his wheelchair, which gave him better function and control in his painting.

ADAPTIVE ART THERAPY AND SENSORY INTEGRATION

Children with physical challenges are often intimidated by art making at first, especially if specific limitations have been issues in creating art in the past. They may feel the pressure to "do something" for the therapist or teacher. When first assessing and working with these children, their play with art materials can help us determine their abilities, limitations, and interests, especially with nonverbal or low-functioning children. Sensory items in art that can be used in this manner include feathers, pom-poms, tissue paper, Crayola Model Magic, foam, fabric, sand (*Note.* sand may be a hazard if there are respiratory issues, or if the child has a tracheotomy, and should be avoided), and a variety of textured media.

"Sensory art therapy" is an approach that allows the children to gain control with the materials, explore their senses, and become familiar with the art therapy session, either individually or in a group. At the same time, the therapist and others can assess the amount of assistance that may be needed for future art therapy directives. For children who have additional developmental disabilities, there may be challenges surrounding sensory activities. "Sensory processing disorder" (SPD; formerly known as "sensory integration dysfunction") is a condition in which sensory signals do not get organized into appropriate responses. Ayres, a pioneering OT and neuroscientist, refers to it as a neurological "traffic jam" that prevents certain parts of the brain from receiving the information needed to interpret sensory information correctly. Children with SPD find it difficult to process and act upon information received through the senses, which creates challenges in performing countless everyday tasks (Ayres, 2005).

Some children with multiple disabilities and medical conditions may exhibit some sensory processing issues; exposing them to the sensory art making may help to desensitize them in these areas. A wonderful, yet simple, sensory art session that we often used at the facility was to create texture collages on Bristol boards (heavyweight paper). A variety of textures (e.g., feathers, sandpaper, crepe paper, cotton balls, and other items with textural and tactile sensitivity) were offered to the children. Children were allowed to feel, toss, and play with the materials before they were invited to create collages with their favorite items (see Figure 1.1).

Another sensory art directive called "swirling colors" (see Figure 1.2) is all about painting with things that roll and having children manipulate the way the paint flows with gross motor movements. We used golf balls in large aluminum pans to conduct the project. In this directive, several areas of sensory stimulation were incorporated:

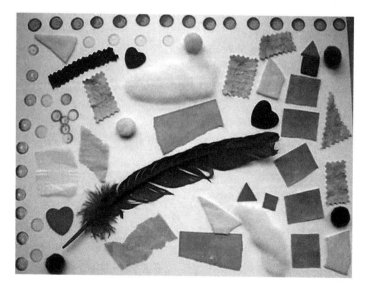

FIGURE 1.1. Example of a texture collage using a variety of tactile and multisensory materials.

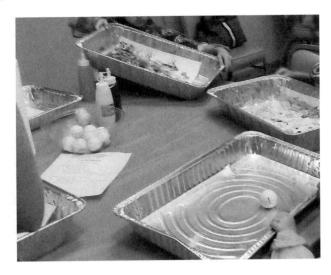

FIGURE 1.2. "Swirling Colors": Rolling golf balls around creates motion, sound, and a multicolor design.

kinesthetic, tactile, visual, and auditory. For children who were impaired visually, the focus was on the tactile and auditory stimulation. For those who had impaired hearing, the visual and the tactile became the dominant senses in the project. All the children enjoyed the swaying (kinesthetic) they needed to do in creating the artwork in this project. The end result was a beautiful abstract painting (see Figure 1.3). Many of the children who participated in this art intervention exhibited a basic memory recall of their sensory experiences despite their limited cognitive functions. When we used this with our lower-functioning children, we were able to assess each child's sensory motor abilities and preferences. One little boy responded to the sounds that the golf balls made on the tray. He laughed and was able to stay focused on the process through the playful exchange with the therapist.

Children in the facility who had limited use of their upper bodies were still able to participate in sensory art therapy with *simple adjustments* that required positioning the workspace. This provided better physical alignment and helped the children sustain the activity for a longer duration. We often incorporated use of the wall to have children experience the tactile feel of the paint and the multisensory experience. Studies have shown that implementing these multisensory experiences increases sustained focus of children with special needs (Thompson, 2011). By combining the multisensory approach and the more comfortable positioning we did see more focus in the children. This sustained focus and engagement ultimately created a sense of accomplishment, pride and cooperation among the children in art therapy.

In addition to simple methods, certain children found success with commercial tools purchased through rehabilitation catalogs. However, overall, we did not need these commercially produced products as much as our own self-created methods and makeshift art tools, like our own hand made cuff for holding paintbrushes (see Figure 1.4).

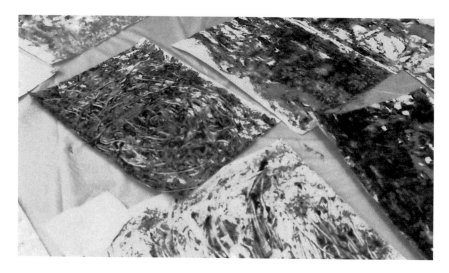

FIGURE 1.3. A finished product from "swirling colors."

Frances Anderson, an art therapist who specializes in adaptive art methods, describes three major categories to consider: "adaptations in the physical environment, adaptations in the art media and tools, and adaptation in the instructional sequence" (1992, p. 271). In *Art for all the Children* (1992), she describes both commercial and homemade adaptive products that, despite the fact that the book was written many years ago, readers can still use it in many contemporary and practical applications.

WHEEL ART: USING WHEELCHAIRS TO CREATE ART

Within the facility approximately 80% of the children were wheelchair-bound. We investigated ways in which we could have the children create art with their chairs. A student intern researched the work of Mary "Mickie" McGraw, an art therapist in Cleveland, Ohio, who is physically disabled and in a wheelchair herself. McGraw (1995) developed "wheel art" for the clients who were also in wheelchairs. In 1967, McGraw started the Art Therapy Studio in an old hospital ward, and it is now part of the MetroHealth

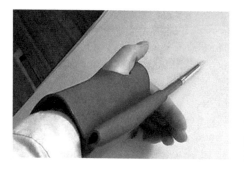

FIGURE 1.4. An example of a "hand-made" adaptive tool to assist children with grasping challenges.

Rehabilitation Institute of Ohio. She developed many creative art therapy methods to use with the patients there, including painting with their wheelchairs. We employed this adaptive approach to art making with the children at the facility, and it was a huge success.

Our own system of "wheel art" developed over time and was refined each year. Every child was given the opportunity to choose a color before it was his or her turn to wheel on the canvas. A large drop cloth was placed over the floor and secured with a lot of tape; then a large canvas was taped down on top on that. We even laid T-shirts along the borders of the canvas so that children could create wearable art. Many student interns and volunteers graciously helped when we scheduled our wheel art day (see Figure 1.5). Most of the children delighted in this project and were able to propel themselves. We had music in the background to inspire "dancing" around the canvas, creating beautiful patterns and textures. Some needed help in moving their chairs and volunteers helped by pushing them across the canvas, paying attention to where the children wanted to go by engaging with them.

In working with wheel art, we discovered an intensity of this directive beyond what we originally imagined. The act of engaging in physical activity allowed the children to feel empowered. It has been suggested that activities such as this (moving physically) also may lessen the feeling of stigmatization by counteracting the negative perceptions associated with individuals with physical limitations (Blinde & McClung, 1997). When the children had a chance to step back and look at the mural a few days later, they were in awe, and their confidence appeared to be enhanced by the experience. The pride and connection that each child made to this piece was powerful. Children would search for their lines and patterns within the whole colorful mural. Because their wheels were, in a sense, "an extension of themselves," it appeared that they gave a part of themselves to the art, and every time they passed it they would see themselves as part of a whole.

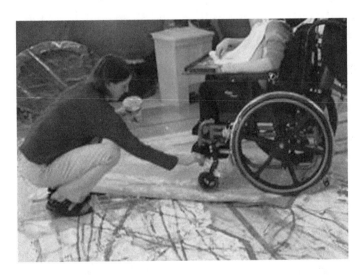

FIGURE 1.5. A student prepping the child to participate in the wheel art project.

CASE EXAMPLE

Occasionally art therapists working in health care settings have opportunities to work with children for extended periods of time or multiple times over repeated hospital admissions. This section presents a case study in which a graduate art therapy intern I supervised was able to work with a child for several months. Adaptive art therapy techniques helped the child create art and helped him to regain self-esteem, confidence, and increased understanding about his condition. This case vignette illustrates some of the therapeutic processes used and demonstrates specific uses of adaptive approaches.

Jorge was a 10-year-old boy with a diagnosis of Duchenne muscular dystrophy. His record also noted that he had attention deficit disorder (ADD) and some developmental and learning delays. He was admitted to the facility and placed in a room with another, much older child with the same diagnosis. Duchenne muscular dystrophy is a neuromuscular disease that is uncommon and terminal, because life expectancy is only to the mid-20s at best, while life expectancy in other forms of muscular dystrophy is longer. "Duchenne's muscular dystrophy is a disease of progressive muscle weakness leading to total paralysis and early death in the late teens or young adulthood. Because it has an X-linked, recessive pattern, the disease affects males almost exclusively" (Lewis, 2003, p. 403). Most children with this diagnosis have to use a wheelchair full-time between the ages of 7 and 14 years. There are stages within this disease that affect the psychosocial lives of the children and their families, including three particular times of crisis for children with Duchenne muscular dystrophy. The first occurs "around the age of five years as the child begins to realize his differences," the second "between the ages of 8 to 12 years when the child loses the ability to walk independently," and the third "during the adolescent years when social activity becomes restricted" (Lewis, 2003, p. 415). It is important to note that psychological responses of the child can be exacerbated by times of transition from one stage to the next and by times of crisis.

Jorge's family situation was that he lived with his grandmother, who had become too ill to care for him. Jorge had been in a wheelchair for the last 3 years and his symptoms were getting worse. When he was first admitted, it was discovered in the initial interview with the psychologist that Jorge had little to no knowledge of his condition. Part of his treatment plan included medical education about his diagnosis. It was recommended that Jorge participate in play therapy and art therapy in order to express emotions regarding his medical condition, social, and family issues. The psychologist reported that Jorge was frustrated by his muscular weakness and socially withdrawn. It was stated in his chart that he had expressed negative feelings of hopelessness and despair to an occupational therapist. He stated, "I wish I were dead," then quickly followed with "No, I'm just kidding" (Eddison, 2005).

Art therapy services were offered to Jorge, and the art therapy intern met with him one to two times per week. The intern made some general observations based on the first several weeks of treatment. The student recalled that in art therapy it was apparent that his thinking was scattered and disorganized. This was reflected in his artwork and his approach to the materials. The adaptive techniques employed in the course of treatment enabled him to think in an organized fashion about creating artwork. The creative process allowed him to experience an ego building success. This adaptive art (approach) paralleled a seemingly new organized way of thinking and outgoing confidence that materialized in Jorge. His thinking became grounded in reality and (within the first few weeks of admission) he emerged successfully into the social milieu of the hospital (Eddison, 2005).

Jorge's initial art making appeared to be regressive, and the intern recalled that although he enjoyed the sensory aspect of this initial phase, Jorge was searching for more meaningful ways to create images as the sessions progressed. Jorge created free and messy finger paintings in the beginning; this piece was the start of Jorge's creative journey (see Figure 1.6). However, after several sessions, the intern sensed Jorge's frustration and decided it was time to introduce some adaptive techniques that would enable him to feel more successful. Before moving forward, the intern did some research and discovered that there was a "virtual" art gallery on the Muscular Dystrophy Association website. She believed that showing this to Jorge would be beneficial and also help to facilitate a discussion about Jorge's diagnosis and inspire him to create a piece of art that would connect him to this community. She was hoping that if Jorge could begin to understand that many other people had this diagnosis, it might normalize his thoughts about the disease and lessen his alienation and stigma. Ultimately it did help Jorge begin to understand his condition and ask more questions about it.

The art therapy intern also presented Jorge with a "drawing kit" that included sophisticated pencils, rulers, cylinders, and stencils. These items served as Jorge's first adaptive devices, because he was unable to draw circles, shapes, or a straight line without them. The intern discovered Jorge's love of baseball and brought in photographs of baseball fields. Jorge wanted to draw a baseball field. Another simple yet essential adaptive technique involved the use of tape. Simply taping the paper to the table gave Jorge the stability to draw with confidence. This was a functional adaptive technique, because it helped Jorge focus and maintain control. The intern noted that these tools gave Jorge

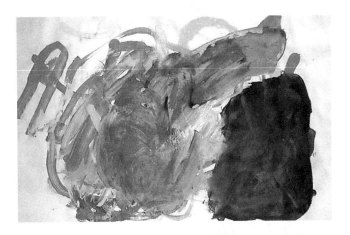

FIGURE 1.6. Jorge's painting.

the self-confidence to keep making art. He was amazed at himself for being able to draw such a large and complex image such as a baseball field (see Figure 1.7). Jorge beamed with pride at his accomplishment and talked about hanging the drawing up in the art room so everyone could see what he made. He seemed to want to use this artwork to make a connection to other people in his environment. The intern and Jorge discussed the future steps he would need to take in order to complete the project. This kind of organized approach made sense to Jorge and provided a context in which he could see how the project would be completed.

Paint was offered for the next session to continue the baseball field project. The intern and I discussed more adaptive strategies that would help Jorge continue feeling successful. The intern showed him the new tempera paint set she brought for him and the special tape he could use again to protect the area he would not be painting that day. Because of some of his prior regressive sessions, she used ice cube trays for the paint to avoid the possibility of Jorge sticking his hands into it and becoming distracted. This was a strategic and functional adaptive technique, because it deterred regression and prevented spills.

As the sessions progressed, Jorge also began to open up with the intern. As he painted, Jorge began to talk about his grandmother and how he missed her. He expressed feelings about being abandoned, as well as fears surrounding his grandmother's health issues. When these more intense sessions occurred, the intern noticed how Jorge wanted to play with the paint and not focus on the ongoing projects. Looking at the totality of

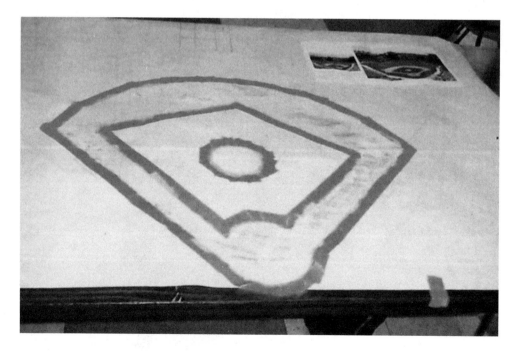

FIGURE 1.7. Jorge's baseball project using reference photos and special tape to assist and control the paint.

Jorge's art therapy treatment, the adaptive art therapy approach allowed him to function to the point of first feeling confident, then safe enough to express more intense feelings and underlying issues that might not have been accessible otherwise. Jorge achieved an understanding about his situation and also had the benefits of discovering the artist within himself.

CONCLUSION

Children with physical challenges and medical issues face daily obstacles and issues that make life situations more difficult and stressful. In addition, being confronted with the stigma of being different affects healthy psychosocial development and self-esteem. By being given opportunities for success in art making, children can begin to feel a sense of pride and achievement. The creative process has the power to rejuvenate and empower these children, as well as tap into their underlying talents and abilities. Therefore, adapting creative activities that allow for small successes, decision making, self-direction, and independence can give children with these challenges a chance to gain control and recognize their abilities. As helping professionals, we want to help them discover these abilities, while recognizing that within this very fragile population, the small triumphs and even limited progress can be big stepping-stones in their lives. As described throughout this chapter, the emphasis of adaptive art therapy is the therapist's ability to bring out children's inner strengths and abilities rather than focus on their disabilities, to be open to adapting methods and materials, and to utilize the assistance and knowledge of other professionals when working with these children.

REFERENCES

Anderson, F. (1992). *Art for all the children: Approaches to art therapy for children with disabilities* (2nd ed.). Springfield, IL: Thomas.

Anderson, F. (1996). *Art centered education and therapy for children with disabilities.* Springfield, IL: Thomas.

Ayres, J. (2005). *Sensory integration and the child.* Los Angeles: Western Psychological Services.

Barg, C. J., Armstrong, B. D., Hetz, S. P., & Latimer, A.E. (2010). Physical disability, stigma, and physical activity in children. *International Journal of Disability, Development and Education, 57,* 371–382.

Blinde, E. M., & McClung, L. R. (1997). Enhancing the physical and social self through recreational activity: Accounts of individuals with physical disabilities. *Adapted Physical Activity Quarterly, 14,* 327–344.

Childress, D. C. (2011). Play behaviors of parents and their young children with disabilities. *Topics in Early Childhood Special Education, 31,* 112–120.

Eddison, M. (2005). *Adaptive art therapy: Case study of a boy diagnosed with Duchenne muscular dystrophy.* Thesis submitted in partial fulfillment of the requirement for the degree of Master in Arts, Steinhardt School of Education, New York University, New York, NY.

Fingerhut, P. E. (2009). Measuring outcomes of family-centered intervention: Development of the life participation for parents (LPP). *Physical and Occupational Therapy in Pediatrics, 29,* 113–128.

Henley, D. (1992). *Exceptional children: Exceptional art.* Worcester, MA: Davis.

Kramer, E. (1986). The art therapist's third hand: Reflections on art, art therapy and society at large. *American Journal of Art Therapy, 24,* 71–86.

Lewis, S. (2003). *Medical–surgical nursing: Assessment and management of clinical problems.* Dallas: Mosby.

Malchiodi, C. A. (1999). Introduction to medical art therapy with children. In *Medical art therapy with children* (pp. 13–30). London: Jessica Kingsley.

McGraw, M. (1995). The art studio: A studio-based art therapy program. *Art Therapy: Journal of the American Art Therapy Association, 12,* 167–174.

Shaw, S. R., & McCabe, P. C. (2007). Hospital-to school transition for children with chronic illness: meeting the new challenges of an evolving health care system. *Psychology in the Schools, 45,* 74–87.

Thompson, C. J. (2011). Multi-sensory intervention observational research. *International Journal of Special Education, 26,* 202–214.

CHAPTER 2

Understanding Children's Drawings in Medical Settings

Margaret Carpenter Arnett
Cathy A. Malchiodi

Learning to understand children's spontaneous drawings in medical settings can add a deeper and important dimension to the healing process of pediatric patients. The medical team is naturally focused on the physical symptoms and treatment of patients; art expression provides a different perspective on patients, including what they may not be expressing verbally. Much like magnetic resonance imaging gives the medical team a look at what is going on inside the physical body to aid in diagnosis and care of the patients, spontaneous drawings can provide ways to understand what is going on in a different way. Through drawings children reveal and convey their fears and concerns that may be a revelation to the staff and caregivers.

In this chapter we discuss spontaneous drawings by young patients and how to use them as a tool for communication with the patients. Case examples are provided to illustrate key points, and suggestions are offered to highlight children's medical challenges and how drawings can facilitate understanding the experiences of illness, death, and dying. Emphasis is on exploration of the meaning of drawings from many perspectives rather than their use as projective tests, underscoring the value of helping children express their experiences of illness, medical treatments, and psychosocial issues through drawings.

SPONTANEOUS DRAWINGS

A spontaneous drawing is a drawing has no external influence and is not directed by the therapist in terms of a theme or topic. One can also broaden the description to include "impromptu" drawings (Furth, 1988), especially when working with children in medical settings. Impromptu drawings allow for simple direction; for example, if children tell the therapist that they are scared when they go for radiation treatment, the therapist might say, "Draw me a picture of yourself having radiation." Both spontaneous and impromptu drawings are accomplished in a short period of time, usually less than 30 minutes, with no preplanning or design.

There are several models to consider when obtaining spontaneous or impromptu drawings from children in medical settings. The first is that when we draw spontaneously the image is prompted by the unconscious mind, as well as the conscious mind; this is based on traditions of psychoanalysis and psychodynamic theory. Visualize an iceberg with one-third showing above the waterline and two-thirds below, with the tip or visible part being the conscious mind, and the submerged part, the unconscious mind; when we draw spontaneously the images arise from both the subconscious and the conscious mind. It is important that we honor this image and not see it as an accident. Consciously or unconsciously, the mind influences the images on the paper in color, form, shape, and content, and these images need to be treated with respect. When someone says to a helping professional, "I don't know why I put that [object] in the drawing, but I had to do it," it is probably something about which the artist is not yet conscious and should be respected as having meaning to the artist even if at first it is not obvious.

Another model for understanding drawings created by young patients involves the idea that the mind–body and psyche–soma are intrinsically linked. In this model, symptoms may be consciously or unconsciously expressed in drawings and art expressions (Bach, 1990). It proposes that patients may include elements that "forecast" aspects of illness, and that these aspects may even reflect patients' internal knowing about the course of disease.

Case Example (Carpenter Arnett)

When I worked as an art therapist many years ago on a pediatric ward, I was initially asked to comment on a 5-year-old child's spontaneous drawing (Figure 2.1). The child had to have his right arm amputated. In his drawing he drew himself with one arm looking normal and attached between the head and body with five normal digits. The other arm he drew coming out of his head just below the ear, and there were five sharp projections on his arm but not attached like normal digits. To me, he was saying in a nonverbal language, "It feels as if my arm is still there but it doesn't work anymore." Amputees often feel that the limb is still there after it has been removed, but a 5-year-old does not go through a long complicated thought process as to how to represent what he is feeling, he just draws.

Looking more closely at the drawing I noticed that he had given particular attention to drawing the ears, which were prominent, with the hair drawn carefully above them, and each had a little dot inside. This focus on the ear, and even the inner ear, made me wonder about the significance of that detail. When I had a chance to talk with him and ask how he was feeling, he said he had been listening to his doctor talk with his parents and some of the things they said were scary and he didn't understand. Additionally, he drew a red line on one ankle, and when I asked him to tell me about that, he said it was his ID bracelet that itched and annoyed him. It could have been be interpreted as a wound if he had not been asked

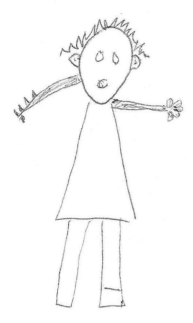

FIGURE 2.1. Five-year-old child's spontaneous drawing of herself.

about it. Here we have a drawing with something obviously odd or unusual in the arms and two other characteristics that were simpler causes for concern but led to productive conversations; each helped me to understand more about this child and his perceptions.

GUIDELINES FOR OBTAINING DRAWINGS

Materials

- White paper, 8½″ × 11″. This is a comfortable size to work with on a bed table or a clipboard, if the child is in a wheelchair. If space allows and a table is available, a larger size paper 12″ × 18″ is sometimes preferable for drawing.

- Crayons, colored pencils, and oil pastels (a minimum of 12 and preferably 24 colors choices are recommended).

- Felt pens (*Note.* Felt pens do not allow for variations in intensity of colors. This can be a challenge to observing intensity and pressure used to create drawings, but children love them!)

Interview

1. "Tell me about your drawing." Allow children tell you about their drawings with as few interruptions as possible initially. Younger children may change their minds about the characters in the drawing even as they talk.

2. "What would you title your drawing?" This provides a general sense of the theme of the drawing and may help some children to communicate more easily.

3. After you feel that the child has said all he or she wants to say spontaneously, then ask questions in response to the information the child has given verbally and based on your own observations.

4. It is important to ask children about their feelings in regard to their drawings. If you sense that the drawing expresses feelings a child is not describing, tell the child how you feel when you look at the drawing. Note any reactions. For example, does he or she agree with or deny those feelings? Give children who are hesitant to talk about themselves the option of talking about the figures, animals, or elements of the drawing in the third person. For example, "What would that cat be feeling right now?" or "If that boy could talk, what would he say?"

5. It is important to know yourself well enough to discern the difference between your own projections and what patients are actually expressing in their artworks. For example, are you reacting from your own past sense of illness or loss, or are you listening to and observing their feelings? Taking a nonjudgmental stance and having a "beginner's mind" (Malchiodi, 1998, 2008) is helpful in staying objective.

Observation

Watching children draw can provide additional insight, especially in the case of very young children as they change images and names of people even as they draw. Sometimes you can see them spend considerably more time on one area than on another. Be discreet in watching, because it may inhibit a child who needs privacy or feels insecure about drawing. Remember that drawing is an individual process for each child; some are more comfortable than others when drawing in the presence of a helping professional (Malchiodi, 1998).

Listening

Good listening skills are imperative in building trust and communication through drawings. After questioning and listening, play back in your own words what the child is saying through words and drawings to obtain clarification for what is expressed. This person-centered approach works well with most children, and also gives you the opportunity to clarify with the child what is in the drawing and any child-initiated narratives that are provided. Finally, while drawings are not a foolproof mirror of a child's mind, a drawing often stimulates conversation and provides something for the therapist and child to talk about in building narratives.

DEVELOPMENT AND CHILDREN'S SPONTANEOUS DRAWINGS

Cox (2005), Foks-Appleman (2007), Malchiodi (2012), and others underscore the importance of familiarity with normal developmental characteristics found in drawings during childhood and adolescence. While the developmental characteristics cannot be covered in this brief chapter, every helping professional who works with medically ill children should have a working understanding of them in order to respond effectively to the content of their drawings. In the same vein, it is also necessary to understand how development impacts children's understanding of their own bodies (see section below for a more detailed discussion).

Developmental influences are also important in understanding how children express the concept of illness in their artwork. Banks (1990) conducted a study of how children ages 3–12 years perceive health and illness, including how colds happen and what germs are. Three age groups of children (3–5 years, 7–8 years, and 9–12 years) completed a drawing task when asked to draw "germs." Predictably, all three groups created drawings with normal characteristics for their age group, and developmental influences were evidence at each age level. The 3- to 5-year-olds drew scribbles and rudimentary forms they called "monsters" or human or animal-like faces or shapes that had "horns" or large, pointed teeth. Monsters also appeared in drawings by the 7- to 8-year-old group, but these children included more elements that looked like cells, demonstrating a growing knowledge of biology and health information. The 9- to 12-year-olds drew cells of one kind or another. Additionally, each group's narratives about "germs" represented a developmentally appropriate perspective; young children believed that external forces (monsters) cause illness, while older children were more likely to give detailed accounts of internal causes of illness (disease-causing elements in the body).

DRAWINGS, SYMPTOMS, AND DIAGNOSES

Many children may express their medical condition, surgery or medical treatments, or symptoms within drawings. Looking at drawings through a "somatic" lens can be particularly meaningful in work with children who have life-threatening illnesses (Malchiodi, 1998, 1999). The term "somatic" is defined as follows: of or relating to the physical body, distinct from the mind and environment. Susan Bach (1975, 1990) is one of few researchers who has studied the somatic content of children's drawings, particularly the spontaneous drawings of terminally ill patients. She observes that spontaneous drawings and paintings may "reflect specific physical illnesses in typical colors, shapes, motifs, etc. . . . Often ahead of recognized symptoms, they may indicate the future development of an illness (1975, p. 87). While no large scale studies have been conducted since Bach's work several decades ago, her contributions provide compelling evidence that there are at least some idiosyncratic characteristics reflective of medical conditions in children's art expressions. Furth (1988), a psychoanalyst who became aware of Bach's work, also proposed the notion that somatic conditions may be communicated by children in their spontaneous drawings. Carpenter Arnett (2011) has also written extensively on connections between art expression and somatic and spiritual aspects.

More recently, those who work closely with children with medical conditions have observed numerous connections between the content of their drawings and illness.

Stafstrom, Rostasy, and Minster (2002) studied 226 children's drawings of their headaches and found that a differential diagnosis for migraine headaches could be made from reviewing the characteristics of their art expressions. In a similar study, Wojacznska-Stanek, Koprowski, Wrobel, and Malgorzata (2008) found some consistency in the content of children's drawings of migraine headaches in comparison to drawings of those diagnosed with tension headaches. Gabriels, Wamboldt, McCormick, Adams, and McTaggart (2000) examined connections between emotional responses and asthma symptoms in drawings by children, while Rollins (1990) and Councill (2012) underscored how young patients depict their experiences with cancer.

Case Example (Malchiodi)

When working with children hospitalized for medical illness, I have observed that they often include content related to their disease, symptoms, and medical intervention. While we are all somewhat biased about what we think we "see" in drawings, the context of illnesses such as cancer, renal failure, cystic fibrosis, asthma, and other conditions does impact what these young patients include in their art expressions. For example, some children who are undergoing treatment for kidney disease or preparing for a kidney transplant may include elements of their experiences with treatment in human figure drawings, reflecting concerns about transplantation and physical reactions to steroids or other medications (Malchiodi, 1998; Figure 2.2).

As early as 1977, Perkins observed that the drawings of children with life-threatening cancer and poor prognoses contained specific color choices and elements. She noted that

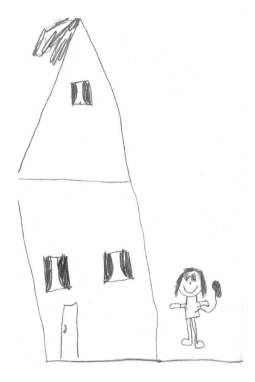

FIGURE 2.2. Child's drawing of her kidney transplantation illustrating the kidney attached to her torso by a string.

the color red was more often used in association with blood, and black was used to represent negative or foreboding events or entities in their drawings and paintings. In the same vein, I have encountered children with leukemia who use the color red in ways specifically related to the course of the disease. For example, a 6-year-old girl with red hemorrhages on her skin repeatedly drew a red-freckled sun and trees losing many red "apples" (Figure 2.3).[1] Other children included figures with "sunglasses" when their eyes became photosensitive during the course of illness.

While not all children universally include characteristics that may be related to their somatic conditions or medical intervention, when they do, we have an opportunity to help them explore their experiences through these drawings. In the brief examples described, each drawing provided a way to learn more from the young patient about the challenges of cancer or other diseases through child-friendly means of communication.

Case Examples (Carpenter Arnett)

A 6-year-old boy, hospitalized when he had been playing swords with his brother and the stick had punctured his right eye, drew an image of GI Joe with a heavily crayoned black patch over his right eye. Rather than draw himself, he chose GI Joe, a combative figure who also has the capacity to fight for him and protect him, and in this case "help me get better." Other children may emphasize areas of a drawing that cause concern or anxiety.

A 13-year-old adolescent being treated for leukemia was admitted to the hospital for observation with a fever of unknown origin. The first time he drew an image for me, he filled the entire page with a rocket ship that was drawn in red crayon with great attention

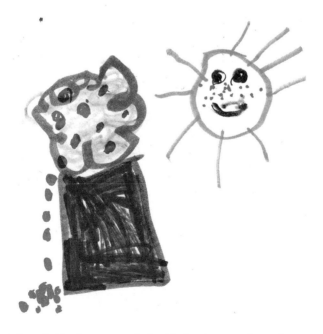

FIGURE 2.3. Child's drawing with freckled red sun and tree losing red apples.

---

[1]Original art in this chapter was in color. It is reproduced here in black and white.

to detail, and depicted as taking off. Initially this seemed to be an aggressive, energetic, and masculine symbol, but there was a heavily shaded black area that stood out in contrast to the rest of the drawing. As I looked more closely at the drawing I noticed that the rocket looked very like a human form with fins where the arms would be and rocket boosters for legs; in that case, the black area would correspond to the upper chest (Figure 2.4). Tests and observation determined that there was an infection around the site of his Hickman catheter (temporary intravenous line for medications, fluids, and transfusions) inserted in the upper chest wall to facilitate treatment. Unconsciously he emphasized the initial site of infection in his drawing. While diagnoses and symptoms are not always present in spontaneous drawings, when they do appear they are powerful reminders of the mind–body connection and its expression through imagery.

END-OF-LIFE ISSUES

Death and dying may affect the content of children's drawings; this includes both children with a terminally ill parent or sibling and children who themselves are terminally ill. Children may not be able to express their feelings with words alone, but they may be able to relate unexpressed fears, questions, or worries through drawings (Malchiodi,

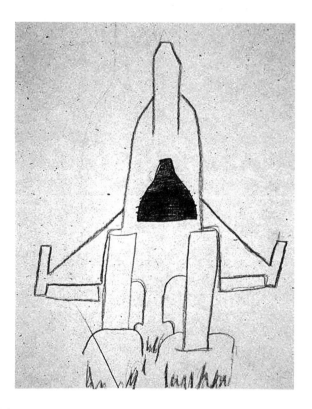

FIGURE 2.4. Adolescent's drawing of a rocket with a black area possibly representing infection.

2008). Bach (1990), mentioned earlier in this chapter, noted a specific configuration of elements that appeared in the drawings of children who were close to death. Based on her studies of Jung and psychoanalysis, she proposed that the upper left-hand quadrant of a drawing or painting held special significance in relation to both spiritual issues (beliefs in God or life after death) and the process of dying and bereavement.

Case Example (Carpenter Arnett)

A 7-year-old boy whose mother was dying of cancer drew many family pictures but consistently did not include his mother in his drawings. There was some concern about how he was dealing with the thought of losing her, but he would not talk about it. The next time he drew, I asked if he could include his mother in the picture; he did so but drew a strange green creature standing next to her. Asked who the green creature was, he said it was "E.T.," who was going to take his mother to play in the other world. This was when the movie *E.T.: The Extra Terrestrial* was popular. He was quite happy about the arrangement and was ready to let her go, while the adults were worried about his seeming disinterest. They were concerned that he did not want to talk about his mother and her illness, but at an inner level, he had already thought about it and found a resolution that satisfied him at the time. This also illustrates how young children (Bach, 1990; Coles, 1990; Landy, 2001) are usually quite comfortable with the concept of a spirit world.

Working with children who are in the process of dying is a difficult situation, but one that can benefit from the use of spontaneous drawings and the art therapist's understanding and compassion. Communication with the family members at that time is important, and they also may benefit from drawing. We prepare for birth with great care, and the same should be true for the end of life. Here the art therapist can do much to bring love and strength on that journey.

For the therapist observing a child's drawings through countless admissions and discharges, the child's drawing style becomes familiar and the physical and emotional ups and downs of disease can be tracked within the images. When children are feeling healthy they draw with more energy and enthusiasm, use a larger variety of colors, and draw with pressure on the pencil. When they are tired and physically depleted, they draw with paler colors, less variety, and less intensity of pressure, sometimes leaving a line or image unfinished.

Case Example (Carpenter Arnett)

An 8-year-old girl with cystic fibrosis completed numerous drawings and wrote poems, spreading much joy to family and friends through her art and writing. She enjoyed the creative process and sometimes expressed what was going on physically and emotionally. One particularly graphic image during hospitalization included an apple with brown spots and facial features, with a large worm eating right through the middle of it, with the word "AOOOOA" beside it in large letters (Figure 2.5). This girl's sister also had cystic fibrosis but a much milder case; these sisters shared an important relationship. A picture the girl drew

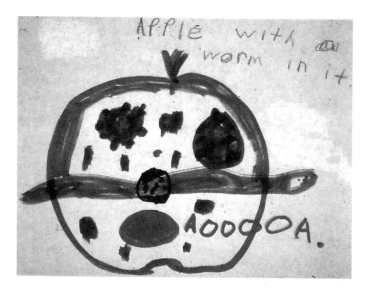

FIGURE 2.5. Eight-year-old cystic fibrosis patient's drawing of an apple being eaten by a worm.

of them on a swing described this relationship. She showed her sister sitting squarely on the swing, drawn in realistic color, but she drew herself as almost transparent, colored entirely in purple, as if floating on the swing seat. A slide drawn between them and colored heavily in grey seemed to form a barrier between them, curved to protect her sister even though they were united on the swing set.

As she became weaker, the girl talked about heaven as a beautiful place just round the corner and said she had friends there. The last drawing she made was a balanced design unlike most of her drawings that contained mostly random elements; in this drawing each side matched perfectly. A large tree with a large trunk was drawn in the center and had many cracks in it, as if it were falling apart. The top part of the tree had a smiling face and the words, "Hi, my name is Spring" (at the time it was winter). There was a ground line across the bottom of the page with three blooming flowers on each side. In the sky were two faint clouds, one on each side with smiles on them, and between the flowers and the smiling cloud were two girls, one on each side. The one on the left was drawn in purple, and the one on the right was drawn in golden yellow and wearing a crown. In poems, the girl wrote that she had a "friend" in heaven who, she said, knew how she felt and understood her; I believe this drawing was her friend accompanying her on her way. While it was not spring at the time, I think that the words on the tree and flowers represented new life to her. The support and devotion of a loving family that colored her short life and made all the difference was always reflected in her drawings.

A 15-year-old who was admitted with cancer was not as fortunate. In fact, the lack of family support or interest led the staff to recommend that I see her to determine whether she was interested in drawing. I worked with this courageous young woman over a period of 15 months and in that time her drawings were key in resolving different emotional issues as she battled with the physical challenges and side effects of treatment. When she was feeling well she loved to draw, and though there were times she did not feel up to it, the connection we had formed through her art enabled her to talk openly as well.

She drew spontaneously for me on my first visit in delicate but realistic colors a view of a mountain stream with pine trees, which she said was a favorite place to go with her boyfriend that made her feel better. What stood out in the drawing were three large black rocks in the stream, and the two of them standing on the bank holding hands and looking at the rocks in the foreground. The next day her physician told me that he was afraid she did not understand the gravity of her situation, but I showed him the drawing and said I thought some part of her knew.

A year later she drew a picture of herself and her boyfriend silhouetted against a sunset at the beach (Figure 2.6). Swimming in the background was a whale, connector to the deep and unknown, and in the foreground, a green turtle emphasizing her slow progress. This time, however, there were six large black rocks. The cancer had returned and spread. To support her treatment I talked to her about positive imagery and how it might help. She understood the concept but had a hard time and stopped before completing a positive image. On one occasion she drew a sad-looking tree on the left-hand side of the page, but all the leaves were falling off in a pile on the ground and the rest of the page was empty. Another time she drew a crab that was going to eat her cancer cells. Again, she stopped, after drawing the crab, which looked small and powerless on the page, and said she couldn't do any more. On better days this adolescent could draw really well, and on one occasion she proudly showed me a beautiful color drawing of two lovebirds that she said represented herself and her boyfriend.

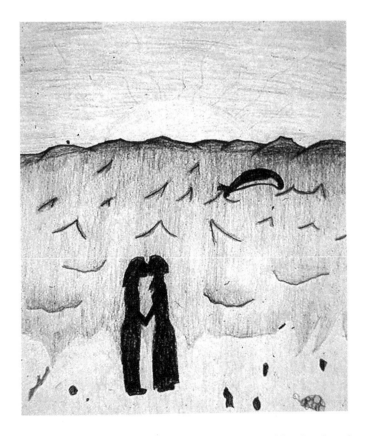

FIGURE 2.6. Adolescent's drawing of herself and her boyfriend.

Because he was the only person who visited regularly, he was her sole source of support and was often featured in her artwork.

Her first admission and ensuing treatment kept her hospitalized for 2½ months, and during that time we began to discuss some important issues that engendered her fears of both cancer and death. After a grey and gloomy drawing of herself with her boyfriend with a barrier between them, I knew there was a problem. As we began to talk about the drawing I found out they were having problems, because he believed he had caused her illness because they had had sex, and had brought on her cancer for which they were being punished. She said she did not believe that, but her boyfriend was influenced by friends who attended a Fundamentalist church. I told her that this was not my personal belief and was able to reassure her, but I also reported the situation to her physician so he could talk to her boyfriend and remove his fears of causing her cancer.

When this issue was resolved, it was as if a big burden was lifted, and she was much more relaxed and cheerful. Without the drawing we would never have known the burden they were carrying. When she was discharged in the spring, she drew a picture of herself and her boyfriend having a picnic in a beautiful meadow under a willow tree, with a big basket of food, because her nausea was gone. But in the background loomed a large black rock like a mountain. At the time they were planning a trip to Disneyland during the summer or fall, but they were never able to make it, which did not surprise me after seeing the other rocks in her art. Bach (1990) felt that the process of decline in illness, as well as healing, can be seen in graphic images and originate from the child's "inner knowingness." The image this adolescent had created appeared to reflect a possible decline in health, as noted by Bach. The girl was in and out of the hospital with treatments for the next 6 months. Sometimes she felt too ill to draw, but she always looked forward to art therapy visits. One time she drew a picture of the hospital at the end of a dead-end street with large revolving doors, which illustrated her relationship with the hospital. Many of her drawings were forecasts in a way, though one never knew until after the event.

During her illness she had courses of radiation and chemotherapy, as well as surgery, and she handled them all with courage and optimism, and hopes for a future with her boyfriend. One time she drew a picture of her dream house, complete with a picket fence. There was a fruit tree in the yard with grass and flowers; a lamp in the large window, with curtains on either side; and a toy ball in the yard. Looking with the intention of carrying myself into the picture I realized that the fence formed a solid barrier across the bottom of the picture and there was no path, door, or sign of access. In reviewing the drawing after she died 9 weeks later, I noticed that there were nine bricks on the chimney and the toy ball was balanced precariously on the ninth picket of the fence. Repetitive numbers in a drawing can be connected to some aspect of the drawer's life. Again, one only sees that later, and it cannot be used as a prognosis, but it is valued in retrospect as evidence of that connection between the unconscious and what we know that we don't know.

During her last month in the hospital, when she was on pain medication and becoming weaker, she drew for me a picture of herself entirely in a pale blue crayon. For the first time she depicted herself in a dress with one arm longer than the other, and she only had a tuft of hair. When people use a blue color in this end-of-life situation, it has been observed that it is like fading away (Furth, 1988).

A week before she died she made me a bookmark with a moon and stars, but soon after that sank into a light coma. However, one of the things she liked when she was feeling stressed was for me to stroke her arm, so she could drift off to sleep. I had asked to be called to her bedside when the end was near. As I was driving in to the hospital I remembered her blue picture with the longer arm, so when I sat by her bedside, with her boyfriend on the other side and she partially opened her eyes, I felt she knew I was there, so I began stroking her arm. Within 10 minutes she drifted peacefully away.

POSITIVE IMAGERY

As well as giving insights to the medical team, drawings can be extremely helpful to children and adolescents in developing positive imagery to support the healing process (Klein, 2001). Most health care professionals now recognize the importance of positivity during illness and recovery for individuals of all ages. For example, guided imagery or guided visualization can help patients create and focus on positive images that can affect many physiological systems, including immune functioning, metabolism, blood pressure, and overall health (Duke University Integrative Health, 2012). In a similar way, drawings of positive imagery, when appropriately introduced, can help to remove fears, enhance the effectiveness of treatments, and give the child a feeling of control.

Case Examples (Carpenter Arnett)

A 12-year-old girl with a brain tumor had a positive outlook and usually drew happy pictures in our sessions. However, one day she told me that she did not feel like drawing because she had to go for radiation that day and did not like her radiation treatments. I asked her to draw a picture of what that was like. She first drew what looked like a large camera lens (the radiation equipment), but the way she depicted herself on a table floating insecurely in midair led me to discuss her feelings about it. She responded that she was afraid in the dark during her radiation treatments.

I talked to her about using her imagination to develop positive images to visualize during the treatment that would help her with her fears. Horses were her passion, so we drew many horses, all carrying cancer cells and galloping away with them into the distance. Normally I do not help with a drawing, but she had some motor impairment that made it hard to get the details the way she wanted, so this one drawing became a collaborative project. She took this picture with her during treatments and used it to think positively about her cancer cells being removed and therefore worried less about the process. She said it really helped to think about the horses and she was much happier with the technicians. Eventually she went into remission and continued with her art making after she left the hospital, sending me drawings from time to time.

A 10-year-old boy with leukemia liked to draw Pac-Men devouring his cancer cells. The first time he did this we counted the good cells he had drawn in one color and the Pac-Men in a different color, and found that there were more cancer cells than Pac-Men. The next time he saw me as an outpatient he made a drawing with himself as a clown on the left side of the paper, which was a spontaneous image, and the same Pac-Men and cancer cells on the right side of the paper. However, this time there were twice as many Pac-Men as cancer cells, and he said that now the Pac-Men could win! This, of course, was a conscious choice to take part in his healing process. Clowns are a favorite in children's drawings, but I have often found that, like a mask, they relate to covering hidden fears but showing a cheery face.

As I went to present the positive image concept to another patient one day, I was duly humbled. This 13-year-old had been hiking in the mountains with his Boy Scout troop and had fallen and suffered a bad break to his leg that required surgery and pinning. I began to explain about helping his healing process and he cut me short. "Oh, like this," he said, producing a detailed pencil drawing of two separate bone ends. The bottom bone looked like a cross section, complete with bone marrow. Being delivered by rocket were assortments of vitamins B and C, calcium, and other healing help. I told him he was way ahead of me! Later he made a second pencil drawing called "The Welding of a Bone." It showed a side view of the two bone ends almost healed together, with pins securing it on the left and a helmeted figure rappelling down the bones on the right, with tanks and a welding torch completing the healing on the right. The area in the center was not quite joined yet. His surgeon, upon seeing the drawing, commented that it was amazingly accurate, and that the center area would be the last to heal.

Being able to draw these images as metaphors gives the child some control in a situation where he or she has little control, but to be effective the imagery must appeal to the child; for example, if the child were afraid of horses it would not work to have them carrying the cancer cells away. The use of positive imagery has to be part of a child's own sense of good helpers to remove fears, boost self-confidence, and enable the child to trust in treatment.

CONCLUSION

Spontaneous and impromptu drawings have great potential in medical settings to improve care by giving children the opportunity for emotional expression, self-efficacy, and opportunity to build trust with health care professionals. In addition, the art therapist and staff can gain valuable insight into psychosocial aspects not necessarily offered through talking alone. While deciphering the content of pediatric patients' drawings is not hard science, it does offer additional and valuable information on children's experiences of serious illness, as well as an avenue for exploration of positive imagery that both supports recovery and provides comfort at the end of life.

REFERENCES

Bach, S. (1975). Spontaneous pictures of leukemic children as an expression of the total personality, mind and body. *Acta Paedopsychiatrica, 41*(3), 86–104.

Bach, S. (1990). *Life paints its own span.* Einsiedeln, Switzerland: Daimon Verlag.

Banks, E. (1990). Concepts of health and sickness of pre-school and school-age children. *Children's Health Care, 19*(1), 43–48.

Carpenter Arnett, M. (2011). *The art of the inner journey.* Bloomington, IN: Xlibris.

Coles, R. (1990). *The spiritual life of children.* Boston: Houghton Mifflin.

Councill, T. (2012). Medical art therapy with children. In C. A. Malchiodi (Ed.), *Handbook of art therapy* (2nd ed., pp. 222–240). New York: Guilford Press.

Cox, M. (2005). *The pictorial world of the child.* Cambridge, UK: Cambridge University Press.

Duke University Integrative Health. (2012). *Mind–body services.* Retrieved January 25, 2012, from *www.dukeintegrativemedicine.org/patient-care/mind-body-services.*

Foks-Appleman, T. (2007). *Draw me a picture.* Nuenens, Netherlands: Foxap-Scriptus.

Furth, G. (1988). *The secret world of drawings.* Boston: Sigo Press.

Gabriels, R., Wamboldt, M., McCormick, D., Adams, T., & McTaggart, S. (2000). Children's illness drawings and asthma symptoms awareness. *Journal of Asthma, 37*(7), 565–574.

Klein, N. (2001). *Healing images.* Madison, WI: Inner Coaching.

Landy, R. (2001). *How we see God and why it matters: A multicultural view through children's drawings and stories.* Springfield, IL: Thomas.

Malchiodi, C. A. (1998) *Understanding children's drawings.* New York: Guilford Press.

Malchiodi, C. A. (1999). *Medical art therapy with children.* London: Jessica Kingsley.

Malchiodi, C. A. (2008). Creative interventions and childhood trauma. In C. A. Malchiodi (Ed.), *Creative interventions with traumatized children* (pp. 3–21). New York: Guilford Press.

Malchiodi, C. A. (2012). Developmental art therapy. In C. A. Malchiodi (Ed.), *Handbook of art therapy* (2nd ed., pp. 114–129). New York: Guilford Press.

Perkins, C. (1977). The art of life-threatened children: A preliminary study. In R. Shoemaker & S. Gonick-Barris (Eds.), *Creativity and the art therapist's identity: The proceedings of the Seventh Annual Conference of the American Art Therapy Association.* Baltimore: American Art Therapy Association.

Rollins, J. (1990). Childhood cancer: Siblings draw and tell. *Pediatric Nursing, 16*(1), 21–27.

Stafstrom, C., Rostasy, K., & Minster, A. (2002). The usefulness of children's drawings in the diagnosis of headaches.*Pediatrics, 109*(3), 460–472.

Wojacznska-Stanek, K., Koprowski, R., Wrobel, Z., & Malgorzata, G. (2008). Headache in children's drawings. *Journal of Child Neurology, 23*(2), 184–191.

CHAPTER 3

Art Therapy and Child Life

*An Integrated Approach to Psychosocial Care
with Pediatric Oncology Patients*

Cathy A. Malchiodi
Ellen Goldring

Pediatric oncology patients range from newborns to young people in their early 20s. No matter the age, the diagnosis of cancer is devastating to patients and families. The presence and treatment of pediatric cancer is often associated with profound psychosocial challenges, and young patients' lives are dramatically altered. Additionally, patients and families suddenly confront coping with new situations, uncertainties of prognosis, and unpredictable distress and trauma responses.

To address the psychosocial needs of these individuals, art therapists and child life specialists provide intervention from the time of diagnosis, during treatment, and posthospitalization that includes issues associated with end of life and bereavement. In most settings, art therapy and child life services complement each other in order to meet patients' and families' needs and provide integrative treatment; in many cases, art therapists may also be well versed or credentialed in the area of child life. Above all, art therapists and child life specialists provide interventions designed to mediate the psychosocial impact of medical illness, to enhance children's adaptive coping skills, and to help patients and families develop resiliency and posttraumatic growth.

This chapter explores how art therapy and child life issues intersect to benefit children and adolescents with cancer and to address psychosocial goals and objectives. It clarifies the role of art therapy and child life issues in pediatric oncology, and how these fields complement and strengthen pediatric patient services in supporting children's self-expression, self-efficacy, and coping during medical treatment through end-of-life care. It also highlights the importance of resilience building in the treatment of young patients and families challenged by a diagnosis of cancer and invasive medical treatment, demonstrating applications of art therapy and child life approaches.

CHILDREN AND CANCER

Childhood cancers are actually rare, making up less than 1% of all cancers diagnosed each year (American Cancer Society, 2012). Because of major treatment advances in the last two decades, about 80% of children with cancer now survive 5 years or more, although the rate varies depending on the type of cancer. However, after accidents, it still is the leading cause of death in children younger than 15 years (American Cancer Society, 2012).

Types of cancers that occur in children are different than those in adults and include leukemia, brain and nervous system tumors, neuroblastoma, Wilms's tumor, lymphoma, retinoblastoma, and bone cancer. Treatment options include chemotherapy, surgery, radiation, and combinations of other treatments. Most childhood cancers respond well to treatment, because these cancers tend to grow quickly, and chemotherapy is effective with those types of fast-growing cells. Children are also more physically resilient than adults and can take higher doses of chemotherapy and more intensive treatments. There are still side effects, however, and they can be both short and long term depending on the patient and the balance of medical intervention.

To address illness, a team includes pediatric oncologists, surgeons, nurses, and radiation oncologists who specialize in using interventions to treat children with cancer. In addition, childhood cancer treatment includes many professionals in allied health fields. Most hospitals treating pediatric patients also provide psychosocial care (see the next section for more information) for both children and their families; these teams may comprise a variety of mental health and allied health professionals, including psychologists, social workers, health educators, rehabilitation therapists, child life specialists, and creative arts therapists (e.g., art or music therapists).

WHAT IS PSYCHOSOCIAL CARE?

Psychosocial care focuses on psychological and social aspects of cognitive and emotional growth and development. Children's and adolescents' psychological development includes the ability to perceive, learn, express, analyze, and experience emotion. Social aspects include the capacity to form attachments to caregivers, family members, and peers; to maintain relationships; and to learn the behaviors of one's cultural system. Children who have a healthy psychosocial status generally are able to attune to others, form stable and secure attachments to parents or caregivers, develop relationships with peers, feel a sense of belonging, perceive a sense of self-worth, trust others, and have hope and optimism in the future (Ganz, 2007; Malchiodi, 2008; Steele & Malchiodi, 2011).

Psychosocial care underscores the connection between children's feelings, perceptions, and thoughts and overall social development, emphasizing that reactions to extreme situations vary because of individual and personal characteristics and environments. The overall goal of psychosocial care is to support and enhance children's growth and recovery by addressing emotional, cognitive, and social needs of individuals. In particular, developmental characteristics are central to successful intervention with pediatric patients, including those with childhood cancer. Rollins and Mahon (2011) provide a developmental perspective of childhood illnesses, central issues of each stage, possible responses and recommended areas for intervention that complement art therapy, and child life services with pediatric patients (Table 3.1).

In most cases, young patients with cancer suddenly must cope with new situations, frightening and possibly painful symptoms, uncertainty about the future, and changes in social and familial relationships. It is particularly important that they receive not only emotional and social support from family but also active intervention from mental health and health care professionals. Additionally, parents and caregivers need support to cope with distress associated with their responsibilities as primary sources of psychosocial care for their children. Finally, successful psychosocial care requires that allied health professionals (including art therapists and child life specialists), medical professionals, and nurses work together to enhance emotional and social treatment objectives for young patients and families facing a diagnosis of cancer.

ART THERAPY AND CHILD LIFE COLLABORATION

In many hospitals, art therapists and child life specialists work in tandem to address psychosocial needs of children and adolescents who have cancer. In some allied health, activity, psychiatric, or creative arts therapies departments, the art therapist and child life specialist may be the same person, having fulfilled education and qualification requirements in both areas of expertise. Rode (1995) introduces the concept of child life and art therapy as a dual profession to help children and adolescents cope with medical illness, treatments, and hospitalization. She notes, "Child life and the creative arts therapies as interconnected, parallel professions can build bridges within the culture of the medical environment to meet the psychosocial needs of hospital children and their families through art and play" (p. 105). More than just "art cart ladies" or "play people," art therapists and child life specialists form a powerful combination of services that encourages a less stressful and more effective hospital experience for pediatric patients and their families. In order to help readers understand the scope of the practice of child life and art therapy, this section defines each profession and central approaches to psychosocial care, and discusses areas of integrative and complementary intervention in medical settings with pediatric patients.

Child Life Specialists

A child life specialist has either a bachelor's or master's degree, with an education emphasizing child development and family systems. The Child Life Council (2011) website describes the profession as follows: "Child life specialists promote effective coping through play, preparation, education, and self-expression activities. They provide emotional support for families, and encourage optimum development of children facing a broad range of challenging experiences, particularly those related to health care and hospitalization."

The central focus of the child life profession is to help to decrease pediatric patients' distress related to medical procedures, to maximize development and familial strengths, and to navigate the ups and downs of the medical experience. Child life specialists work to normalize the hospital experience, to make it patient-friendly, to help children feel more comfortable and safe, and to imprint some positive memory associated with the hospital stay or visit. They are knowledgeable about child and adolescent development and how this relates to the medical experience. Therapeutic play is the central focus for child life specialists' work with younger patients; therapeutic play generally includes creative expression through toys, props, art, music, books, and expressive activities.

Child life specialists use a variety of play techniques, including *familiarization*, *expressive*, and *diversionary* approaches. For example, familiarization play often involves actual medical supplies and "play" medical kits as part of the process to help patients and families become more familiar with medical procedures; the goal is to reduce anxiety and fears, and to increase a sense of self-efficacy. In order to prepare children psychologically for medical experiences the child life specialist works in tandem with the medical team to educate and prepare young patients, and provides familiarization play. Expressive play using toys, props, or art supplies may encourage children to communicate feelings through dramatic enactment, rhythm instruments, clay, or other media. Finally, diversionary play includes games and other activities that can help relax pediatric patients and literally divert their attention from stresses of hospitalization.

Like others involved in pediatric psychosocial care, child life specialists focus on understanding the coping style of the patient. For example, does the child want to watch medical procedures? Does the child want more information about procedures or other aspects of treatment, or is the patient overwhelmed by excessive information? Would the child cope best by being distracted during the procedure? Child life specialists may also teach patients and families how to engage in self-advocacy, focusing on the family members' strengths and enhancing their ability to feel confident within the hospital setting. The intention is to reinforce patient- and family-centered care in which patients and families are viewed as partners in their medical treatment.

Art Therapists

Art therapists are professionals with master's-level specific education and experience in psychotherapeutic application of art media to treatment of patients. While child life

TABLE 3.1. Understanding Children Who Are Ill: A Developmental Perspective

	Erikson	Piaget	Issues	Possible troublesome responses	Interventions
Infant	Trust versus mistrust • To get • To give in return	Sensorimotor • Exploration of physical self and environment • Object constancy • Cause and effect	Separation Lack of stimulation Pain	Failure to bond Distrust Anxiety Delayed skills development	Maximize parental involvement Maximize parental information Provide stimulation; visual; auditory; tactile; kinesthetic vestibular
Toddler (1–3)	Autonomy versus shame and doubt • To hold on • To let go	Sensorimotor Preoperational (preconceptual phase) • Can hold and recall images • Increasing use of symbolization • Highly egocentric perception of world	Separation Fear of bodily injury and pain Frightening fantasies Immobility/ restriction Forced regression Loss of routine and rituals	Regression Uncooperativeness Protest (verbal and physical) Despair Negativism Temper tantrums Resistance	Maximize parental involvement Maximize parental information Provide medical and therapeutic play Foster environmental exploration Provide routine and ritual Encourage self-expression
Preschooler (3–6)	Initiative versus guilt • To make (going after) • To "make like" (playing)	Preoperational (preconceptual phase) Preoperational (intuitive phase) • Transition period between depending solely on perception and depending on truly logical thinking • Better able to see more than one factor at a time that influences an event	Separation Fear of loss of control, sense of own power Fear of bodily mutilation or penetration by surgery or injections, castration	Regression Anger toward primary caregiver Acting out Protest Despair and detachment Physical and verbal aggression Dependency Withdrawal	Maximize parental involvement Maximize parental information Provide medical and therapeutic play Environmental exploration Routine and ritual Self-expression

Stage	Psychosocial	Cognitive	Fears/Concerns	Behavioral Responses	Interventions
Schoolager (7–12)	Industry versus inferiority • To make things (completing) • To make things together	Concrete operations • Increasing ability to think logically in the physically concrete realm • Understands the meaning of series of actions of order and sequencing	Separation Fear of loss of control Fear of loss of mastery Fear of bodily mutilation Fear of bodily injury and pain especially intrusive procedures in genital area Fear of illness itself, disability, and death	Regression Inability to complete some tasks Uncooperativeness Withdrawal Depression Displaced anger and hostility Frustration	Maximize parental involvement Maximize parental information Continue education Provide medical play/information Provide therapeutic play Foster self-expression, skills building, and meaningful projects Encourage group activities/peer support
Adolescent (12–18)	Identity and repudiation versus identity diffusion • To be oneself (or not to be) • To share being oneself	Formal operations • Deductive and abstract reasoning • Can imagine the conditions of a problem—past, present, and future—and develop hypotheses about what might logically occur under different combinations of factors	Dependence on adults Separation from family and peers Fear of bodily injury, pain, and loss of identity Body image/sexuality Concern about peer group status after hospitalization	Uncooperativeness Withdrawal Anxiety Depression	Encourage peer activities/visits Provide privacy Foster independence (choices) Encourage self-expression Address body image/sexual and future concerns Offer medical preparation Continue education

Note. Adapted with permission from Rollins and Mahon (1996, p. 24).

specialists may use art activities in their work, art therapists have more in-depth knowledge of a wide array of visual media and techniques. Their approaches are specifically adapted to the needs of pediatric oncology patients to enhance visual and tactile experiences and support psychosocial goals. Councill (1999) observes that "creating art in the medical setting brings familiar and usually pleasurable materials into an unfamiliar and sometimes threatening environment. The child artist also gains an import measure of control, as he or she is the creator and foremost expert on his or her art" (p. 81). Councill also notes that "when art therapy is partnered with medical treatment children can begin to develop ways to meet the challenges of serious illness" (p. 75). Art therapy in the form of what is often called "medical art therapy," continues to grow in hospital settings, particularly in the area of pediatric and adult oncology treatment (Malchiodi, 1999, 2012).

In particular, art therapists' approaches include *manipulative, expressive,* and *symbolic* art expression. Manipulative art therapy capitalizes on developmental and psychosocial use of art materials to help children control and master their environment (in this case, the hospital setting). While helpful with patients of all ages, it is particularly useful with young patients who may need to learn and practice age-appropriate developmental tasks. In play-based approaches, children might be encouraged to work a puzzle or put together a gadget; art therapy may direct the child to build an object with clay, to learn how to hold a syringe filled with paint and create an image on paper, to create a wooden sculpture with tongue depressors, or to glue objects on a mask. Sometimes art therapy or play is helpful simply as a form of energy release; an anxious 5-year-old patient might need to pound a piece of clay or pretend to hammer nails into wood with a toy hammer. The overall goal is to enhance a sense of empowerment and self-efficacy during hospitalization, when children often feel less in control of their environment because of constant medical intervention.

Expressive art therapy focuses on providing not only strategic and specific art materials for patients to express feelings but also a variety of psychotherapeutic and counseling approaches to address anxiety, fears, and trauma reactions. For example, art therapy may involve a specific directive, such as using felt markers to depict "mad, scared, happy, sad," followed by verbal exploration of these feelings with the child; depending on the art therapist, a person-centered, solution-focused, or other approach may explore the content of the artwork and assist the child. Art therapists may also use guided imagery and mind–body stress reduction and relaxation techniques that capitalize on art making and imagination to help support children's adaptive coping skills to address worries, enhance resiliency, and reduce trauma reactions (Malchiodi & Rozum, 2012). Finally, symbolic approaches may evolve from patients' self-expression through art expression. Art therapists working on pediatric units are well versed in evaluating the content of children's art expressions and how they may communicate perceptions and experiences with hospitalization, illness, and death and dying (Councill, 2012; Malchiodi, 1998). They may also use art-based assessments to contribute information on psychosocial aspects of patients to the medical treatment team and patients' records.

ART THERAPY AND CHILD LIFE PSYCHOSOCIAL CARE

All psychosocial care begins with an evaluation of patients' capacities and capabilities through art and play, including but not limited to the following:

1. *Developmental.* What is the child's developmental level in terms of age-appropriate physical, cognitive and social skills?
2. *Affect.* Is the young patient generally happy or is his or her affect flat or sad? Does the child's mood change rapidly and without logical connection to something in the environment? What is the child's overall temperament?
3. *Interpersonal.* Does the child actively engage with others (treatment team, family, and visitors) or does he or she seem withdrawn or passive?
4. *Previous stress or trauma.* Has the child experienced any traumatic events prior to the current hospitalization? Events can include nonmedical ones such as abuse, separation from parents or caretakers, or death of a family member.
5. *Coping skills.* Does the child handle stresses easily (appropriately request help from adults or use relaxation skills) or does he or she use developmentally earlier forms of coping (crying, hypervigilance, clinging to parents, aggression, or pouting)? Does the child cope through avoidance or display fright, flight, or freeze responses to uncomfortable or threatening situations?
6. *Self-efficacy and self-concept.* Does the patient readily engage in activities or does he or she need excessive encouragement or approval from others? Does the child make positive statements about self or display actions that demonstrate self-confidence and independent choices? Is the child able to bond appropriately with helping professionals, or is he or she overly cautious, fearful or disengaged?

Councill (1999, 2012) recommends several art-based tasks in evaluation, including the following: (1) free (no directive given) drawing or painting; 2) drawing "a bridge and where you are on the bridge" to understand the child's feelings about the present and expectations of the future; and (3) the Person Picking an Apple from a Tree assessment (Lowenfeld, 1957) to evaluate development and coping skills. Play activities that are useful in evaluation include dramatic play with puppets, which are also effective as part of an overall assessment.

To illustrate integrative applications of art therapy and child life approaches to psychosocial care of pediatric cancer patients, the following case example is provided.

Case Example

Five-years-old Jeanette was diagnosed with neuroblastoma (malignant tumor found in nerve tissue). Despite her diagnosis, the art therapist/child life specialist noted that she was bright, positive, charming, and easily able to interact with the therapist and her family. However, when asked how she felt about getting injections, she replied, "Oh, I like them." Her inappropriately positive response to a painful procedure may have been for the benefit of her family, herself, or helping professionals; when asked about this response, Jeanette began to cry uncontrollably and was inconsolable. It was evident there were underlying difficult emotions related to being in the hospital for such an extended time and having to undergo medical procedures on a recurring basis. Yet Jeanette needed to maintain her sense of positive outlook and not directly confront these other emotions.

At a subsequent session, the art therapist/child life specialist introduced a medical art collage. Medical supplies, including syringes of all sizes, were displayed as creative materials for use. A variety of art supplies was available, including paints of diverse colors. Jeanette approached this art therapy/child life activity with absolute enthusiasm. She opened numerous Band-Aids, applied them to the paper, and taped down the largest syringe. Then she painted them, first blue then red, eventually covering the page with red paint in broad energetic strokes. Jeanette knew when she was finished and maintained control and the ability to make decisions throughout the session. Jeanette loved her finished collage, as did her family, but she never discussed the syringes or any feelings related to them. However, the process appeared cathartic for Jeanette and enabled her to play with these medical materials in a structured and safe art activity. It also provided a release of feelings by facilitating personal expression with both the medical and art supplies Jeanette experienced during her hospital stay.

In cases like Jeanette's, both art therapists and child life specialists are familiar with the emotional and developmental needs of children with this particular diagnosis undergoing cancer treatment. They have medical knowledge about typical treatments and prognoses. This information helps them to develop a psychosocial treatment plan based on what a child may experience physically and emotionally as a result of types of chemotherapy and surgeries, duration of hospitalization, whether medications will be administered, whether the child is an outpatient or inpatient, and the total predicted length of medical intervention. Child life specialists and art therapists have experience with coping styles and a range of responses, and can differentiate the levels of distress related to the illness.

In this case scenario, the art therapist/child life specialist evaluated and determined that Jeanette's reactions fell within the normal range. She understood a typical 5-year-old's reactions to daily injections and emotional effects of cancer treatment. As an art therapist, she was able to select developmentally and psychosocially appropriate art materials to complement the treatment plan and meet both child life and art therapy objectives. For example, the use of medical supplies in art allowed Jeanette to gain control over these items used during her hospitalization.

Additionally, the art therapist/child life specialist designed interventions to help Jeanette understand medical procedures and address questions she might have about being ill. Specifically, art therapy assists children like Jeanette in self-expression, drawing from the child's emotional style and comfort with art materials. In this case, paint was the primary art material for Jeanette, because it facilitated emotional release, and was visually pleasing and fluid. Even when the 5-year-old was not able fully to control the paint, she was proud of her painting and the outcome. In brief, the child life specialist/

art therapist was able to encourage Jeanette to experience some degree of catharsis, as well as a sense of empowerment.

RESILIENCY AND PSYCHOSOCIAL CARE

Children and adolescents with cancer and their family members are confronted by threats to physical health and quality of life. In order to help patients and families, the art therapist/child life specialist works to enhance patients' and families' capacity for resilience. Resilience helps patients adjust more positively to their experience with a life-threatening illness. It assists them in utilizing already achieved coping skills and promotes openness in attaining new abilities to deal with the stressors and fears of diagnosis and treatment.

When confronted by an initial diagnosis or recurrence of cancer, some children are better able to cope adaptively than others. These different reactions are the result of many factors, including family support, past experiences, previous trauma, and personal temperament. To describe children who seem able to cope more easily than others, we often use the word "resiliency," because they are able to draw on internal and external resources to adapt successfully. Research indicates that resilient children and adolescents share certain characteristics, including but not limited to the following: (1) stable attachment to caring adults and peers; (2) ability to interact successfully with adults and peers; (3) ability to request help from others when necessary; (4) positive role models; (5) adaptability to changing circumstances; (6) sense of self-efficacy and internal locus of control; (7) engagement in active play; (8) interests in hobbies or activities; and (9) optimism and hope for the future (Ganz, 2007; Malchiodi, 2008; Tedeschi & Kilmer, 2005).

A number of factors can impact children's resilience when confronted with a cancer diagnosis. For example, children's adjustment to illness is directly affected by their parents' and families' coping behaviors. The level of parental support, parental optimism, and communication with health care providers are all associated with improved coping among pediatric oncology patients (Suzuki & Kato, 2003). Role models, including parents, caregivers and helping professionals, are particularly important in resiliency enhancement for children and adolescents; a positive relationship with adults is one of the most powerful factors in trauma recovery in children, including those experiencing life-threatening illnesses (Tedeschi & Kilmer, 2005).

Adopting a focus on resiliency in planning art therapy and child life interventions for pediatric cancer patients is helpful for two reasons. First, it emphasizes children's and adolescent's strengths, assets, and capabilities for growth over pathology and redirects treatment goals to activities that capitalize on capabilities rather than disabilities. Also, resiliency provides the opportunity for a hopeful perspective rather than a trauma-laden and problem-focused viewpoint. This encourages patients and families to identify their strengths and competencies at a time when they are most needed.

One way to build resiliency in children and teens is to nurture a healthy self-image even when patients lose their hair, experience body changes, miss school, and have low energy and limited social interactions. Both art therapists and child life specialists can rehearse behavioral coping techniques and encourage empowerment self-advocacy with patients and families. The art therapist/child life specialist utilizes art activities designed to produce positive outcomes when patients need to develop a sense of self-worth. A successful art experience reassures children and adolescents that what they produce is valuable and that they can remain active even when they cannot attend school or participate in sports or other activities because of illness, hospitalization, or medical interventions. In brief, art making, including crafts, provide a sense of accomplishment and achievement of a tangible goal, a key factor in resiliency enhancement. The following case example demonstrates building resiliency with an adolescent patient.

Case Example

Maddy, a teenager hospitalized for a bone marrow transplant after chemotherapy failed to eradicate her cancer, was a pretty and popular girl and before her illness, an accomplished athlete, and a star on the school basketball team. Academics came easily to her and she was recognized as a good student. Maddy was well-liked by peers, teachers, and coaches because of her optimistic, friendly, bubbly personality. However, she was sick for a prolonged amount of time and in the hospital frequently after her transplant. Her optimism waned as a result. She lost all her hair, had skin sores on her face, inside her mouth, and down her digestive tract.

Maddy was in constant discomfort and did not choose to have friends visit; her mood had changed along with the changes in her body. Staff noted that she was withdrawn and had lost her enthusiasm for life, choosing to remain mostly in bed. Maddy was skilled at art, although it was not an activity she pursued outside of the hospital. An evaluation by the art therapist/child life specialist determined that because Maddy could not be successful personally and in a social context, she had lost a central part of herself. Knowing Maddy's competence with art materials, with the art therapist/child life specialist introduced mask making. Maddy worked diligently on the mask; she sat up in bed, which was a step forward, then moved to the chair to create her piece.

Maddy's affect changed with the completion of her mask, and she showed it to everyone who entered her room. She also got out of bed to leave her room to show the mask to staff and patients on the unit. By sharing her creative work with others, she became more confident and started to perceive herself as a success, proving to herself that she was not a failure. In spite of her illness and effects of treatment, she was still able to be an accomplished young woman. Maddy regained her capacity for resiliency through art therapy, even though her battle with cancer was often arduous and at times debilitating.

END-OF-LIFE CARE

Art therapy and child life services often have to address end-of-life care for pediatric patients and their families, particularly those who have had repeated hospitalizations for cancer. Like other aspects of patient care, there is often an overlap with other professionals, including social workers and nurses. Social workers generally provide supportive counseling for the family and help with the practical aspects of bereavement, including financial arrangements, and advocate for family needs, wishes, and choices. Nurses may also provide supportive intervention, along with explaining end-of-life issues and procedures to family members. Art therapists and child life specialists support the services provided by others on the psychosocial team, including preparation of the family for visitation, and supportive activities for memory-making and grief interventions. At this point treatment may become less focused on the young patient and more on family members, especially siblings. For example, the art therapist/child life specialist may help prepare the patient's brothers and sisters for a visit. This preparation may involve therapeutic medical play and include a developmentally appropriate description of how the patient looks, the equipment in the hospital room or intensive care setting, and how the patient may react to visitors.

Preparation of young patients for their own death is one of the most difficult challenges for all helping professionals. One common child life and art therapy intervention involves "legacy building," a process that helps a dying patient create art, poems, journals, or other tangible items by which the patient can be remembered. For example, making a simple scrapbook can be a way for patients to express feelings, reflect on memories of family members, and say goodbye.

Patients' family members often express their gratitude at being able to leave the pediatric intensive care unit (PICU) after the death of their child with some type of tangible memento. For example, a plaster handprint from the patient is one item that is routinely offered to families. Although greatly appreciated by the families, handprints can be a challenge to make; the art therapist/child life specialist's understanding of end-of-life issues and psychosocial care becomes critical in facilitating this process. Many PICU units have a "bereavement cart" (a portable cart that can be taken to bedside) that contains materials for creating mementos, such as handprints or memory boxes to hold a patient's lock of hair, or identification bracelet (for more information on pediatric care and end-of-life issues, see Chapters 2, 6, 20, and 21, this volume).

CONCLUSION

Art therapists and child life specialists continue to expand the parameters of their roles in work with pediatric oncology. Dual training allows the art therapist/child life specialist to provide developmentally appropriate care to children and adolescents with cancer to reduce potential stress and achieve psychosocial objectives with a wider array of methods than are possible with either approach. Whether supporting recovery from pediatric cancer, adaptive coping with medical intervention, or resiliency building or easing the stresses that accompany end-of-life issues, art therapy and child life services provide an essential component of patient care that not only gives children and adolescents an opportunity for self-expression but also provides a developmentally relevant way of confronting and overcoming the challenges of cancer and hospitalization.

REFERENCES

American Cancer Society. (2012). *Cancer facts and figures*. Retrieved May 1, 2012, from *www. cancer.org/research/cancerfactsfigures/index*.

Child Life Council. (2011). Definition of child life specialist. Retrieved November 14, 2011, from *www.childlife.org/the%20child%20life%20profession*.

Councill, T. (1999). Art therapy with pediatric cancer patients. In C. A. Malchiodi (Ed.), *Medical art therapy with children* (pp. 75–93). London: Jessica Kingsley.

Councill, T. (2012). Medical art therapy with children. In C. A. Malchiodi (Ed.), *Handbook of art therapy* (2nd ed., pp. 222–240). New York: Guilford Press.

Ganz, P. (Ed.). (2007). *Cancer survivorship: Today and tomorrow*. New York: Springer Science.

Lowenfeld, V. (1957). *Creative and mental growth*. New York: Macmillan.

Malchiodi, C. A. (1998). *Understanding children's drawings*. New York: Guilford Press.

Malchiodi, C. A. (Ed.). (1999). *Medical art therapy with children*. London: Jessica Kingsley.

Malchiodi, C. A. (Ed.). (2008). *Creative interventions with traumatized children*. New York: Guilford Press.

Malchiodi, C. A. (2012). Using art therapy with medical support groups. In C. A. Malchiodi (Ed.), *Handbook of art therapy* (2nd ed., pp. 397–408). New York: Guilford Press.

Malchiodi, C. A., & Rozum, A. L. (2012). Cognitive-behavioral and mind–body approaches. In C. A. Malchiodi (Ed.), *Handbook of art therapy* (2nd ed., pp. 89–102). New York: Guilford Press.

Rode, D. (1995). Building bridges within the culture of pediatric medicine: The interface of art therapy and child life programming. *Art Therapy: Journal of the American Art Therapy Association, 12*(2), 104–110.

Rollins, J., & Mahon, C. (1996). *From artist to artist-in-residence: Preparing artists to work in pediatric healthcare settings*. Washington, DC: Rollins & Associates.

Rollins, J., & Mahon, C. (2011). *Therapeutic activities for children and teens coping with health issues*. New York: Wiley.

Steele, W., & Malchiodi, C. A. (2011). *Trauma-informed practices with children and adolescents*. New York: Taylor & Francis.

Suzuki, L., & Kato, P. (2003). Psychosocial support for patients in pediatric oncology: The influences of parents, schools, peers and technology. *Journal of Pediatric Oncology Nursing, 20*(4), 159–174.

Tedeschi, R., & Kilmer, R. (2005). Assessing strengths, resilience, and growth to guide clinical interventions. *Professional Psychology: Research and Practice, 36*(3), 230–237.

CHAPTER 4

Art Therapy with Children and Adolescents Who Have Epilepsy

Janice Havlena
Carl E. Stafstrom

Medical professionals and advocacy groups have endeavored to dispel the myths and misperceptions that have surrounded epilepsy for centuries. However, children and adolescents with this illness continue to face many challenges. Over the last decade, numerous studies have examined quality-of-life issues for young people with epilepsy and their families. Among the findings, a lack of knowledge about epilepsy by mental health, education, and health care professionals persists (Fernandes, Snape, Beran, & Jacoby, 2011), as well as a poor understanding of the interplay between the features of epilepsy and the social and emotional development of children as serious concerns that should be addressed (Wu et al., 2008). Our aim in this chapter is to provide a foundation of knowledge about epilepsy and its impact on the adjustment of children and adolescents, along with practical suggestions as to how art therapy can be applied to intervene with some of these issues and enhance quality of life. This discussion has been culled from our ongoing consultation and research collaboration combining neurology and art therapy.

WHAT IS EPILEPSY?

"Epilepsy" is a neurological disorder characterized by seizures. A "seizure" is a transient disruption of the brain's electrical function caused by neurons firing abnormal electrical discharges. In a seizure, rather than firing single electrical impulses, neurons fire rapid barrages of impulses. This abnormal neural firing causes clinical symptoms that can range from a brief staring spell to a full-blown convulsion with stiffening and shaking of all extremities. The manifestations of a seizure depend upon the part of the brain involved and the extent to which the seizure spreads from its site of initiation in the brain ("focus") to other brain areas (Figure 4.1). The occurrence of a single seizure can represent the brain's response to an acute, temporary insult in an otherwise healthy individual (e.g., high fever or excessive alcohol ingestion); such a "reactive" seizure might be an isolated event or the sign of impending epilepsy. "Epilepsy," defined as the condition of having recurrent seizures, reflects altered underlying brain function and can occur as a consequence of brain injury or genetic predisposition. The physiological hallmarks of epilepsy are brain "hyperexcitability" (the tendency of neurons and networks of neurons to fire discharges in response to little or no provocation) and "hypersynchonicity" (the

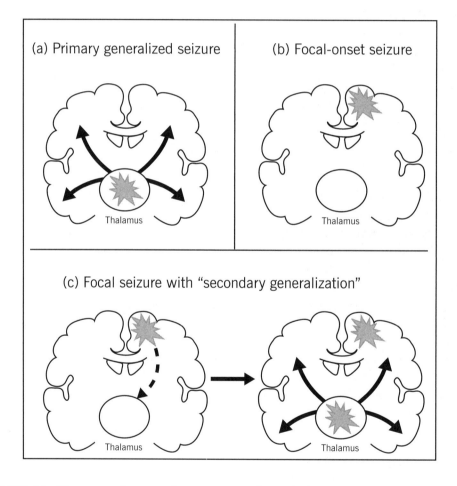

FIGURE 4.1. Illustration depicting the initiation and spread of seizure activity in the brain. Pictured are coronal sections of the brain. (a) Generalized seizure begins deep in brain (thalamus) with spread to superficial cortical regions (arrows). (b) Focal-onset seizure begins in one area of the brain (star); it may spread to nearby or distant brain regions. (c) Focal-onset seizure that "secondarily generalizes" by spreading first to thalamus (left panel) then to widespread cortical regions (right panel).

tendency of neurons and networks of neurons to fire together rather than individually) (Stafstrom, 2006)

WHAT ARE THE TYPES AND CAUSES OF EPILEPSY?

Causes of epilepsy are either "idiopathic" (cause unknown) or acquired. Many idiopathic epilepsies have a genetic basis, and the majority present during childhood, thereby affecting individuals only during a particular time window. For example, absence epilepsy in childhood, which manifests as brief, 5- to 15-second staring spells without motor involvement such as shaking, convulsions, or falling, is typically outgrown during adolescence. Therefore, these children are perfectly healthy and have normal neurological development—they just have unpredictable staring spell seizures. The challenges faced by such youngsters include the need to take antiepileptic medication (at least for several years), the potential embarrassment of "zoning out" while talking to friends, and the all too common stigma of being labeled as "epileptic" (Fernandes et al., 2011). Of course, an adolescent with uncontrolled absence seizures cannot drive, putting a crimp on the teen's social life, and the ability to obtain employment and participate in sports. Comprehensive care of such patients necessarily involves more than simply writing a prescription for antiepileptic medication—the individual's global daily function must be considered.

Acquired epilepsy (also called "symptomatic") has numerous causes—essentially, anything that can injure the brain can lead to epilepsy (Shorvon, 2011). Examples of such causes include lack of sufficient blood flow or oxygen during the birth process (which also commonly leads to cerebral palsy) or later in life (stroke), traumatic brain injury, infection of the brain (e.g., meningitis or encephalitis), and congenital abnormalities of brain development (which lead to areas of abnormal neural circuits, small or large, that endow the brain with hyperexcitability and hence, epilepsy). In addition, many other medical conditions include epilepsy as part of the disorder. For example, a brain tumor causes both seizures and neurological dysfunction, because the tumor mass presses on adjacent brain structures, and metabolic disorders characterized by energy failure cause severely low muscle tone and dysfunction of multiple organs, such as the heart, as well as seizures. A further comment regarding head injury is warranted here due not only to the common occurrence of such injuries in motor vehicle accidents, but also the huge increase in violence-related head injuries among both civilians and military personnel (Risdall & Menon, 2011) The onset of epilepsy caused by head injuries is often delayed months or even years after the initial injury. During the latent period between injury and epilepsy, the brain is undergoing structural and physiological changes that lead to hyperexcitable, hypersynchronous firing (Giza, 2010). For this etiology, we therefore have an opportunity to intervene, both medically and psychosocially, *before* the epilepsy develops. Because epilepsy, especially the acquired type, can involve *progressive* brain dysfunction, affected individuals are at risk for ongoing intellectual and cognitive dysfunction, memory loss, affective and mood disorders, and psychosocial difficulties. Table 4.1 summarizes some of the medical and psychological challenges of common epilepsies.

TABLE 4.1. Some Common Types of Epilepsy in Childhood

Epilepsy etiology	Epilepsy syndrome	Seizure types within the syndrome	Age of onset	Psychosocial challenges[a]
Generalized[b]				
Genetic (idiopathic)	Childhood absence epilepsy	Staring spells	5–10 years	Normal development, might lose track of conversations during absence seizures
	Juvenile myoclonic epilepsy	Staring spells and generalized tonic–clonic convulsions	12–18 years	As above, plus stigma of unpredictable convulsions
Symptomatic	Infantile spasms	Abrupt "startles" with head nod and extension of flexion of trunk and extremities	3–9 months	Prognosis related to etiology of the spasms, often leads to severe epilepsy and cognitive decline
	Lennox–Gastaut syndrome	Prolonged staring, tonic, clonic, or generalized tonic–clonic	2–4 years	Intellectual disability, seizures respond poorly to medications
Localization-related[b]				
Genetic (idiopathic)	Rolandic epilepsy	Usually twitching of face/neck, drooling, speech arrest but maintained alertness	7–11 years	Embarrassment of acute seizures
	Occipital epilepsy	Usually visual symptoms such as blurring	3–10 years	As above; can lose vision temporarily
Symptomatic	Temporal lobe epilepsy	Altered awareness, automatisms, fumbling movements; may secondarily generalize to generalized tonic–clonic (convulsion)	Any, depending on injury onset; typically teen–young adult	As a progressive condition—cognitive impairment, difficulty with employment, relationships, etc.

[a]All types of epilepsy might include dulling of affect, drowsiness, depression, anxiety, low self-esteem, and so forth, due to either the brain dysfunction itself or to medications used to prevent the seizures.

[b]Generalized epilepsy involves seizures that start in the entire brain at the same time; can lead to either staring or generalized convulsion. Localization-related epilepsy is also called "partial" epilepsy, since the seizures start in a specific *part* of the brain. A seizure that begins in one part of the brain can spread to other parts of the brain and even to the whole brain (generalized), at which time the seizure is called "secondarily generalized."

WHAT ARE THE PSYCHOLOGICAL AND SOCIAL CHALLENGES OF EPILEPSY?

In epilepsy, the abrupt and unpredictable occurrence of seizures can wreak havoc on a person's daily life. Several comorbid factors contribute to the often used clinical mantra that "in epilepsy, seizures are just the tip of the iceberg." Other complicating aspects of epilepsy (the part of the iceberg below the surface) include the need to take antiepileptic medications with their attendant side effects (drowsiness, fatigue, etc.); progressive cognitive impairment; psychological comorbidities, including depression, anxiety, and low self-esteem; and social barriers to employment, driving, interpersonal relationships, and ability to obtain health care, including insurance coverage (Hamiwka & Wirrell, 2009). Obviously, people with epilepsy face formidable challenges. While not every person with epilepsy exhibits all of these comorbidities, and many lead perfectly normal lives, a significant proportion of epilepsy sufferers requires multidisciplinary assistance with life's demands.

Epilepsy can begin at any age, from infancy to old age. Children encounter particular obstacles in coming to terms with their chronic, often lifelong disorder. It is well established that children with epilepsy, regardless of cause, suffer from increased rates of depression, anxiety, academic difficulty, social stigma, and isolation. Controlling seizures, usually with one or more antiepileptic medication, is the first step in preventing seizures and the potentially stigmatizing public embarrassment of having a seizure at school, at the mall, or on the playground. However, to optimize the functioning of children with epilepsy, it would be ideal to provide assistance and support on a variety of other fronts, to build their self-esteem, enhance scholastic performance, and improve social skills. In this regard, art therapy may have an important role to play (Stafstrom & Havlena, 2003).

HOW IS EPILEPSY DIAGNOSED AND TREATED?

Epilepsy is suspected initially based on clinical aspects of the "spell" or episodic neurological dysfunction reported by the patient or caregiver. As clinicians, we are mindful that there is a wide variety of causes for a person to shake, stiffen, lose awareness, or fall, many of which are not epileptic in nature. Physicians are assisted in the clinical evaluation by "electroencephalography" (EEG), a noninvasive test that records brain electrical activity by means of small electrodes attached to the scalp. Many epilepsies have distinct EEG patterns even between seizures (called the "interictal period"). If one is fortunate enough to record an actual seizure during an EEG, additional information is gleaned from the location of onset of the electrical seizure activity, clinical signs and symptoms that accompany the seizure, the type of discharges recorded, and how they spread from one brain area to another, and so forth. If a brain structural anomaly is suspected, imaging in the form of brain magnetic resonance imaging (MRI) is performed. The MRI is very sensitive to structural abnormalities such as tumors, scars, hemorrhages, calcium accumulation, and abnormal brain development (Richardson, 2010). Genetic testing is proving invaluable in uncovering mutations that may lead to epilepsy (Helbig, Scheffer, Mulley, & Berkovic, 2008) Finally, neuropsychological testing measures numerous aspects of memory, cognition, and affect that accompany epilepsy (Jones-Gotman et al., 2010) .

The most common epilepsy treatment is medication, the choice of which is determined by the specific epilepsy syndrome that is diagnosed. While it is beyond the scope of this chapter to elaborate on particular drugs, suffice it to say that each drug has potential side effects that can alter a person's cognition and mood (Cavanna, Ali, Rickards, & McCorry, 2010). For patients who do not respond to medication, more "advanced" epilepsy treatments might include specific diets (e.g., the high-fat, low-carbohydrate ketogenic diet), electrical stimulation devices (e.g., the vagus nerve stimulator), and, for very selected cases, epilepsy surgery. These latter therapies are considered only when a patient's seizures are not responsive to several medication trials; people warranting these treatments typically have severe epilepsy and even greater psychological comorbidities.

APPLICATION OF ART THERAPY WITH EPILEPSY

Background

The art therapy focus groups and approaches described in this section are derived from our research study (Stafstrom, Havlena, & Krezinsky, 2012), which investigated the graphic features of drawings made by children with epilepsy, the usefulness of seizure drawings to understand the experience of children with their illness, and the efficacy of art therapy groups to address quality-of-life issues related to childhood epilepsy.

Art Therapy Focus Groups

We believe that there is no upper limit on enhancement of self-esteem for developing children, and all children with epilepsy may benefit from opportunities to participate in programs that promote positive adjustment to their illness. As a component of our research on the use of drawings to assess children and adolescents with epilepsy, we also conducted multiple series of art therapy focus groups for participants over the course of 2 years. Participants ranged in age from 7 to 18 years and were drawn from throughout the region, with some traveling as much as 3 hours round-trip for the weekly sessions. All participants had active epilepsy, with no other serious health, psychological, or cognitive impairments. Our focus groups were structured by age range and approximate level in school: upper elementary school, middle school, and high school. Sessions were held once a week for 4 consecutive weeks, for approximately 1½ hours per meeting. The choice of four weekly sessions was made to ensure consistent attendance. The series were scheduled to fall between major holidays and school semester vacations to minimize disruption of family plans. Four weeks seemed to be the most practical and realistic commitment for most families given the constraints of competing schedules and travel distance for many of them.

The primary purpose of the art therapy focus groups was to explore a few, key quality-of-life concerns of youth with epilepsy. We hoped to enhance participants' adjustment to epilepsy while learning more about each child's functioning, including his or her strengths, within a relatively short time frame. The four sessions were strategically designed and structured to allow enough interaction to develop a positive group membership dynamic and address important topics productively. The series of meetings allowed for the development of trust and rapport among group members, with open communication and sharing of feelings. Topics progressed developmentally from introductions to exploration of challenging feelings, to identification of individual resources for coping with illness, to reflection on visions for the future. Emphasis was on helping children to access their capacity for creative self-expression in the here and now as a means of discovering each person's unique resources. Themes and media were chosen to be engaging yet adaptable to the various age ranges, while keeping the weekly content essentially the same across age groups for the purpose of comparisons within our study. Specific directives for themes and art processes were modified in complexity for the different age groups.

Most of the time within each session was devoted to making art, following an introduction to the weekly topic and materials. To share the artwork, all pieces were always displayed to the entire group and placed in front of each child, so that all work would be seen at the same time before discussion began. Children were taught how to look at the art as a body of work—first to notice any similarities in shapes, colors, objects, or use of art materials, then to appreciate how each piece was unique. This technique seems to reduce any tendency to compare one's skills negatively with others, and also to keep the artwork, and hence the immediacy of the thoughts and feelings involved in the art process, accessible to each participant. Individuals were then encouraged to say whatever they would like about their work, and as a group, to discuss the weekly topic in more depth. The pace and emotional intensity of each session and of the series as a whole were regulated, in part, by carefully constructing directives for art processes and questions for sharing. In this approach, children's defenses are anticipated and appreciated as naturally occurring responses that are useful to children in their everyday functioning and should not be dismantled abruptly. Art process and art production are considered both for their uniquely nonverbal and metaphorical capacity to practice new ways of looking at problems and as practice in making choices that improve self-confidence.

Weekly Topics and Art Processes

First Group

This opening session served as orientation to the focus group series, to art therapy, and to the confidentiality and other behavioral expectations of the group. We acknowledged that all participants had epilepsy—perhaps different types and with different symptoms—and that they would have a chance to talk about that more in the following week. This session, however, would be spent getting to know one another with one of our favorite art processes. Here, the abbreviated presentation about epilepsy was an intentional means both to establish common ground and support individuality; to capture participants' uneasiness and resistance about what they might be asked to discuss during the art groups; and to offer the possibility that discussion of a difficult topic could be viewed as "a chance"—an opportunity—that might be a positive experience. Shifting from this introduction into the art process was a deliberate move designed to replace any lingering uneasiness with a more interesting and enjoyable creative activity. The introductory session also gave participants some time to prepare themselves for more difficult work.

For this session, group members were invited to create individual collage boxes that would serve to introduce themselves to the group (Table 4.2). The box in this exercise functioned as a metaphor for the self. Portrayal of personal interests, qualities, abilities, likes, and dislikes reinforced a holistic model of the self rather than one defined solely by their medical condition. The metaphorical implications of containers and their applications within art therapy are diverse (Farrell-Kirk, 2001). The box and lid used here were very important components in the process. The inside–outside theme opened discussion about a public and a more private self. A range of shapes, sizes, and types was essential, so that each participant could choose a box he or she found appealing, one that would stand in place of the self. They could explore and portray whatever they choose in their artwork, while maintaining control over what they would share with the group and what would be kept private. Lids to the self-portrait boxes could be open or closed. Creating opportunities like these for choice and control in the art process is especially critical for children receiving art therapy in medical settings, where medical interventions and treatment must take precedence over other needs (Councill, 2012).

TABLE 4.2. First-Week Art Process

Theme and Media: "Self-Portrait, Inside–Outside Box"; collage and drawing media.

Purpose/rationale: Introduces self to others; reinforces sense of self not defined solely by medical condition; opens discussion of public and more private information.

Introduction: Choose a box that you like. You will use it to introduce yourself to the group. On the outside, show things about yourself that are easy for people to know about you. On the inside, show things about yourself that are harder for people to know, or that you keep more private. When we share our work you will have a chance to say whatever you like about what you worked on.

Directions: Start anywhere. Draw or write on your box; use magazine pictures and words, or both. Decorate it if you like.

Materials:
- Boxes with lids—variety of shapes, styles, and sizes, including recyclable gift boxes and cardboard craft boxes
- Magazines—assortment of family, news, sports, nature, children's and teens' titles—typical "waiting room" titles
- Decorative papers, trim, ribbon, string, yarn
- Glue sticks
- Scissors
- Markers

Finishing techniques: Participants can place anything inside their boxes to save or to work on later in another session if time permits.

Sharing: Who is willing to go first? Show us your box, and tell us about how you worked on it. What is one important part?

The self-portrait box project functioned very well as an introductory exercise for several reasons. Group members could quickly learn what they had in common, as well as the ways each was a distinct individual. The box also provided several levels of engagement. Some children began by decorating the outside of their boxes with designs, then slowly became more comfortable with the idea of sharing information about themselves. Figure 4.2 illustrates how one young adolescent chose a mailbox for his self-portrait project, then decorated it in bright colors. On the outside, a cartoon snake is coiled and a monkey "chews on something." He explained that he likes to "joke around with his friends." Although the box was wide open, he said nothing was inside—"yet." This piece may suggest that while he was alert and wary in this first session and perhaps not taking things too seriously, he also was "open" to both incoming and "outgoing" communication.

Children who did not have confidence in their drawing ability were able to select photos and text from magazines. Images could contain symbolic content that was not only personally meaningful but also could be kept private. For example, both younger children and adolescents in different groups placed magazine photos of beds inside their

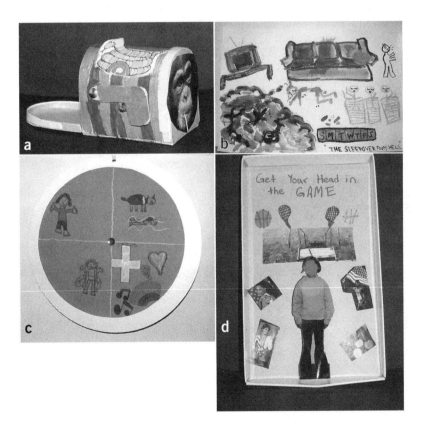

FIGURE 4.2. Art processes from each weekly session. (a) "Self-Portrait Inside–Outside" collage box; (b) "Memory or Feeling about Epilepsy" painting; (c) "Mandala of Personal Symbols"; (d) "A Dream or Goal for My Future" diorama.

boxes but chose not to comment on them. Some types of epilepsy may lead to early morning seizures, falling out of bed during a seizure, or loss of bladder control during nighttime seizures. Any of these associations may or may not have had relevance for those participants, but their choices to include the image without an explanation were respected. Throughout our sessions, most participants included in their collage box at least one image that they chose not to discuss openly.

Second Group

While the first session established parameters for personal choices and group safety, the second session was designed to assist participants directly with work on a personal experience or emotion resulting from their illness. Group members were asked to recall and portray through drawing and painting an incident that focused attention on their epilepsy, a memory or dream about having epilepsy, or a difficult feeling they would be willing to explore. The purpose of this activity is to acknowledge a feeling that is troublesome or a challenge that is a current concern, and to provide an opportunity for closure on an incident that may have caused psychological distress. Exploring these topics allowed group members to reach an empathic understanding, as well as to problem solve with same-age peers who had similar experiences (see Table 4.3).

TABLE 4.3. Second-Week Art Process

Theme and media: "A Memory or Feeling about Epilepsy"; crayon-resist and watercolor

Purpose/rationale: Provides an opportunity for participants to "tell their stories." Externalizing experience may help to provide closure on a difficult incident. Opportunity for empathic sharing with same-age peers. Crayon-resist is a two-step process that provides structure and slows down the process to promote reflection. Drawing with crayon on watercolor paper requires some physical exertion, releasing physical tension that may be evoked by the topic. The second step, painting, is fluid and promotes relaxation and release.

Introduction: Think back on a memory about your epilepsy. This could be something that happened, or a feeling that comes up for you that might be hard to talk about.

Directions: When you decide what to show, draw it out first with crayons, then paint it. It is important to press fairly hard so the wax in the crayon will stick to the paper. If you use a very light color crayon, the drawing will be invisible until you paint over it.

Materials:
- Crayons
- Watercolor paints and brushes
- Watercolor paper 12″ × 18″
- Oil pastels (for drawing over finished paintings and adding titles)

Finishing techniques: Mount on colored paper.

Sharing: Give your painting a title; write it on the front or back. Somebody get us started: Tell us the title and what is happening in your painting.

Although the primary emphasis in the art therapy group series was on nurturing strengths, this session provided a structured opportunity for participants to "tell their story." As our first study indicated, children's experiences of their epilepsy may be more intense than would be anticipated by their medical symptoms alone (Stafstrom & Havlena, 2003). The effects of trauma among children with medical illness in hospital settings has been an area of both research and treatment in art therapy (Chapman, Morabito, Ladakakos, Schrier, & Knudson, 2001). In a study on art therapy and trauma resolution with adolescents experiencing posttraumatic stress disorder, individuals with a "serious medical problem" constituted more than one-third of study participants (Lyshak-Stelzer, Singer, St. John, & Chemtob, 2007). Exercises in recounting individual experiences are seen as an essential step in the art therapy trauma healing process and are carefully integrated into the therapy (Gantt & Tinnin, 2009; Malchiodi, 2012). In their work with art therapy and trauma, Gantt and Tinnin note that "an exclusive focus on teaching coping skills can delay or even ignore trauma processing altogether. Such a delay can be misinterpreted by the patient as the therapist's unwillingness or inability to deal with the actual event, reinforcing the idea that the trauma itself is [too difficult to deal with]" (p. 151). This particular art therapy exercise offered several options for interpretation of the directive, as well as choice in the detail of disclosure, so that each young person could participate at his or her own level of readiness.

Crayon-resist watercolor paint and oil pastels on watercolor paper were used for this process. Drawing first with crayon then painting over the lines allows the image to emerge slowly. This process affords control over the rate and degree of visual contrast and the intensity of the image. Some areas of the painting can be soft or ambiguous, while others can be more clearly defined, reworked, or even covered over with paint or water-soluble oil pastels when the paper has dried. The media and techniques used here support a thoughtful engagement with the directive and a regulation of emotion during reflection on the event and accompanying feeling states. Kaplan (2007, p. 96) describes the transformative and calming effect of art making on the emotions as the "shift occurs in the brain so that internal babble is suppressed while sensory modules are activated."

When completed, participants were asked to give the picture a title and to record it directly on the painting as a departure point into discussion of the artwork. Individual responses to this process often were poignant. Stories included injury from falls during a seizure, the sensation of walking in a thick fog and losing one's way home from school, and embarrassment about taking medication at school. A common theme was disappointment about exclusion from peer-group activities for fear of a seizure—activities that could potentially be too dangerous such as amusement park rides or driving. This process sparked much spontaneous discussion and exchange among group members. Through this art piece children and adolescents have shared many of the challenges of epilepsy—their experiences with seizures on field trips or family outings, worries about participating in activities that make them feel vulnerable, and the burden of medication compliance when away from home. In "The Sleepover from Hell," Figure 4.2, an adolescent recounted the consequences of forgetting to take her medication during a sleepover with friends. In her painting, she feels a seizure begin and searches for her bags to locate her medicine. Her friends, asleep, do not hear her, so they cannot help. Some older adolescents depicted difficult choices between "having a social life" and a healthy lifestyle—getting sufficient sleep, eating healthy foods, and abstaining from alcohol—that their epilepsy demands but to which few of their peers adhere.

Deliberations about how and with whom to share their epilepsy came up in every series through this second group session art process. When one participant described his efforts to conceal his need for medication from his classmates, another expressed surprise that it would even be possible, because everyone in her class had witnessed her seizures. One child described how he had been teased by a friend, to whom he had previously confided about his epilepsy, after an argument on the playground. Another girl in the group then labeled the friend's behavior as bullying and ticked off the steps her school endorsed for dealing with bullies. Children who chose not to share their epilepsy with even close friends learned how other children informed their classes about their epilepsy with the help of their teacher at the beginning of the school year.

Although this topic brought up the most difficult material, participants worked hard on the art process and were earnest in their contributions to group discussion. Some of the behavioral changes observed after this session included easier separation from parents at the start of group the next week; more informal conversation with the art therapist facilitators and other group members before, during, and at the conclusion of the sessions that followed; and more forthcoming conversation with parents about what participants were doing in the group.

Third Group

Mandalas bearing symbols of empowerment were the art process for this session. Group members were guided to identify personal sources of strength that would positively underscore their individuality, and promote reciprocity and a sense of belonging in relationships. This art process was designed to support the development of resilience by assisting children in identifying resources to draw upon in their everyday lives (e.g., family and friends), their beliefs and values system, the natural world, and their participation in the broader community. The mandala functions as a symbol of wholeness in this exercise, and each quadrant focuses on a different area: important relationships; values or beliefs that are good for the world; a place or part of nature that is special; and things participants do well that make a contribution or things they can do for others (Table 4.4). Taken together, the areas make up a balanced sense of self and life.

Participants were encouraged to draw shapes and symbols, and to include text and colors that held personal significance for them by conveying just the most important features. A favorite quotation or slogan could be incorporated as well. Loumeau-May (2008, p. 90), in her art therapy grief work with children, observed that "through development of imagery and symbolism, meaning is given to experience, sometimes highly personal, and sometimes numinous and spiritual." The mandalas created in our groups commonly depicted religious beliefs and church activities, and many children drew themselves

TABLE 4.4. Third-Week Art Process

Theme and media: Mandala of personal symbols; mixed drawing media.

Purpose/rationale: Identifies individual resources; mandala serves as a symbol of wholeness.

Introduction: Each section of the mandala is for a different part of your life. Use simple drawings, symbols, and colors that will help you to show:
- Your important relationships—people you love and care about and who feel that way toward you.
- A value or belief you have that is good for the world.
- A favorite place or part of nature—also can be an animal or even a favorite season.
- A skill, activity you really enjoy doing, or something you can do for others.

Directions: Symbols are what people, communities, and cultures use as reminders of what is important to them. Begin by deciding what symbols you will use for each section. Symbols can be made by first sketching out ideas. Then make a simple drawing by using just the major shapes and lines. Next, choose a color circle you like, or that has special meaning for you, for the background. Draw your symbols on it, then glue the circle to the cardboard disc.

Materials:
- Cardboard circles, 12″ diameter
- Precut colored art paper, cut into 10″ circles and divided into quadrants with pencil lines
- Markers, oil pastels
- Assorted collage items such as gems, mirrored shapes
- String, yarn
- Glue sticks, tacky glue
- Hole punch
- Scissors

Finishing techniques: Think of a title, maybe a quote or words from a song for your mandala. Write it in the space around the circle. Punch a hole in the top; add string or yarn loop to hang.

Sharing: Read us your title and point out some symbols that go with it. Is there anything that you didn't know was important to you, or forgot about, until you worked on this project?

helping someone in response to the question about what they could do well or do for the world. Figure 4.2 depicts how a young adolescent symbolized her beliefs and values of happiness, love, and faith with music notes, hearts, a rainbow, and a cross; how swimming and the pet animal she raises connect her to nature; how her mother is "always there for her"; and how an older adult in a wheelchair represents her volunteer work in a nursing home. She enjoyed this service work and said she might like to work in a hospital when she grows up.

Frequently, the quadrant of the mandala that explored important relationships more often emphasized closeness to parents and pets than to friends. These responses may convey unanticipated effects on children as a result of facing challenges associated with their illness—close relationships with parents, a developed belief system, and appreciation for the important roles of caregivers and service professionals.

Fourth Group

This final session explored ideas about the future. The group members were asked to envision themselves achieving a desired goal. Photos, drawing, collage media, and shallow boxes were available to construct dioramas. Through this process children and adolescents were able to share their thoughts about the future, identify a goal or dream, and imagine themselves achieving it. Use of digital portraits in this project reinforced the idea of self-identity and self-confidence. During the previous session, photos were taken of each young person, including a whole-body shot and striking a pose he or she wanted to use for this project. They also had a chance to prepare for this photo—to wear a favorite shirt, a hat, or to hold a treasured object.

This session allowed participants to acknowledge their hopes and dreams, and to voice their doubts or limitations, while "working on the future" symbolically. Photo portrait outlines were cut and glued to cardstock so the figure could stand independently and literally be placed into the scene (Table 4.5). A bridge toward optimism was provided by asking participants to think through their vision for themselves, to create it, and to "take their place" in the world. Last, a title, a phrase of encouragement, or an affirmation was recorded somewhere on the diorama.

This project was, by far, the favorite art therapy process of most children. Some common themes included their future selves as independent adults who were married, traveling, or living in another part of the country. One teen remarked that this art piece "asked us to think about our future, which we don't do at school, and I liked that." Many

TABLE 4.5. Fourth-Week Art Process

Theme and media: "A Dream or Goal for My Future"—diorama with digital photo and mixed media.

Purpose/rationale: Provides an opportunity to identify and explore a goal. Placing your self-portrait photo in the scene is a chance to "rehearse" for a decision or next step toward a goal.

Introduction: Imagine yourself doing something that is important to you in your future. The future time could be next month, next year, or when you are older.

Directions: Use drawing, painting, collage, and mixed media to create the scene within cardboard box. Attach the inverted lid to the bottom, extending it in front to make a platform or stage. Cut around outlines from digital photos of participants and reinforce with cardstock, leaving a tab at the bottom to make a stand.

Materials:
- Shallow boxes with lids—smaller sizes work best
- Magazines—nature, travel, sports, news, people, professional
- Glue sticks, tacky glue, glue guns
- Natural materials, shells, stones, twigs, moss

Finishing techniques: What words of encouragement or inspiration will help you to work toward this dream? Write those words somewhere on your scene.

Sharing: What is going on in your future? What sights and sounds do you notice in your scene? How does it feel to be there?

of the dioramas involved scenes that tested the young people physically, challenged their skills, or placed them near settings (e.g., waterfalls or hiking trails) that they had been restricted from exploring in the past, because of the potential danger. Other scenes represented current decisions they were contemplating, including extracurricular activities for the upcoming year or what to do after high school. In a diorama titled "Dedicated," a young adult described her plans for the future—going to college, returning to her birthplace, pursuing adventures in wilderness areas, and finding "that perfect match." She was philosophical and planned to savor experiences while they lasted, and to push past setbacks such as the one in her self-portrait photo for this project—sports training despite an injury. A younger adolescent announced that she would try out for the swim team after all, despite her former fears that she would always come in last. Swimming lanes, sports figures, and "Get Your Head in the Game" surround her self-portrait (Figure 4.2). Other affirmations from this process included "Be Yourself," "Live Life," "Be the Change You Want to See in the World," and "Just Try It." In this final session each member also selected one piece of artwork to revisit in a group image review; all work was returned, and participants were encouraged to share their artwork with their parents.

SYMPTOM-RELATED GRAPHIC CONTENT

Representation of visual phenomena of epileptic seizures or symptom-related experiences are often incorporated into the artwork of children and adolescents with epilepsy (Naitove, 1983; Stafstrom & Havlena, 2003). While graphic features such as quality of line, color, and thematic content may have multiple layers of intention and meaning in any client artwork, it is important for the art therapist to understand how physiological experience might be portrayed in a particular piece. Some symptom-related content noted in the artwork from our focus groups included blurry or fog-like scenes, halos of light and colors, and depictions of crying eyes. In several drawings, participants represented themselves with smiles or neutral expressions but simultaneously with tears streaming from their eyes. These drawings perhaps could be interpreted to suggest denial or a defense against conflicted emotions in relation to other content in the drawing. In each case, however, the young person contextualized the drawing as the uncontrolled crying he or she experiences following a seizure. They also shared their feelings of awkwardness about what appears to be crying in public, and frustration about their inability to control the tears. Examples of how variations on a specific visual phenomenon experienced by one participant have been incorporated into a series of artwork are presented in Figure 4.3. A drawing of a sphere of light and color is for this child a familiar visual image "that makes everything else go away" (Figure 4.3). Next, the sphere of colors fills the space between this child and his teacher during a seizure at school (Figure 4.3). A smaller and more manageable ball is seen in his choice to create a colorful planet Earth with land, water, and clouds during free time in the group (Figure 4.3). In his last project (Figure 4.3), "The Whole Wide World"—a diorama project depicting a goal or dream for the future—he is a pilot. The sphere of colors and planet are now in the background as he

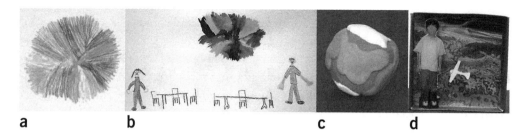

a   **b**   **c**   **d**

FIGURE 4.3. Symptom-related graphic content. Visual phenomena of seizure depicted in art processes: (a) seizure drawing; (b) "Memory or Feeling about Epilepsy" painting; (c) free-clay activity; (d) "Dream or Goal for My Future" diorama.

flies over coastal waters. The sphere may have become the backdrop that he flies above, and perhaps masters, in the future.

CONCLUSION

One of the striking findings from our focus groups was that the vast majority of the children had never met another person with epilepsy prior to participation in the group. For the young adolescents transitioning into middle school, the timing of the focus group seemed particularly appropriate. Middle school is a challenging time when many young people experience social awkwardness or believe they do not quite fit in, or that they are flawed in some way. The transition to a new school, new teachers, and a new and perhaps larger peer group may intensify their concerns about their symptoms and how they will negotiate management of their epilepsy in the new setting. As the middle school group gathered in the waiting area for the first art therapy session, it was interesting to observe group members glancing around expectantly, trying to pick out who else in the room might have epilepsy, then to see the surprise register as they learned that all of the young people there would be joining the group.

The length, pace, structure, and topics of the art groups and their intersections with the specific goals of the series seemed to coalesce well to address our overarching objective to enhance the adjustment to illness of children and adolescents with epilepsy, and to understand more about how they experience themselves. Fernandes et al. (2011) found that in adult narratives "some portray epilepsy as a journey, or transition, in which lessons have been hard earned, whereas others view it as an end in itself. As such, stories reflect both changes in identity and in perception of time" (p. 59). Through the artwork and narratives in our art therapy groups, we heard the voices of a broad range of young lives in progress—sometimes humorous and playful, other times frustrated or confused, and almost always empathetic and hopeful. This diversity of expression perhaps served more than any other single influence to reduce their isolation in connection with epilepsy, which appeared to be a major outcome for many of the young people in these groups. Perception, or fear of stigma, whether directly experienced or not, may be linked to isolation and other dimensions of quality of life (Jacoby & Austin, 2007). Reduction of perceived stigma associated with epilepsy and improvement in quality of life has been increasingly confirmed by research (Fernandes et al., 2011). Over the 4 weeks of our art therapy group sessions, we observed improved comfort and animated conversation among group members. Similarly, parents reported that their children had become more open and willing to talk about their experiences in the sessions, and about their epilepsy in general. The children and adolescents across all age groups consistently demonstrated engagement in the art processes and discussions. Identification with their art products appeared to be strong: artwork was completed, well-cared for, and taken home. The art therapy groups provided the impetus and the focus for self-discovery at a critical time in the unfolding of their stories, and the art served as a record of that growth. Future research will entail analysis of art therapy as a function of epilepsy type and syndrome, epilepsy duration, epilepsy severity, age, and correlation of medical outcome with qualitative art expression.

REFERENCES

Cavanna, A. E., Ali, F., Rickards, H. E., & McCorry, D. (2010). Behavioral and cognitive effects of anti-epileptic drugs. *Discovery Medicine, 9*(45), 138–144.

Chapman, L., Morabito, D., Ladakakos, C., Schrier, H., & Knudson, M. M. (2001). The effectiveness of art therapy intervention in reducing posttraumatic stress disorder (PTSD) symptoms in pediatric trauma patients. *Art Therapy: Journal of the American Art Therapy Association, 18*(2), 100–104.

Councill, T. (2012). Medical art therapy with children. In C. A. Malchiodi (Ed.), *Handbook of art therapy* (2nd ed., pp. 222–240). New York: Guilford Press.

Farrell-Kirk, R. (2001). Secrets, symbols, synthesis, and safety: The role of boxes in art therapy. *American Journal of Art Therapy, 39*(3), 88–92.

Fernandes, P. T., Snape, D. A., Beran, R. G., & Jacoby, A. (2011). Epilepsy stigma: What do we know and where next? *Epilepsy and Behavior, 22*(1), 55–62.

Gantt, L., & Tinnin, L. (2009). Support for a neurobiological view of trauma with implications for art therapy. *The Arts in Psychotherapy, 36*(3), 148–153.

Giza, C. C. (2010). Posttraumatic seizures and epileptogenesis: Good and bad plasticity. In J. M. Rho, R. Sankar, & C. E. Stafstrom (Eds.), *Epilepsy: Mechanisms, models, and translational perspectives* (pp. 181–208). Boca Raton, FL: CRC Press.

Hamiwka, L. D., & Wirrell, E. C. (2009). Comorbidities in pediatric epilepsy: Beyond "just" treating the seizures. *Journal of Child Neurology, 24*(6), 734–742.

Helbig, I., Scheffer, I. E., Mulley, J. C., & Berkovic, S. F. (2008). Navigating the channels and beyond: Unraveling the genetics of the epilepsies. *Lancet Neurology, 7*(3), 231–245.

Jacoby, A., & Austin, J. K. (2007). Social stigma for adults and children with epilepsy. *Epilepsia, 48*(9), 6–9.

Jones-Gotman, M., Smith, M. L., Risse, G. L., Westerveld, M., Swanson, S. J., Giovagnoli, A. R., et al. (2010). The contribution of neuropsychology to diagnostic assessment in epilepsy. *Epilepsy and Behavior, 18*(1–2), 3–12.

Kaplan, F. (2007). Art and conflict resolution. In *Art therapy and social action* (pp. 89–102). London: Jessica Kingsley.

Loumeau-May, L. (2008). Grieving in the public eye: Art therapy with children who lost parents in the World Trade Center attacks. In C. A. Malchiodi (Ed.), *Creative interventions with traumatized children* (pp. 81–111). New York: Guilford Press.

Lyshak-Stelzer, F,. Singer, P., St. John, P., & Chemtob, M. C. (2007). Art therapy for adolescents with posttraumatic stress disorder symptoms: A pilot study. *Art Therapy: Journal of the American Art Therapy Association, 24*(4), 163–169.

Malchiodi, C. A. (Ed.). (2012). *Handbook of art therapy* (2nd ed.). New York: Guilford Press.

Naitove, C. E. (1983). Where ignorance prevails: An art therapist's approach to the epilepsies. *The Arts in Psychotherapy, 10*, 141–149.

Richardson, M. (2010). Update on neuroimaging in epilepsy. *Expert Review of Neurotherapeutics, 10*(6), 961–973.

Risdall, J. E., & Menon, D. K. (2011). Traumatic brain injury. *Philosophical Transactions of the Royal Society B: Biological Science, 366*(1562), 241–250.

Shorvon, S. D. (2011). The causes of epilepsy: Changing concepts of etiology of epilepsy over the past 150 years. *Epilepsia, 52*(6), 1033–1044.

Stafstrom, C. E. (2006). Epilepsy: A review of selected clinical syndromes and advances in basic science. *Journal of Cerebral Blood Flow and Metabolism, 26*(8), 938–1004.

Stafstrom, C. E., & Havlena, J. (2003). Seizure drawings: Insight into the self-image of children with epilepsy. *Epilepsy and Behavior, 4*(1), 43–56.

Stafstrom, C. E., Havlena, J., & Krezinsky, A. (2012). Art therapy focus groups for children and adolescents with epilepsy. *Epilepsy and Behavior, 24*(2), 227–233.

Wu, K., Lieber, E., Siddarth, P., Smith, K., Sankar, R., & Caplan, R. (2008). Dealing with epilepsy: Parents speak up. *Epilepsy and Behavior, 13*(1), 131–138.

CHAPTER 5

Art Therapy with Children Who Have Asthma
A Randomized Clinical Trial

Anya Beebe

Many children with chronic asthma face both the physiological and psychological challenges of having a major illness. In addition to facing the physical challenges of a disease, children with asthma often have a strong need for psychological support as well. Art therapy has proven to be a beneficial modality of therapy to help children cope with the emotional aspects of having a chronic illness. More prevalent now in hospitals around the country, art therapy has become a valuable adjunct therapy in the treatment of asthma and many other chronic conditions.

This chapter provides an overview of a clinically randomized trial conducted at National Jewish Health in Denver, Colorado. In this study, art therapy was shown to be an effective way to reduce anxiety significantly, improve quality of life, and strengthen self-concept for children with chronic asthma (Beebe, Gelfand, & Bender, 2010). Children in this study were able to find solutions through art therapy to help them overcome their fears and barriers, and to manage the emotional arena of their illness. Research has indicated that emotional regulation is an important factor to consider when treating asthma, and further information related to the mind–body connection in healing for these children is explored as well.

CHILDREN WITH ASTHMA

Asthma is a complicated condition that involves a chronic inflammatory disorder of the airways which causes recurrent episodes of coughing, wheezing, chest tightness, and difficulty breathing (*www.cdc.gov/asthma*). Asthma affects nearly 4.5 million American children a year, and an estimated 1,000 of these children die from the disease (Welch, 2011). The severity, acuteness, triggers, and symptoms of asthma vary considerably and can range from mild shortness of breath to a complete blockage of the airway (Welch, 2011).

To keep children with severe asthma safe from triggers, many have restricted levels of activity and reduced exposure to environments that may increase their symptoms. Unfortunately, these restrictions may interfere with children's education, acceptance by peers, and participation in extracurricular activities (Bender, 1995). When children are not able to participate in typical childhood experiences and social activities they often get excluded and left behind. These limitations may hinder their psychological development, as well as development of healthy self-esteem and self-concept (Bender, 1995). Not surprisingly, these factors also lead to increased rates of anxiety, depression, stress, and emotional dysregulation in children with asthma (McQuaid, Kopel, & Nasasu, 2001). For some children, the emotional stress of having a chronic illness can be as taxing to manage as their medical symptoms (Beebe et al., 2010).

Children with asthma face many challenges, and understandably, one of the biggest challenges is the fear of not being able to breathe. Often, this fear is so great for these children that it can contribute to ongoing feelings of anxiety. Heightened levels of anxiety and stress are a concern for children with asthma, as emotional dysregulation may bring on an attack or worsen an existing mild episode (Blackman & Gurka, 2007). In turn, when children are anxious and perceive their asthma to be severe and life-threatening, they often have increased depression rates as well (Blackman & Gurka, 2007). Complicating things even further, depression in children and adolescents with asthma has been linked to noncompliance with medications, as well as an increased mortality rates (Bender & Zhang, 2008). Understanding this information, it is apparent that the connection between emotions and asthma is too significant to be ignored.

Although the disease of asthma is physiologically based, evidence shows that heightened levels of stress, depression, and anxiety are often linked to asthma attacks (Bender & Zhang, 2008; Wambolt, Bender, & Rankin, 2011; Wood et al., 2007a, 2007b). Advanced research explains that psychobiological pathways and internal physical mechanisms closely link emotions and stress with disease reactivity (Wright, Cohen, & Cohen, 2005), and that there is a clear relationship between dysregulated emotional states and the severity and intensity of asthma exacerbations (Koinis-Mitchell et al., 2009; Bender, 1995). Emotions and physical symptoms are so closely connected that in one research study, airway constrictions could be brought on by suggestion in most asthmatic children (Mrazek, 1985). Wood et al. make an important point regarding the treatment of asthma and explain that it is becoming fully recognized that the mind and body interact and influence the severity of asthma symptoms. In fact, emotional triggering related to anxiety and depression have become too important to ignore in the treatment of asthma (Wood et al., 2006; also see Sternberg, 2000). Given this knowledge, it seems clear that helping asthmatic children manage and cope with their internal emotional states may be just as important as providing them with medical treatment.

ASTHMA AND ART THERAPY

More and more medical centers and hospitals have come to recognize the importance of the mind–body connection in illness, and alternative therapies that help patients improve their mental health are becoming more prevalent. Art therapy in particular has become increasingly common in pediatric hospital settings and provides many avenues of healing for patients with chronic illness (Malchiodi, 1999). Children who are given art materials and support from an art therapist to express themselves have an opportunity to examine and explore their personal emotional worlds. Through art making, hidden inner experiences are brought forward for further contemplation (Franklin & Siemon, 2008) and can be expressed and understood in more objective way. Art making also gives physically ill children the ability to establish distance between themselves and their medical concerns. By processing their feelings through art, children often come to understand that their problems are separate from themselves and that they have an identity outside of their illness (Rubin, 1999).

Children also tend to have a very positive response to art therapy. Expressing feelings through creative exploration and play comes naturally to most children; therefore, art making can be a safe way to explore what might otherwise be overwhelming feelings (Malchiodi, 1999). Art therapy is also particularly effective for children, who do not have the same ability to articulate their emotions, perceptions, or beliefs that adults do (Malchiodi, 1999). In one study, drawings were shown to be a valuable clinical tool in helping children with asthma express feelings about their illness that they could not otherwise verbalize (Gabriels, Wamboldt, McCormick, Adams, & McTaggart, 2000). By providing a means to communicate their feelings through art therapy, children are given an opportunity to express, face, and cope with feelings that might be to challenging to communicate verbally. Once they express themselves in the art, children are often better able to understand and come to terms with feelings about their illness and are better able to move forward with increased resilience.

ART THERAPY RESEARCH STUDY
FOR CHILDREN WITH ASTHMA

Research Objectives

Since the early 1980s, art therapy groups have been a part of the pediatric services at National Jewish Health and have been considered one of the most integral elements of a child's treatment. At National Jewish Health, known globally for its advanced research in treating asthma, it is understood that a close collaboration between physical and mental health treatment is vital in the stabilization of the disease.

Many very important, well-researched case studies and quasi-experimental studies have been published in the field of art therapy. However, there have been very few randomized clinical trials involving art therapy, and at the time of this study none were found involving research with asthma. Understanding the benefit of art therapy in helping children with asthma, and the need for clinical validity in this field, a randomized clinical study at National Jewish Health was designed to determine whether art therapy could be clinically proven to be an effective means of helping children with emotional regulation. This study was conducted in the hope that if art therapy could be proven clinically to improve emotional resilience in children with chronic illness, then more hospitals might offer art therapy services to their patients.

Methods

The participants of the study were enrolled from a school for children with asthma, located on the campus of National Jewish Health. The twenty-two 7- to 14-year-old children enrolled in the study had a diagnosis of persistent asthma that required daily treatment. Once consent was obtained, participants were randomized to either an active treatment or wait-list control group. Participants completed all measures immediately before the first art therapy session, immediately after the last art therapy session, and then again in 6 months, after the sessions had concluded. Children assigned to the wait-list control group completed all evaluations at the same intervals as the children receiving art therapy, but did not receive the art therapy interventions. After all the data were collected and the study was complete, children in the control group were offered the same series of art therapy sessions as a way of thanking them for their participation in the study.

Instruments and Measures

To assess accurately the broad range of feelings and behaviors of the children in the study, four measures were used: the Beck Youth Inventories (Beck, Beck, & Jolly, 2005), the Pediatric Quality of Life Asthma Module (Varni, Burwinkle, Rapoff, Kamps, & Olson, 2004) for children, as well as the module for parents; and the Formal Elements Art Therapy Scale (FEATS) applied to the Person Picking an Apple from a Tree (PPAT) assessment (Gantt & Tabone, 2003). Although there are many art therapy assessments, the PPAT was chosen due to its well-researched reliability and measurable consistency in scoring.

Participants who were randomized to the active group met weekly for a 1-hour art therapy session, for seven weeks. The art therapy sessions were facilitated by a trained art therapist and took place in the Creative Arts Room at National Jewish Health. These sessions included specific art therapy tasks designed to encourage creative expression related to the challenges of having a chronic illness. Each art therapy group included an opening activity, discussion of the weekly topic and art intervention, art making, an opportunity for patients to share their feelings related to the art they created, and a closing activity.

Art Therapy Session Content

Session 1: "Who Am I?"

To begin the first art therapy session, the group started with an opening activity called the Jewels Within. This activity was introduced with the metaphorical explanation that we all have "jewels" inside of us, and our jewels are the good feelings we have about ourselves. The group members were encouraged to think about three characteristics about themselves that made them feel proud and good. A tray of colored glass jewels was presented, and the children were asked to pick three jewels to represent these three characteristics. The tray of jewels was passed around the circle, and the children took turns choosing jewels, then sharing if they wanted to do so. During circle time, it was understood that each person could share whatever he or she chose, without judgment from others. All of the children were given a satin bag in which to keep their jewels, and they added three more jewels every week during this repeated opening activity.

The topic of the first session was "Who Am I?," and the group members were asked to think about how they felt about themselves in relation to their illness. Several group members explained that they felt their illness defined who they were and wished they could be "normal" like other kids. The group members were asked to give their asthma a voice and express through art what their illness felt like for them. In Figure 5.1, a girl expresses all the ways that asthma, allergies, and acid reflux affect her body. She even

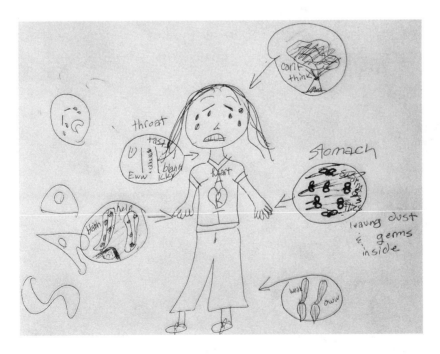

FIGURE 5.1. A 10-year-old girl shows how her illness affects her physically and emotionally.

acknowledges that the illnesses cause her to be unable to think clearly and to have pain in her legs. In Figure 5.2, A 7-year-old describes that when her condition acts up, she feels as if she has a "ladder" in her chest. After making the art, she explained that she did not realize that her asthma and reflux felt this way until making the art. This visual information helped in her treatment as the image was indicative of her reflux levels. As this artwork shows, children often have unique and specific ways of expressing their physical symptoms that might only emerge through visual expression.

After acknowledging their feelings that asthma is indeed a part of their lives, group members were then urged to look at other aspects of their personality as well. They were given an art directive to draw or make an art piece of their choosing that expressed the many facets of their personalities and the qualities that made them who they were. Through the art making and in sharing their experience, the children in the group were given the opportunity to discover that their illness was separate from their identity. For many children, this may have been one of first times they were able really to look at themselves as an entire person, not just a child with asthma. When children are able to focus on activities that help them feel good and less anxious, their condition often improves. In Figure 5.3, the same girl who drew the previous image explained that when she does fun things that help her feel happy, like dancing, her chest does not hurt as much. She added that the love and good feelings (depicted in the picture as hearts and

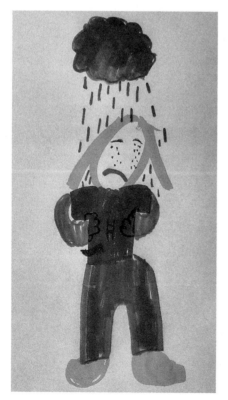

FIGURE 5.2. Unique imagery, as shown in this picture, often gives clues to the underlying medical condition.

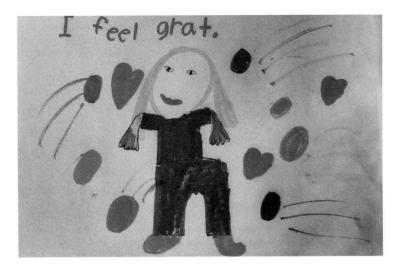

FIGURE 5.3. "Feeling Great": A 7-year-old girl focuses on feeling good.

colored circles) she receives from being with family and friends helps her feel better as well.

At the end of the session, the group gathered for a closing activity called Transformation. To begin this activity, group members were given a clear piece of cord and asked to pick two beads to put on the cord. It was explained to them that the beads signified their involvement and importance in the art therapy group. This became the weekly closing activity, allowing the children to add two beads to their cords each week.

Session 2: "Feelings Related to Illness"

In the second session, the art therapist explained that most children experience many different feelings about having a chronic illness. The group members were asked to think about and write down their feelings in two columns: one that represented how they felt when they were sick, and another that represented their feelings when they felt healthy. The group members were then given two papier-mâché masks to paint, one to represent how they felt when they were sick, and the other to show how they felt when they were healthy.

Some of the group members created two very different masks, clearly showing how they felt when sick and when healthy. Some of the children explained that they had a difficult time showing what if feels like to feel healthy. One boy shared, "I don't even know what if feels like to feel healthy and good because I always have problems with my asthma." Instead, he decided to make a mask to represent what he *imagined* it felt like to be healthy. After sharing their feelings about their masks, the group members were encouraged to think further about how they might transition emotionally from feeling sick to feeling better.

Session 3: "Healthy Expressions of Anger"

In the third art therapy session, we discussed that all feelings are okay and there are many ways to use art to express feelings. The group members talked about how being sick, at times, might make them feel mad or angry. To help the group members understand a positive way to channel anger through art, each was given a block of clay and a wooden mallet. They were encouraged first to think about any angry feelings they might have about their asthma, then to pound, poke, tear, or do whatever they wanted to get their anger out using the clay. This seemed to be a very cathartic experience for the group and most children were very expressive as they pounded and smashed their clay. One boy expressed that he was able to "show the clay what if felt like to be a kid with asthma." After talking about the experience, group members were then asked to reform their clay and shape it into a volcano that would later be a container for their anger.

In addition, some children also chose to draw a volcano to express their feelings more clearly. One girl expressed how she often held her anger in and "cried on the inside" (Figure 5.4). After understanding that it was all right to be angry about her

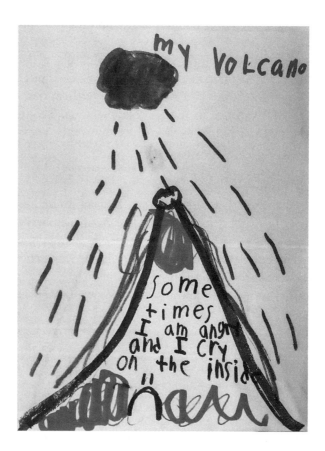

FIGURE 5.4. "Sometimes I Cry on the Inside": A powerful example showing the emotional effects of having a physical illness.

illness and to express the full range of her feelings, she was able to open up more and vocalize her feelings in a more productive way. Holding feelings in can be very common for children with asthma, and art therapy can be a very effective tool to assist in healthy emotional expression. Image making gives children the ability to explore feelings that are buried deeper and harder to access on a conscious level. When these hidden feelings are brought to the surface, children like the girl who made this image are then able to express, process, and cope with their feelings with greater resilience.

Session 4: "Transforming Anger"

In this session, the group continued the previous week's discussion of ways to manage and cope with anger and other overwhelming feelings. For the first part of the art activity, the group members were asked to paint an "angry" image. Then with paint colors of their choosing, they were asked to transform the image in some way that felt good to them. The group discussed this process and one girl whose angry image was a monster explained, "As soon as I put cool blue on the monster I created, I felt better, safe and calm." We talked about how sometimes when we can feel, express, and accept our feelings, especially the more difficult ones, and how sometimes they can then transform and change.

For the second part of the art activity, group members were asked to revisit the clay volcanoes they made the week before. The volcanoes had been fired in the kiln and were now ready to paint. It was suggested that group members could paint their volcanoes any way they chose, and that they might decide to transform some volcanoes into something else. Group members were reminded of their first art piece of the day and that sometimes feelings change, and can be transformed with colors. The group members were assured that any way they chose to paint their clay piece was perfectly all right and was their choice. One boy decided that his volcano looked more like a birthday cake and that is what he chose to transform it into. He excitedly explained to the group that he didn't feel as mad as he used to, and now he wanted to think about and do more fun things, like going to birthday parties. Several other children decided that their volcanoes had transformed into "strong mountains."

Group members were also offered the idea that their clay sculptures could be used in a manner similar to a "God box." In the future, if they felt upset or troubled, they could write down their feelings on pieces of paper, put them inside their clay piece, then let their worries or troubles go. It was again emphasized that expression of all feelings helps us feel better and that it was healthier to express than to hold in feelings of stress, worry, anger, and sadness.

Session 5: "Painting the Worries Away"

In the fifth session, patients were asked to think about what it feels like to have an asthma attack, or to be worried about an attack. Group members shared their worries and fears related to their illness, as well as things that help them calm down and feel better. After this discussion, group members were given pallets of soothing hues of paints and were asked to pretend they were younger and were just discovering how to use paint. They were encouraged not make any particular image, just to fill the paper with color and paint in silence for 5 minutes. This exercise was repeated six times using different selections of colors. After the paints were cleaned up, group members were asked to think about how they felt doing this exercise and what colors helped them feel best. Further discussion focused on how certain colors can help to soothe people and make them feel better. The children were asked to imagine their favorite soothing color enveloping them like a soft blanket and helping them feel good. They were reminded that they could use this image in the future to help them feel calm and better when feeling ill, worried, or upset.

Session 6: "What Makes Me Feel Good"

In this session, the group talked about examples of how negative emotions and stress can sometimes affect the severity of an asthma attack. The group revisited the importance of processing and expressing overwhelming feelings through art, talking to someone, journaling, or any other ways that might feel helpful. The concept of negative self-talk was explained, and the children explored ideas to counteract negative self-talk and ways to focus on positive thoughts that made them feel good inside. The group was given an art therapy activity to decorate paper stars, butterflies, or kites, then write personal, affirmative statements on the images.

One of the group members shared that when she felt an asthma attack coming on in the future, she was going to think of the positive words she had written on the butterflies to help her calm down. She said she was then going to imagine that the butterflies were going to fly up inside her chest to open her airways and help her breathe better. Another boy explained that he was going to hang his kites above his bed to make him feel better at night, when his asthma was the worst.

Session 7: "Taking Care of Myself"

In the final session, the group began with a brief review of the different topics and art therapy interventions from the previous sessions. The children then moved on to their regular opening activity that included choosing three jewels. This time, they talked about the three pieces of artwork from the last 7 weeks that made them feel the most proud and added the jewels to their satin bags. The group members were encouraged to continue this practice of acknowledging their accomplishments at home and were given extra jewels to take with them.

For the main activity in the last session, the children discussed self-care and the importance of taking medications and seeing their doctors when they felt sick, as well as for regular checkups. The children were asked to make an art piece of their choosing in relation to the medical treatment of their asthma. Some children drew pictures of themselves using their inhalers and medicines (Figure 5.5); others made three-dimensional

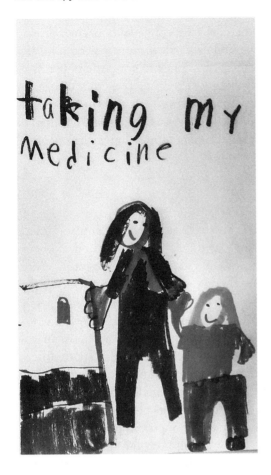

FIGURE 5.5. This drawing depicts one child's understanding of the importance of taking her medicines.

sculptures using medical supplies. One of the group members made a peak flow monitor (a device used to measure airflow) to remind her of the importance of checking her airflow on a regular basis.

At the end of the final session, the group members gathered for the closing activity. The children put their last two beads on the cord to which they had been adding beads every session. In addition to the beads, each child was given a charm of his or her choice to add to the cord as well. Once the beads and the charm were secured, it was revealed that what they had made was actually a suncatcher. The children were asked to hold their suncatcher up to the window to see that the beads they had put on the cord now changed color and turned bright when exposed to the sun. The group was encouraged to think of how, like the beads, they had transformed their relationship with their asthma.

Summary of Art Therapy Group Sessions

The members in the active treatment group seemed clearly to benefit from and enjoy the art therapy groups. Most of the children were very engaged in the process, and many seemed to learn to accept and come to terms with their asthma. Creer and Bender

(1995) explain that patients' ability and willingness to accept the reality of their disease lead to more positive outcomes in treatment, as well as a reduction in severity and frequency of asthmatic episodes. The group members also seemed to grasp the importance of expressing their feelings, as well as understanding the significant role that emotional distress has on their asthma. It has been shown that improved emotional regulation is vital in controlling and minimizing asthma episodes (Beebe et al., 2010), and children in the group demonstrated that art therapy was a key component in helping them improve their ability to cope with their illness.

Results

After the art therapy groups were concluded, both the active and the control groups completed another round of measures. To ensure that the data were unbiased, the scoring was completed by a clinician blinded to treatment and control group status. When the scores of the active group that received art therapy were compared to the control group that did not, a significant difference was noticeable between the two groups. In the active group, a reduction was seen in both the parent- and child-reported worry scores from the Pediatric Quality of Life questionnaires; a decrease was seen in the Anxiety score and an increase in the Self-Concept score from the child-reported Beck Inventories; and improvements were seen in the color, logic, and details scores from the PPAT. Measures were again collected 6 months after completion of the therapy (with no further art therapy given in between), and the benefits persisted. Compared to the control group, the treatment group continued to have improved parent- and child-reported Worry and Total scores from the Pediatric Quality of Life questionnaires; a reduced Anxiety score from the Beck Inventories; and higher color and detail scores from the PPAT.

The results of this randomized clinical trial were enlightening and inspiring; furthermore, the benefits from the art therapy groups continued when participants were retested 6 months after treatment. This study demonstrated that art therapy effectively reduces anxiety and improves quality of life and self-concept in children with asthma. In addition, this study clinically determined that art therapy for children with severe, chronic asthma is of significant benefit.

Although this study was not designed to establish whether art therapy can reduce asthma episodes or the need for medical treatment, this would be an interesting follow-up study to consider. More clinical research would be beneficial in the area of medical art therapy and asthma to foster additional clinical information regarding the effects of mental wellness and emotional regulation on physical health.

CONCLUSION

In summary, this encouraging research clearly indicates that the emotional health of chronically ill children may be improved using art therapy interventions. Coping with anxiety is a key factor in managing the physiological response of asthma, and this study was able to demonstrate the positive impact of using art therapy to reduce anxiety in children with asthma.

Evidence from this study also shows that art therapy improved both self-concept and quality of life for the participants in the active group. Results of this study were encouraging from a data perspective, but most importantly from the perspective of observed changes in children's positive affect after completing the art therapy groups. It was evident that art therapy helped these children feel better about themselves as well improve their relationship with asthma, and thus, their overall quality life. As Van de Wetering, Bernstein, and Ley (2010) explain, clinical studies indicate that patients who feel positive about themselves and have a more optimistic outlook on life have a stronger immune functions when faced with stress. Research also indicates that people with higher-functioning immune systems have a lower occurrence of physical and chronic illness, and an increased recovery rate as well (Achtenburg, 2002). In other words, when a patient is given the opportunity to feel better about him- or herself and improve feelings about quality of life through art therapy, the body's natural healing mechanism, the immune system, has a greater ability to ward off and overcome illness. If art therapy can contribute to this outcome, it seems reasonable that it is worthy of serious consideration as a complementary healing modality for more people with chronic illness.

It is apparent that treatment of both the physical and emotional health of patients with asthma is valid and important. As demonstrated by the research presented in this chapter and in so many other very important studies and publications, art therapy is more highly regarded as an effective healing modality in modern medicine. More medical professionals have come to understand that illnesses not only affect the body but also influence, and are influenced by, the psychological health of the person (Achterberg, 2002). This growing acceptance of mind–body healing in health care creates a greater potential for more patients with chronic illness to benefit from art therapy. As McNiff (1992, p. 11) has stated, "Art is a medicine," and in some cases art making may be the ideal adjunct medicine a patient needs to promote healing. Through art therapy, we offer patients a creative form of medicine to help them heal in a more integrated way and bridge the gap between mental health and physical well-being.

REFERENCES

Achterberg, J. (2002). *Imagery in healing.* Boston: Shambhala.

Beck, J., Beck, A., & Jolly, J. (2005). *Beck Youth Inventories* (2nd ed.). San Antonio: NCS Pearson Education.

Beebe, A., Gelfand, E., & Bender, B. (2010). A randomized trial to test the effectiveness of art therapy for children with asthma. *Journal of Allergy Clinical Immunology, 126*(2), 263–266.

Bender, B. (1995). Are asthmatic children educationally handicapped? *School Psychology Quarterly, 10*(4), 274–291.

Bender, B., & Zhang, L. (2008). Negative affect, medication adherence and asthma control in children. *Journal of Allergy and Clinical Immunology, 122*(3), 490–495.

Blackman, J., & Gurka, M. (2007). Developmental and behavioral comorbidities of asthma in children. *Journal of Developmental Pediatrics, 28,* 92–99.

Creer, T. L., & Bender, B. (1995). Recent trends in asthma research. In A. J. Goreczzy (Ed.), *Hanbook of health and rehabilitation psychology.* New York: Plenum Press.

Franklin, M., & Siemon, T. (2008). Toward an understanding of the fundamental healing and therapeutic qualities of art. *Journal of Thai Traditional and Alternative Medicine,* 6(3), 269–273.

Gabriels, R., Wamboldt, M., McCormick, D., Adams, T., & McTaggart, S. (2000). Children's illness drawings and asthma symptom awareness. *Journal of Asthma, 37,* 565–574.

Gannt, L., & Tabone, C. (1998). *The formal elements art therapy scale: The rating manual.* Morgantown, WV: Gargoyle Press.

Koinis-Mitchell, D., McQuaid, E., Seifer, R., Kopel, S., Nassau, J., Klein, R., et al. (2009). Symptom perception in children with asthma: cognitive and psychological factors. *Health Psychology, 28*(2), 226–237.

Malchiodi C. (1999). *Medical art therapy with children.* London: Jessica Kingsley.

McNiff, S. (1992). *Art as medicine.* Boston: Shambhala.

McQuaid, E., Kopel, S., & Nasasu, J. (2001). Behavioral adjustment in children with asthma: A meta-analysis. *Journal of Developmental Behavioral Pediatrics, 22,* 430–439.

Mzarek, D. (1985). Childhood asthma. *Advanced Psychosomatic Medicine, 14,* 16–32.

Rubin, J. (1999). Foreword. In C. A. Malchiodi (Ed.), *Medical art therapy with children.* London: Jessica Kingsley.

Sternberg, E. (2000). *The balance within: The science connecting health and emotions.* New York: Freeman.

Van de Wetering, S., Bernstein, D., & Ley, R. (2010). Imagery, cerebral laterality, and the healing process: A cautionary note. In A. Sheikh (Ed.), *Healing images: The role of imagination in health.* Amityville, NY: Baywood.

Varni, J., Burwinkle, T., Rapoff, M., Kamps, J., & Olson, N. (2004). The PedsQL in pediatric asthma: Reliability and validity of the Pediatric Quality of Life Inventory Generic Core Scales and Asthma Module. *Journal of Behavioral Medicine, 27,* 297–318.

Wambolt, F., Bender, B., Rankin, A., (2011). Adolescent decision-making about use of inhaled asthma controller medication: Results from focus groups with participants from a prior longitudinal study. *Journal of Asthma, 48,* 741–750.

Welch, M. (2011). *Allergies and asthma, what every parent needs to know.* Elk Grove Village, IL: American Academy of Pediatrics.

Wood, B., Cheah, P.A., Lim, J., Ritz, T., Miller, B., Stern, T., et al. (2007a). Reliability and validity of the Asthma Trigger Inventory applied to a pediatric population. *Journal of Pediatric Psychology, 32*(5), 552–560.

Wood, B., Cheah, P.A., Lim, J., Ritz, T., Miller, B., Stern, T., et al. (2007b). Family emotional climate, depression, emotional triggering of asthma, and disease severity in pediatric asthma: Examination of pathways of effect. *Journal of Pediatric Psychology, 32*(5), 542–551.

Wright, R. J., Cohen, R. T., & Cohen, S. (2005). The impact of stress on the development and expression of atopy. *Current Opinion in Allergy and Clinical Immunology, 5,* 23–29.

CHAPTER 6

Expressive Arts with Grieving Children

Rebekah Near

The experience of death is a painful time for anyone, yet for children this occurrence and the grief that follows can be filled with uncertainty. When death enters the lives of children we are often left speechless, scurrying around to find the "right words." Exploration about death and grief among children and adolescents should be encouraged within the field of health care. Tapping into children's creative energy can help them gain understanding, enabling them to access their feelings. Creating through the arts utilizes the intuitive and emotional aspects of a child's self. The expressive arts become an outlet for the troubling emotions that are often associated with grieving. The metaphoric value of creative expression can help to free the inner emotions associated with this major life experience.

The creative process of generating art during a traumatic time of loss offers an opportunity for transformation and making connections. Children lost in grieving, daunted by it, or blocked by the denial of it, can find their way back into the world through the arts. Sharing art making and experiences of children's grief exposes readers to new ways to be in relation with grief and with one another. This chapter explores developmental factors of child and adolescent grief, presents a description of expressive arts as an intermodal approach, and shows how use of expressive arts is an effective method for working with children and adolescents in a hospice setting. Examples show how the expressive arts currently may be used in response to grief as part of an interdisciplinary hospice team.

Transformation cannot happen, personal or communal, unless we are in contact with "what is." Using the arts to dialogue with grief releases the vitality children need to carry on living. This chapter is part of the ongoing effort to explore the value of the expressive arts in the field of thanatology (Near, 2012).

CHILDREN AND GRIEF

Death is a complex concept. Children's conceptualization of death is dependent on many factors. How children comprehend, accept, and actually grieve depends on their chronological age and developmental level. The mental age of a child has a major impact on his or her understanding of death (Nguyen & Gelman, 2002).

General concepts involved in the understanding of children dealing with death include irreversibility, universality, nonfunctionality, and causality (Balk, 2007; Silverman, 2000; Speece & Brent, 1996). "Irreversibility" is a concept about the finality of death. Young children between ages 2 to 7 typically do not understand that death is irreversible (Malchiodi, 2003). "Universality" means the child comes to understand that no one can predict when death will happen, and that all things must die. Members of the 7- to 11-year-age group realize that death is irreversible and a universal occurrence (Malchiodi, 2003). Children actually begin to develop a very crude awareness about death as early as infancy (Wolraich et al., 2000). "Nonfunctionality," is the concept that a once living thing is dead, all of its bodily functions cease, is difficult for children to understand. In learning about "causality," a child comes to understand what happens to bring a living thing to death. This notion evolves throughout the adolescent years. Older children can comprehend more abstract concepts in relation to death. Spiritual and religious perceptions aid in their understanding of death (Malchiodi, 2003).

The difficulty of the grieving process can be identified by the following circumstances: the cause of death, the length of the dying process, and the means by which the loss occurred. Accidental, suicidal, and violent deaths are usually the most difficult, because the survivors are not able to say goodbye to their loved ones (Clements & Burgess, 2002). Social structures and supports are additional factors that have an effect on a child's grieving process (Balk, 2007; Romanoff & Terenzio, 1998). These components refer to the way each individual is positioned in the family system and his or her relationship to the departed. A need exists for the bereaved child to maintain a connection to the deceased. The loss of a parent is often traumatic due to the loss of emotional and psychological support (Christ, Siegel, & Christ, 2002; Stokes, Reid, & Cook, 2009).

Children have psychosocial and physiological responses to death. Birenbaum (2000) reported that children's psychosocial reactions to bereavement included guilt, anxiety, anger, fear, sadness, hopelessness, worry, and depression, and feelings of rejection, self-doubt, inferiority, isolation, and deprivation. Negative effects of bereavement include low self-esteem and excessive guilt (Quarmby, 1993; Stokes et al., 2009). Buxbaum and Brant (2001) reported that the bereaved child's psychosocial reactions can create problematic social responses, such as poor school performance and strained family relationships. Childhood physiological responses, as reported by Birenbaum (2000), included enuresis, stomach pains, convulsions, asthma, and psychosomatic complaints. The death of a loved one can impede a child's capacity to move forward developmentally and emotionally (Christ et al., 2002).

Since dying is inevitable, children need to be able to deal with the feelings and emotions associated with death. Children need a caring, nurturing environment to foster healing. A child's grief is often mistaken or over looked. Children grieve differently from adults due to their psychosocial and developmental level. Conversely, how children express their grief is both parallel to and different from adult grief (Corr, 2010). Typically in the aftermath of a death, adults have been programmed not to express their grief in certain situations, such as at work, or when some time has passed. Children are not always aware of these social constrictions and might begin freely asking questions about death (Corr, 2010). Although differences occur between adults and children, grief work has the same underlying component. A child needs the go-ahead to grieve. Familiar routines help children feel secure to go forward in their grief.

Children who are grieving can integrate into the world through the arts. It has been acknowledged that talk therapy is not always the most suitable intervention for bereaved children (Silverman, 2000; Wood & Near, 2010). The use of expressive arts offers another way of engaging children and their concerns that is open to the diversity of their experience. When the grieving child moves among the art modalities, he or she is able to deepen understanding of his or her lived experiences. The emerging arts are a response to life.

EXPRESSIVE ARTS THERAPY: AN INTERMODAL APPROACH

The concept that art making can be helpful in a time of loss is certainly not new. However, exploration of the implementation of the expressive arts in working with grieving children and adolescents is just emerging (Wood & Near, 2010). Expressive arts integrate the visual arts, movement, drama, music, writing, play, and other creative processes to foster personal transformation. As with any approach in therapy, central to the process is receptivity to what the client is communicating, then development of an intervention that suits the individual's needs and objectives (Malchiodi, 2003). Expressive arts therapy is moment- and person-specific. The expressive arts therapist is the facilitator of inquiry into the intermodal transfer (moving from one art modality to the next).

Expressive arts therapy invites a person to move flexibly among media, following his or her creative instincts and interests. Expressive arts therapy directly engages auditory, visual, and kinesthetic senses, as well as emotions (Knill, Levine, & Levine, 2005; Wood & Near, 2010). Expressive arts therapy is a field rooted in philosophy, psychology, and the intermodal use of the arts (Knill et al., 2005; Wood et al., 2010). The expressive arts field grounds itself in phenomenology, the lived experience. One clearly understands that the expressive arts fall under the canopy of creative arts therapy, sometimes referred to as expressive therapies (Figure 6.1). Under this umbrella are the fields of art therapy, movement/dance therapy, music therapy, poetry therapy, drama therapy, and expressive arts therapy.

Expressive arts therapy distinguishes itself from the closely related disciplines of art therapy, music therapy, dance/movement therapy, poetry therapy, and drama therapy by being grounded in the interrelatedness of the arts (Estrella, 2005). It is in this integration of the visual arts, movement, drama, music, writing, play, and other creative

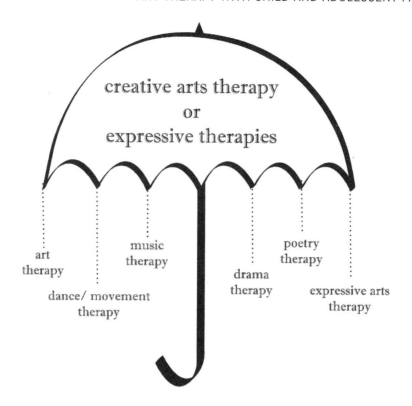

FIGURE 6.1. The canopy of creative arts therapy or expressive therapies.

processes that personal transformation is fostered. The expressive arts refer to the inter-modal use of the art disciplines working together in moving from one art medium to the next. "Intermodal" refers to the shift from one art form to the next during a session. Intermodal shift uses an art experience to build on another art experience. Through creative expression and tapping into the imagination, individuals can examine their bodies, feelings, emotions, and thought processes (Knill et al., 2005; Wood et al., 2010). The expressive arts are used with a variety of populations and encompass therapy, coaching, and social change. This chapter highlights expressive arts therapy and its use with grieving children in a hospice setting.

USING EXPRESSIVE ARTS WITH GRIEVING CHILDREN IN A HOSPICE SETTING

Hospice is a concept of care that provides a team-oriented approach of trained professionals to support patients and their families dealing with an end-of-life illness (Hospice Foundation of America, 2011). In recent years the term "hospice" has embraced the use of creative arts in the field as part of an interdisciplinary team effort. Within a hospice program each interdisciplinary team addresses the issues of end-of-life care based on its own expertise. The doctor and nurse address the medical components of pain management. The social worker takes care of services and emotional well-being. The chaplain addresses the spiritual care of patients and their families. The expressive arts therapist is able to use the arts to access the thoughts and feelings of children and family members, and bring them from the literal reality of the world to its imaginable possibilities (Levine, 2009). The patient or family member might not always want to talk about the current situation or have the words to express his or her thoughts. As the expressive arts facilitator decenters (guides into art-making experience) both patient and therapist are able to be present with the uncertainty of death. "Being present is understood as being courageous to 'step forth' into decentering. We step forth even though we are ourselves helpless to fix the problematic, helpless situation of the client, while still trusting in the process of facilitation through the arts" (Knill et al., 2005, p. 168). Working through the expressive arts can support the hospice team in developing a plan of care. The creative methods may bring to light obstacles that might not have surfaced using traditional resources. This is illustrated below in the Torres case.

Torres Family

Expressive arts therapy enabled Ryan, a young boy with a brain tumor, and his entire family to deal with the pain as they mourned their mother's death and prepared for Ryan's impending death. I worked with Ryan, age 12; and his three siblings: Maria, age 14; Kyle, age 10; and Anna, age 8 to create their visual image of heaven. This artistic venture was sparked by the children's curiosity about heaven. While the children worked, music was playing in the background. Ryan and Maria were singing along to the song. The song they were singing provided the opportunity to shift from one art modality to another (intermodal transfer, Knill et al., 2005, p. 125). This intermodal transfer brought the children to a deepening of their creative realism. Together we began to play with sounds and words. As the decentering continued these are the improvised lyrics that emerged:

NO PAIN
NO MORE BAD RELATIONSHIPS
NO MORE SICKNESS
NO MORE BEING IN THIS BED
I JUST WANT TO LET GO

When we harvested the images and music the children discovered that they believed Ryan would not go to heaven because he was not baptized. Ryan believed this to be true as well. The arts allowed the children to explore this imaginary reality and then bring it back to their everyday circumstances. With the children's permission I shared their concerns with their father and the hospice team. Even though members of the hospice team had visited the Torres family on numerous occasions they were surprised to learn of the children's concerns. The expressive arts allowed an opening for this information to surface. The chaplain went out a few days later and baptized Ryan. A week later Ryan died (Wood & Near, 2010, p. 387).

Currently, in hospice settings, various creative arts therapies are being used with children to address issues of grief. Expressive arts therapy offers a distinct approach that differs from the traditional creative art therapies. Unlike other creative arts therapies that concentrate on a single artistic mode, expressive arts therapy combines multiple arts to expand the range of expression and imaginative potential (McNiff, 2009; Thompson & Berger, 2011). Through the intermodal transfer, grieving children can release the wide range of emotions in their realm of reality. It is in the interconnection of the arts that children are free to move through their grief. By its very nature, grief is a multi-dimensional, open-ended state of being, one that eludes any predetermined expressive form. The emotions accompanying grief vary from person to person and may shift from moment to moment. The expressive arts speak to this variability by engaging children wherever they are in their grief process and transforming the grief. The very nature of the intermodal nature of expressive arts gives children another way to work with their stories of grief. The intermodal shift allows the griever to discover new insights into the grief story. The use of expressive arts can offer a way of engaging children and their concerns that is open to the diversity of their experience. The freedom to move from one expressive mode to another allows the senses to be engaged (Thompson & Berger, 2011).

> Intermodal expressive arts integrate the properties of the various art forms to serve the goals of the therapeutic work. Using arts experiences to "decenter" from a presenting problem, the client is then able to refocus his or her attention, to recognize internal and external resources, to imagine new possibilities and to bring new learning to bear on the life situation at hand. (Atkins & Williams, 2007, p. 3)

The case study of the Swartz family illustrates how a teenage girl redefined her life after the death of her father. The expressive arts helped to refocus her attention and enabled her to discover the abilities she already possessed.

Swartz Family

I was working as part of an interdisciplinary hospice team as the expressive arts therapist and bereavement coordinator, when the chaplain asked me to work with a family that had four children. I remembered him noting that the family was very private and probably would not let me work with them. The chaplain already had a connection with the family, and he accompanied me on my first visit. My job was to facilitate the meeting between the children and the arts.

The Swartz family included Edmir, age 45, the adored father who was dying from cancer; Anna, age 45, his beloved wife and devoted mother to Jonah, age 18, Sadie, age 17, Shira, age 15, and Neal, age 14. The Swartz family was Syrian American Orthodox Jews. The family follows the laws of the Torah and the customs of their heritage. They keep a strict Kosher household, following Jewish dietary laws. The women dress modestly. The men wear a *kippah* (head covering) and *tallit* (prayer shawl) at all times. According to Orthodox Jewish tradition, men and women are not permitted to touch except as husband and wife. I met the Swartz family in the last few weeks before Edmir died. Typically, hospice care is facilitated within the home.

The first session was arranged in the living room around the coffee table. While I worked with the children, the chaplain attended to the needs of the rest of the family in an adjoining room. Although skeptical, the children were willing to try what I was asking of them. During our meeting I provided an array of art materials: paper, pastels, markers, colored pencils, and scissors. I asked the children to create "something they wanted me to know about them." I left this intervention open so the children could direct what they wanted to divulge. The children were quiet as they diligently worked on their pieces. Once finished, I invited them to share. Sadie was the most talkative and seemed to be the dominant voice among her siblings. Shira's image (Figure 6.2) and storytelling conveyed what life had been like since the onset of her father's illness. The ups and downs of his illness mirrored the ups and downs of Shira's emotions. Jonah, Sadie, and Neal chimed in, revealing similar feelings. As Shira shared her narrative, her siblings added their own stories. Shira's courage to express became the catalyst for her siblings to release their own feelings. This session gave the children a start. It was an opening for them to communicate with each other the thoughts and feelings they had all been experiencing but not sharing.

Over the course of the next year and a half I facilitated Shira's grieving process through expressive arts therapy sessions. It was advised by the Rabbi that Jonah and Neal should work with a male counselor. Sadie worked with a religious counselor from her community. On a weekly basis Shira would come to my office to engage in the arts as she processed her grief.

Six months into our sessions Shira created a mandala, a circular image. The mandala was the result of a movement warm-up exercise we did together. Shira had come to the office talking about the grief she felt was stuck in her body. I suggested that we explore the grief sensation she was feeling. I asked Shira to place her hands on the grief. She positioned her

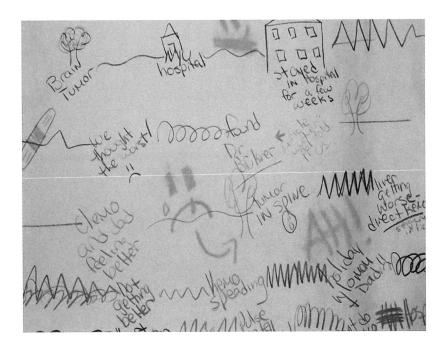

FIGURE 6.2. Shira's timeline of grief.

hands over her heart and then proceeded to slide them down, where they rested on her belly. We took a deep breath together. "Do you experience grief anywhere else in your body?" I asked. Shira took another breath, breathing deeply into her grief. Once she experienced where her grief was stuck I asked her to find a movement that encompassed her grief. With her hands clutching into her heart and stomach she hunched over. I asked Shira to continue to repeat the hunching motion that she distinguished to be her grief. Then I invited her to explore a movement that could possibly release her grief. Shira's arms immediately shot out from her body and whirled in the air. She danced around the room, engaging her whole body in the releasing. In the intermodal shift from movement to visual art, I asked Shira to choose two pastels, one for each hand, while still staying with her movement. The next maneuver involved transferring her movement to paper. Shira took a green and a blue pastel and began to thrust the colors in an outward–inward motion. Shira's visual image emerged as seen below in Figure 6.3.

The second intermodal shift occurred when Shira did a "free write" (writing anything that comes to mind) about her mandala. The second intermodal shift was from visual art to writing. With the free write completed, I asked Shira to circle eight words that stood out in her writing. I encouraged her to play with the words to create a poem. Here is Shira's poem.

What is true happiness?
An A on a test?
Friends?
Family?
Truth
Fear
Grief
Thoughts
All come from within yourself

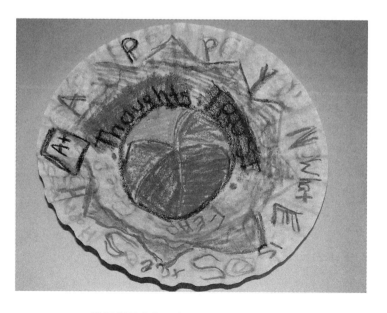

FIGURE 6.3. Shira's mandala image.

It's up to you
Do you want to be happy?
It's all up to you

The final phase of the expressive arts therapy session was to "harvest" the arts, helping Shira bridge her lived experience to her present-day reality. I prompted Shira to make a connection from the arts to the actuality of her situation. Working through the arts, Shira came to be aware that she possessed the tools to release her grief. In the course of harvesting she realized that happiness was within her reach.

During our last session together Shira and I worked in tandem to create a collective piece of art. This image would act as a transition piece and a tangible reminder of the growth Shira achieved during our sessions together. Shira wanted to create with paint. We filled our palettes with acrylic paint colors. With color on our brushes and closed eyes we began to paint while soft music played in the background. The initial brush strokes that we made with our eyes closed acted as inspiration for our image. When we opened our eyes we continued to create by rotating the paper. This allowed us to paint from many perspectives. A face began to emerge in the painting. Shira quickly decided to make it more pronounced with highlighting and was satisfied with the results.

She named the face that emerged from the painting "Good Grief Gary" (Figure 6.4). This was the beginning of an intermodal shift: visual into drama. A place was designated in the room to be our stage. I advised Shira to construct questions for interviewing Good Grief Gary. I encouraged Shira to play the character Good Grief Gary, while I played the interviewer. Shira held the painting over her face like a mask while I asked the questions. As she developed the character, Shira morphed her voice to have a low-toned quality, making it distinct from her own. I asked, "Where are you from?" Good Grief Gary responded, "I am from the land of grief. I have not always lived there, but I made it my home after my father died." As my final interview question I asked, "What advice do you have for us as we leave the land of grief?" Good Grief Gary responded, "Blow away the sadness: Even when you feel hopeless, know that *you* have the power to blow away the sadness."

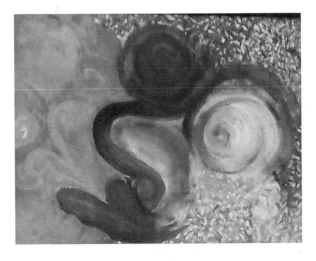

FIGURE 6.4. "Good Grief Gary."

As we worked with the experiences of this session Shira came away with an understanding that the arts could hold her grief. The expressive arts were a vessel, a place to deposit her grief, and to release it. The expressive arts nourished her spirit in the depths of despair and helped to her to create life again.

BENEFITS OF USING EXPRESSIVE ARTS WITH GRIEVING CHILDREN

What understanding lies beneath the words we use to describe grief? Our lived experiences pierce the superficial surface of grief to help children discover what is their own truth. How can children connect to their grief? Through the arts! Exploring the phenomenon of grief via the arts permits children to traverse the language of mourning. Through the intermodal shift children can explore the phenomenon of grief. The shaping of experiences through the imagination allows the client/artist to receive gifts from the emerging creations. The act of creating crystallizes client grief and allows him or her to see grief in a new light (Near, 2012). Thompson and Berger (2011, p. 305) state that "images of grief and loss are allowed to take shape in whatever artistic medium is indigenous to the experience and consonant with the particular circumstances and needs of the individual or community. This freedom to move from one expressive mode to another prompts shifts in the articulation and elaboration of images as more of the senses are engaged." The process of making art is the cathartic value of the expressive arts. It allows children to engage their awareness through sight, sound, and touch.

"Children grieve cyclically—moving in and out of their grief"(Toray, 2010, p. 250). Advancing from one art modality to another in the expressive arts echoes the grieving process, moving from one emotion to the next. As previously illustrated, Shira was able to engage in a full range of emotions as she participated in the expressive arts. Through this interaction Shira relinquished her grief.

Imagination and play are an integral part of the expressive arts. Children learn naturally during play. While engaging in play children become aware of their surroundings. Children often communicate their feelings through play (Webb, 2008). Guided by the client/artist's self, the expressive arts replicate the child's individual grief process. The expressive arts meet a child where he or she is and build on that foundation. Expressive arts clinicians do not interpret the arts; rather they help to facilitate poesies—learning through making. The expressive arts allow children to access what they know and what is in their unconscious by making and creating.

Working within a family system, the method of creating art together fosters empathy and a continuing connection (Parashak, 2008). I have found that the expressive arts are able to connect the child with his or her parents and siblings in coming to some understanding about each others' personal struggles with grief and hopes for the future (Wood & Near, 2010). When the expressive arts are used, they assist the family in understanding a child's experience as it relates to the family system. As the expressive arts and experiences of grief are shared with others in the family, the arts promote a deeper knowledge, as well as a way to be in relation with one another.

Children can honor their grief through the arts. It is not so much the art itself, as it is that through the arts they are able to revere grief. The expressive arts help children to connect with their grief. They can unite with their deepest pain reservoir. When we talk about grief, it is easy to intellectualize. However, the arts allow us to integrate our grief, building a bridge between our intellect and emotion, allowing them to play together to discover the mutual comprehension of one another's nature. Grief is not a singular emotion, but an assemblage of emotions. Through the artistic arrangement of emotion the expressive arts are a porthole into grief.

CONCLUSION

Children conceptualize death distinctively from adults. The developmental level of children has a large impact on how they understand their grief. How children grieve is greatly influenced by how those around them grieve. The expressive arts can help children and adults integrate into everyday life as they move through their grief. Intermodal shifting of the arts echoes the changes of grief. Expressive arts offer a way to converse in the language of mourning. The benefit of the expressive arts comes in not just seeing or listening to the arts, but in creating them.

The expressive arts can be the springboard that catapults children into the exploration of their grief. It is the comingling of visual arts, music, drama, movement, poetry, and play—commonly referred to as the expressive arts—that provides a valuable modality for the expression of grief. The importance of the expressive arts in the health care system cannot be overlooked. The expressive arts as a healing agent should continue to be supported within the hospice community and health care system at large.

In my work and personal life I use the expressive arts as a way to respond to loss and grief. In the opinion of Grainger (1999) expressive arts methods are used "not so one can abandon that [painful] experience but in order to change it by revisiting it from 'somewhere else'" (p. 14). He goes on to state that healing should not be seen as something produced "but as something that emerges. . . . From this point of view, the healing function of the arts therapies is to create contexts for existential change" (p. 130). The expressive arts are about connecting creatively, allowing oneself to be moved by the practice of creating within the arts. "The therapeutic power of the arts rests not in its elimination of suffering but rather in its capacity to hold us in the midst of that suffering so that we can bear the chaos without denial or flight" (Levine & Levine, 1999, p. 31, quoted in Estrella, 2005, p. 188). I have been honored to be witness to children who have used the arts to transform their grief and allow the unknown to come to light. It is in this witnessing of one's own grief and that of others that transformation has emerged.

REFERENCES

Atkins, S., & Williams, L. D. (2007). *Sourcebook in expressive arts therapy*. Boone, NC: Parkway.

Balk, D. E. (2007). Working with children and adolescents: An overview of theoretical and practical issues. In K. J. Doka (Ed.), *Living with grief: Before and after the death* (pp. 209–227). Washington, DC: Hospice Foundation of America.

Birenbaum, L. K. (2000). Assessing children's and teenager's bereavement when a sibling dies from cancer: A secondary analysis. *Child Care, Health and Development, 26*, 381–400.

Buxbaum, L., & Brant, P. M. (2001). When a parent dies from cancer. *Clinical Journal of Oncology Nursing, 5*(4), 135–140.

Christ, G. H., Siegel, K., & Christ, A. (2002). Adolescent grief: It never really hit me until it happened. *Journal of the American Medical Association, 288*, 1269–1278.

Clements, P., & Burgess, A. (2002). Children's response to family members homicide. *Family Community Health, 25*(1), 32–42.

Corr, C. A. (2010). Children, development, and encounters with death, bereavement, and coping. In C. A. Corr & D. E. Balk (Eds.), *Children's encouters with death, bereavement, and coping*. New York: Springer.

Estrella, K. (2005). Expressive arts therapy: An integrated arts approach. In C. A. Malchiodi (Ed.), *Expressive therapies* (pp. 183–209). New York: Guilford Press.

Grainger, R. (1999). *Researching the arts therapies: A drama therapist's perspective*. Philadelphia: Jessica Kingsley.

Hospice Foundation of America. (2011). What is hospice? Retrieved from *www.hospicefoundation.org/whatishospice*.

Knill, J., Levine, E. G., & Levine, S. K. (2005). *Principles and practice of expressive arts therapy*. Philadelphia: Jessica Kingsley.

Levine, S. K. (2009). *Trauma, tragedy, therapy: The arts and human suffering*. Philadelphia: Jessica Kingsley.

Levine, S. K., & Levine, E. G. (Eds.). (1999). *Foundations of expressive arts therapy: Theoretical and clinical perspectives*. London: Jessica Kingsley.

Malchiodi, C. (2003). Using creative activities as intervention for grieving children. *Trauma and Loss: Research Interventions, 3*(1), 12–18.

Malchiodi, C. A. (Ed.). (2005). *Expressive therapies*. New York: Guilford Press.

Martin, T., & Doka, K. (2000). *Men don't cry . . . women do: Transcending gender stereotypes of grief*. Amityville, NY: Baywood.

McNiff, S. (2009). *Integrating the arts in therapy: History, theory and practice*. Springfield, IL: Thomas.

Morgan, J. D. (1995). A philosopher looks at children and death. In E. Grollman (Ed.), *Bereaved children and teens: A supportive guide for parents and professionals*. Boston: Beacon Press.

Near, R. (2012). Intermodal expressive arts. In R. A. Neimeyer (Ed.), *Techniques of grief therapy*. New York: Routledge.

Nguyen, S., & Gelman, S. (2002). Four and 6 year olds biological concept of death: The case of plants. *British Journal of Developmental Psychology, 20*, 495–513.

Parashak, S. T. (2008). Object relations and attachment theory. In C. Kerr (Ed.), *Family art therapy* (pp. 65–94). New York: Routledge.

Quarmby, D. (1993). Peer group counseling with bereaved adolescents. *British Journal of Guidance and Counseling, 21*(2), 196.

Romanoff, B., & Terenzio, M. (1998). Rituals and the grieving process. *Death Studies, 22*(8), 697–711.

Silverman, P. R., (2000). *Never to young to know: Death in children's lives.* New York: Oxford University Press.

Speece, M. W., & Brent, S. B. (1996). *Handbook of childhood death and bereavement.* New York: Springer.

Stokes, J., Reid, C., & Cook, V. (2009). Life as an adolescent when a parent has died. In D. E. Balk & C. A. Corr (Eds.), *Adolescent encounters with death, bereavement, and coping* (pp. 177–194). New York: Springer.

Thompson, B. E., & Berger, J. S. (2011). *Grief and expressive arts therapy.* In R. A. Neimeyer, D. L. Harris, H. R. Winokuer, & G. F. Thornton (Eds.), *Grief and bereavement in contemporary society: Bridging research and practice* (pp. 303–313). New York: Routledge.

Toray, T. (2010). Children's bereavement over the death of pets. In C. A. Corr & D. E. Balk (Eds.), *Children's encounters with death, bereavement, and coping* (pp. 237–256). New York: Springer.

Webb, N. B. (2008). *Play therapy to help bereaved children.* In K. Doka & A. S. Tucci (Eds.), *Living with grief: Children and adolescents* (pp. 269–286). Washington, DC: Hospice Foundation of America.

Wolraich, M. L., Aceves, J., Feldman, H. M., Hagan, J. F., Howard, B. J., Navarro, A., et al. (2000). The pediatrician and childhood bereavement. *Pediatrics, 105*(2), 445–451.

Wood, D. D., & Near, R. L. (2010). Using expressive arts when counseling bereaved children. In C. A. Corr & D. E. Balk (Eds.), *Children's encounters with death, bereavement, and coping.* New York: Springer.

CHAPTER 7

Digital Art Therapy
with Hospitalized Children

Cathy A. Malchiodi
Emily R. Johnson

Art therapy, like allied health and mental health fields, is adapting to the influx of electronic technologies for communication and self-expression. The expansion of computer-mediated art therapy is due to the ubiquity of digital technology and electronic communication (Malchiodi, 2000, 2009), as well as a generation of individuals who have experienced its existence since childhood. What children play with is drastically changing, and for today's youth there is no memory of a world without computer screens, smartphones, and handheld electronic devices (Davis, 2011). Adolescents in the United States now use all forms of digital media and online communication as a form of socialization with their peers (Lenhart, Madden, Macgill, & Smith, 2007), and smartphone technology has made it possible for youth to shoot, edit, and transmit images and films almost instantaneously.

Most practitioners agree that technology is influencing the way art therapists practice in a variety of settings, which includes addressing the needs of pediatric patients in a variety of medical settings. Working with young clients who make up a "digital generation" demands that those who provide intervention to children understand the possibilities, challenges, and limitations of digital technology in psychosocial care. Art therapists, play therapists, and other health care professionals who work with children in hospitals or medical settings are already applying various forms of digital media in their sessions. This chapter addresses this emerging approach, reviews commonly used digitally based methods, makes recommendations for applications to practice, and explores ethical issues inherent to using digital media in psychosocial care. Case examples are provided to illustrate ways digital art therapy is being used with pediatric patients in hospitals.

WHAT IS DIGITAL ART THERAPY?

"Digital art therapy," a relative newcomer to art therapy methods and materials, can be defined as "all forms of technology-based media, including digital collage, illustrations, films, and photography that are used by therapists to assist clients in creating art as part of the process of therapy" (Malchiodi, 2012, p. 33). It involves any activities that use computer keyboards and screens or other technological devices for image making within the context of treatment. Equipment used to generate, modify, or manipulate images and electronic methods such as photocopying, filmmaking, videotaping, and photography in various iterations from single reflex devices to digital cameras and smartphones are also part of spectrum of digital art therapy methodologies (Austin, 2009; Malchiodi, 2000, 2012; Thong, 2007).

The current availability of digital technology and media has exponentially increased capabilities to transform preexisting images through advances in scanners, printers, photo enhancement software, and Internet programs that even allow user to "clip" images for use and manipulation. Collages, for example, can be created on a computer screen using programs such as Polyvore (a website offering millions of images for digital use), stored on its website, and printed if needed. There are easily accessible online filmmaking programs and webcams, "flip cams" (pocket video cameras), and smartphones than can both take photographs and make short videos are commonplace. Platforms such as YouTube and Vimeo have increased interest in filmmaking and generated possibilities for sharing film footage that were unimaginable only a decade ago. Digital technology has also brought about social networking, a phenomenon wherein people can communicate in real time over Internet platforms such as Facebook, offering an additional means of instant communication that incorporates text, links to information, images, and films.

DIGITAL TECHNOLOGY AND GENERATION Z

In the early 21st century, most pediatric patients fall into a unique group of individuals with computer-savvy backgrounds because of their age and current cultural influences. "Generation Z" (also known as Gen Z or "digital natives") is a term used to describe people in the United States and Western cultures born from the early 1990s to the present, who have grown up with the World Wide Web, instant messaging and texting, mobile phones, and digital technologies. They are known for their ubiquitous participation in social media (YouTube, Facebook, and Twitter) and frequently share personal information and opinions in public online forums. Members of Gen Z are also multitaskers, who often feel comfortable engaging in several electronic forms of communication and activities at the same time; for example, imagine a teenager simultaneously texting, posting an update on Facebook, and listening to an MP3 player. Additionally, members of Gen Z are adept at performing tasks quickly, appear to thrive on fast-paced experiences, expect instant gratification, and prefer information to be presented in smaller segments (consider the 140-character limit for the current Twitter and the expected word count of blogs).

Most art therapists, play therapists, counselors, and child life specialists who work in hospital settings agree that it is important to "meet children where they are at" by responding with developmentally appropriate experiential interventions; this includes digital media for young patients who are comfortable in using it for self-expression. However, recognition that children and adolescents may feel comfortable with digital technology and computers is not a new concept. In the 1980s, Canter (1989) made a convincing case for why computer-mediated art therapy might be the method of choice with children and adolescents in particular, largely because younger clients came to know and feel comfortable with computers at an early age. She observed that "sometimes it takes a modern tool like the computer to stimulate clients today" (p. 314). Today, there is no argument that digital devices are a part of the day-to-day environment of most children and adolescents, and an expected part of daily life. Practitioners currently encounter digital natives in hospitals and other medical settings, underscoring the need for art therapists and other professionals to consider just how digital media can be successfully applied to psychosocial care.

APPLICATIONS OF DIGITAL ART THERAPY WITH PATIENTS

With digital media as a form of intervention and component of psychosocial care has become more widely used, several areas of application have emerged. These include but are not limited to (1) digital art making and image manipulation; (2) adaptive technology; (3) virtual reality therapy; and (4) social networking. A fifth area addresses how records are stored by practitioners—digital archiving of patient artwork.

Digital Art Making and Image Manipulation

As previously mentioned, digital art making and image manipulation include a wide range of platforms and devices, including drawing and painting software, cameras and webcams, and a variety of apps (short for "applications") with which to create. Digital art making offers many of the same characteristics as traditional media. For example, newer touch-tablet technologies offer patients a chance to experience drawing and painting through hands-on-screen expression. A drawing app or painting software may even provide a range of lines, colors, and textures not found in a set of felt marking pens or acrylic paints. Software, such as Photoshop, and online programs, such as Picassohead, provide opportunities to manipulate a wide range of preexisting imagery that is impossible with scissors and glue (for a list of various digital art making and image manipulation resources, see Table 7.1).

There is one question that continually emerges regarding the nature of digital art making itself: Is it different than the hands-on, creative expression of drawing, painting, clay sculpture, and collage making? Opinion varies widely. Seiden (2001) proposes

TABLE 7.1. Recommendations for Software, Apps, and Devices

It is impossible to list all digital technology that can be used in art therapy with pediatric patients, because new technology is constantly emerging. At the time of this writing, the following recommendations for software, apps, and devices are examples of the current technology that can be applied and adapted to work with children with medical illnesses and/or physical challenges.

Drawing, painting and collage software

Artweaver—*www.artweaver.de/products-en/artweaver-free*. Freeware painting program that is suitable for beginners but also for advanced users.

Tux Paint—*www.tuxpaint.org*. Free drawing program for children ages 3 to 12 (e.g., preschool and K–6). Tux Paint is used in schools around the world as a computer literacy drawing activity. It combines an easy-to-use interface, fun sound effects, and an encouraging cartoon mascot who guides children as they use the program.

Art Rage—*www.artrage.com*. Painting program for many platforms, including iPad.

Dogwaffle—*www.thebest3d.com/dogwaffle/free/index.html*. Paint and animation program.

Gimp—*www.gimp.org*. Free image manipulation program.

Picassohead—*www.picassohead.com/create.html*. Create your own "Picasso" with this free online program.

Apps[a]

SpinArt and SpinArt Studio—User-friendly apps to produce colorful SpinArt designs.

Uzu—Award-winning app that allows users to apply different kinds of touch to create colorful designs.

Virtuoso—Free piano app for music making via virtual piano keys.

Art of Glow—App that allows users to create colorful and relaxing designs.

Thicket—Part toy, part wind chime, and part spider web, this app provides the experience of texture, line, and tone.

Meritum Paint—Popular app and software for digital finger painting.

Pottery HD—Create virtual pottery.

Drawing Pad—Mobile art studio designed exclusively for tablets, using photo-realistic crayons, markers, paint brushes, colored pencils, stickers, and roller pens.

Photowall—Collage app that is easy to use to create images, greeting cards, wallpapers, and screensavers.

Helloflower—App that lets users create their own flowers by shaping petals, choosing colors, and fine-tuning the design.

Communitas—Developed by an expressive arts therapist, this app allows people to create together.

Digital filmmaking

iMovie (Apple platform)

Windows Moviemaker (PC platform)

Movie Maker (app for iPhone)

[a]Short for "applications." There are thousands of apps, and new ones are regularly available. The apps included in this table are popular ones for use with children.

that technology requires a distinctly different sensibility than traditional materials, and emphasizes conceptual and perceptual abilities over manual skills. However, there is emerging evidence that digital media may be beneficial to some young clients because it does not require the same manual skills as a pencil or paintbrush. For example, SketchUp 3D modeling software (Project Spectrum, 2011) has demonstrated that individuals on the autism spectrum actually find drawing a house using this platform to be both less frustrating and more gratifying than drawing with a pencil on paper. They also report that it makes more visual sense to them than a pencil-and-paper drawing. In establishing a computer art program in conjunction with child life program at a children's hospital, Thong (2007) observes that children who engaged in traditional forms of art making (drawing, painting, sculpting) were able to achieve a similar level of creative expression with a computer. She was also able to reach young patients who did not respond to traditional materials and to provide computer-mediated tools that matched individuals' preexisting artistic styles.

Adaptive Technology

For children who have physical challenges due to illness, accidents, or medical treatment, technology may provide necessary adaptations to compensate for any lack of manual skill needed for art making. For example, a "light pen," an input device that uses a light-sensitive detector to select images on a computer screen or make lines or choose colors on a tablet, can be useful because it eliminates the need for hand pressure. Additionally, voice commands can activate devices or be used to choose specific functions.

Weinberg (1985) noted the potential of computers to enhance art therapy with patients with quadriplegia, stroke, and traumatic brain injury (TBI). What Weinberg described at the time would now be defined as extremely primitive technology: an Atari 800 computer with a simple graphics component for drawing and image manipulation. However, she observed that computer-mediated art therapy could offer "an unusually novel and rapid approach to successful art experiences," and that "it has the unique power and advantage to elicit disabled patients' curiosity and motivation" (p. 69). In the 1980s, drawing software programs involved a keyboard or sometimes a light pen to trace images. In the 21st century, drawing can involve a mouse, a stylus, and most often, touch technology, so that the artist can simply draw directly on the screen. The current and ever-evolving technology has opened up far-reaching possibilities for use with patient populations that have physical and cognitive challenges.

Adaptive technology also addresses how art therapy services are delivered to those who may not be able to travel to a hospital or office. Collie and Cubranic (1999) were in the forefront of art therapy and what is sometimes called "telehealth"—health services delivered through computer-mediated and/or digital technology. Their work underscored how art therapy could be provided to patients with cancer and other illnesses in rural areas through synchronous (real time) and asynchronous means to address psychosocial objectives (Collie & Cubranic, 2002; Collie, Cubranic, & Long, 2002; Collie et al., 2007).

Virtual Reality Therapy

"Virtual reality therapy" (VTR) is defined as a type of psychotherapy and is currently applied as part of intervention for trauma symptoms, including posttraumatic stress disorder (PTSD; Macedonia, 2009). VRT is used as a form of exposure therapy and is believed to be a promising method in the treatment of trauma reactions, including PTSD (Hoffman, 2004). Virtual reality (VR) programs provide controlled, technology-driven environments in which patients can experience a situation while learning to cope with overwhelming emotional responses. VR has primarily been used with adult military veterans; studies indicate that after 6 months, participants experience a significant reduction in startle responses, one of the more troublesome symptoms related to PTSD (Reger et al., 2011).

Many researchers and practitioners are optimistic that younger patients who are interested in digital media may find VR helpful. It has been used with children with physical disabilities, including cerebral palsy (Reid, 2005); VR environments allow young clients to practice skills, for example, within a virtual representation of a non-hospital setting such as school or home. Initial findings by Reid (2002) indicate that virtual play activities that are enjoyable and increase play engagement enhance a sense of mastery and self-efficacy in children with physical challenges due to cerebral palsy. Because empowerment and engagement with therapeutic activities are important factors in recovery and in developing a sense of self-efficacy, VR approaches hold promise in addressing the psychosocial needs of patients with illnesses that compromise self-efficacy and a sense of independence.

Social Networking

Seymour (2011) notes that social networking sites have a vast potential to enhance "relationships, and emphasize opportunities to reduce social isolation and promote creativity and play" (p. 16). Rice (2009) observes that the popularity of platforms such as Facebook are due to the capacity to create a sense of belonging through sharing meaningful items, such as photos and images, and to stay in contact with family and friends. Social networking also provides a perceived sense of control, acceptance, and authenticity (Rice, 2009; Seymour, 2011). It is easy to understand that for a homebound or bedridden patient, social media can be a form of social support, especially from other patients who share similar challenges with illness or disability.

There are many specific social networking sites dedicated to relevant issues for youth with a medical illness, particularly cancer. For example, the Starlight Foundation's "Starbright World" uses social media, including Facebook and Twitter, to help teenagers find support and establish meaningful relationships with others their own age who are challenged by chronic and life-threatening illnesses. For individuals who are unable to leave the hospital or their homes, this program provides a way to reengage with peers. There are also multiple ways to connect with others, including a moderated "chat room," discussion boards, surveys and polls, and "e-cards" (an electronic version of a greeting card or postcard). Similarly, programs such as "I'm Too Young for This! Cancer Foundation" offer online support and virtual communities that help teens and young adults meet fellow cancer survivors.

Archiving Artwork

While many medical professionals use digital means to record or update progress notes, art therapists may be the only practitioners who use digital technology for storage of visual images created by patients. In the past, art therapists have had to address ways to store drawings, paintings, collage and three-dimensional objects, such as clay sculptures or assemblages. Depending upon the size of the art expression, storage in a secure setting was often a challenge; photography required development of prints and storage of photographic prints. With the advent of digital cameras it became possible to take a photograph of a patient's art expression and simply transfer that image to a computer, hard drive, disk, or other digital storage device. The secure storage and permanence of digital artwork archiving are current issues that continue to be discussed with regard to ethics and legalities of electronic transmission of records (see additional discussion below).

CHALLENGES IN THE USE OF DIGITAL ART THERAPY

Peterson, Stovall, and Elkins (2005) note that some art therapists believe that computers and digital technology offer benefits, while others feel that digital media may be technologically overloading patients, particularly children (Klorer, 2009). Art therapists themselves give digital technology mixed reviews (Asawa, 2009). Additionally, art therapists themselves are overwhelmed by digital media because technology evolves so rapidly and they lack understanding of social networks and software programs (Malchiodi, 2012). Many therapists lack education on how to use digital technology, are unsure of the ethical and legal limitations (for more information, see discussion below), or are simply afraid of media they do not understand. "Just the thought of operating a computer and mastering equipment such as 'scanners' and 'modems' can baffle, bewilder, and mystify even the most intelligent person" (Malchiodi, 2000, p. 32). Today's technology can be even more baffling because of its rapid development, turnover and operation.

Aside from these challenges, there are practical barriers, too. Because newer technology is often expensive, financial limitations for acquisition of computers, cameras, tablets, scanners, and printer may exist. Unlike a paintbrush or a set of watercolors, digital equipment is not easily replaced when broken or malfunctioning. Ink jet printer ink for printing tangible reproductions of patients' artwork is costly, and ink jet printers often require frequent maintenance if they are used for high volumes of printing. There may also be issues of infection control if the same device is to be used by many children, adding the need for repeated antiseptic measures. Finally, not all equipment is universally adaptable for all patient populations. For example, tablets that operate by touch may be frustrating for some individuals; some may need a "joystick" (a single, vertical stick mounted on a base) or a pointing stick or light pen to be able to use a computer.

DIGITAL TECHNOLOGY IN ACTION ON A PEDIATRIC UNIT

New applications of digital technology are emerging every day and are being appropriated for use in art therapy with pediatric patients. However, two current technologies—digital cameras and tablet technology—are more widely used in hospitals by art therapists, play therapists, and child life specialists.

Digital Cameras

Art therapy programs in hospitals often have digital cameras available for use with patients, and some programs have cameras that can be loaned to families during a child's hospital stay. Digital cameras allow children and family members to take unlimited photos, because there is no cost for film or development. Some art therapists are able to print photos and make CDs of digital images for families to take home. The photos can be sources of images for collage or scrapbooking projects while at the hospital or simply serve as a digital record of the hospital experience after discharge. In choosing a digital camera, it is important to select one that is sturdy, as well as easy to use. For example, some companies make digital cameras that take high-quality photos but can be dropped or submerged in water; these cameras are suitable for younger children, who may not handle equipment with care.

Weiser (1999) has written extensively on the use of phototherapy with people of all ages, including those who have medical illnesses. She notes that "every snapshot a person takes or keeps is also a type of self-portrait, a kind of 'mirror with memory' reflecting back those moments and people that were special enough to be frozen in time forever. Collectively, these photos make visible the ongoing stories of that person's life, serving as visual footprints marking where they have been (emotionally, as well as physically) and also perhaps signaling where they might next be heading" (Weiser, 2012). Weiser (2010) also explains that there is a difference in the practice of PhotoTherapy versus "photo art therapy"; the latter often involves an art therapist facilitating the creation of art as the central part of therapy sessions. Additionally, individuals may use photography as personal therapy, often outside of formal counseling or psychotherapy (Weiser, 2010).

In our experience with pediatric patients, there are many advantages to using digital cameras that integrate the three approaches cited by Weiser, including but not limited to the following:

- Communicates patients' and families' perspectives by literally showing us how they see the world.
- Provides a means of self-reflection and personal understanding.
- Offers a different form of expression and self-reflection than traditional art materials.
- Capitalizes on young people's interest in technology.
- Gives control to patients and families at a time when they have limited choices due to necessary medical treatments.
- Promotes learning opportunities for patients and families to acquire new skills in technology.

- Provides developmentally appropriate mental stimulation for patients when academic education is interrupted by treatments and long hospital stays.
- Creates art expressions that can be shared with others electronically when appropriate.

To illustrate the use of digital cameras with pediatric patients, here are two brief vignettes.

Case Examples

When the art therapist first met 3-year-old Sam, he was reluctant to engage in art making. Sam had recently been diagnosed with cancer and had undergone surgery to put in a "port" so he could receive medications. His mother expressed concern about her son not being himself and not wanting to get out of bed or play. Sam would not respond verbally, but he was interested in the camera when the art therapist presented it and he reached out to hold it. He initially took photos from his bed, including photos of the people around him and his toys in bed (Figure 7.1). The art therapist took this opportunity to ask Sam to take more pictures of things outside his room, which required him to get up and move (Figure 7.2). Sam took the camera and was able to walk down the hall, taking photos on his way and more while in the playroom (Figure 7.3), where he began to play. Being able to use digital media in art therapy with Sam was vital for his reengagement in normal, 3-year-old behavior. Sam did not have to use words, and he was able to explore his surroundings through this medium. The photographs he took were products of that moment in his treatment and were given to his mother on a CD. His mother also used digital photographs to help tell Sam's story through short movies created using filmmaking software. She included photos she had taken of Sam's experiences with treatment, adding statistics about childhood cancer and posting them on social networking platforms to raise awareness about pediatric cancer.

Other children have used digital cameras to document their experiences with cancer. For example, Noah used digital photography to record his chemotherapy (Figures 7.4 and 7.5). After Noah completed his treatment for cancer, the art therapist was asked to assist in a school reentry program and met with Noah to create a slide show of his photos that Noah subsequently shared with his class. Through his digital photos, Noah was able to look back

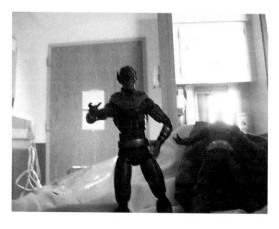

FIGURE 7.1. Sam's photo taken while in his hospital bed.

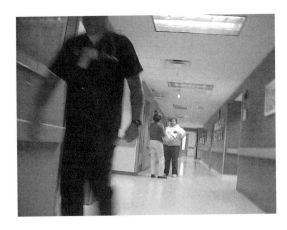

FIGURE 7.2. Sam's photo taken outside his hospital room.

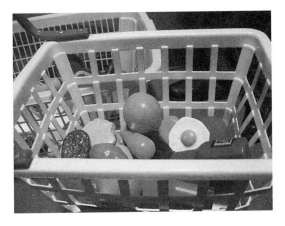

FIGURE 7.3. Sam's photo of the hospital playroom.

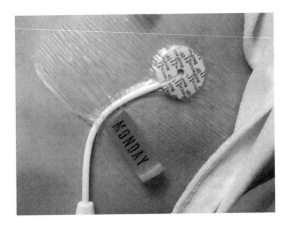

FIGURE 7.4. Noah's digital photography of chemotherapy line.

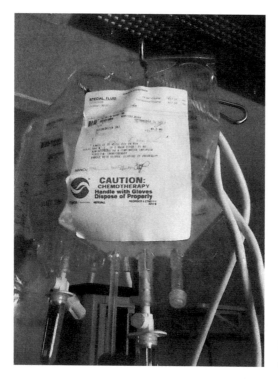

FIGURE 7.5. Noah's digital photography of chemotherapy bag.

over his yearlong treatment for cancer visually, seeing exactly where he had come from and where he was now. He was able to have complete control over what he chose to share with his classmates. The photos also gave him the ability to connect with his peers by illustrating for them exactly what he had been going through over the past year and during the time when he was unable to go to school.

Camcorders, compact "flipcams," and even smartphones with film capabilities offer accessible and user-friendly ways to make movies. Similar to the way they use digital cameras, children and adolescents may be able to record aspects of their hospitalization on film or be the "stars" in art therapist–initiated film projects. Seeing oneself on film played back on a laptop is only exciting for pediatric patients but it also provides another avenue for reflection and meaning making of a hospital experience.

Tablet Technology

Digital media can provide a means of creating artwork that can be shared without putting patients at risk for spreading infection. Many art therapists work with children in isolation, who cannot leave their room due to infectious diseases. In this situation, using an iPad or other tablet technology is one way to overcome challenges of providing art materials that may transmit bacteria or viruses. This is particularly helpful for patients during bone marrow transplant, because they have very compromised immune systems and are not able to leave their room or have visitors other than immediate family.

Under these circumstances, an iPad can become a medium to transmit images from one person to another. For example, a friend of a patient who was very concerned about her well-being was able to make her a "digital" art gift. Because of the risk of bringing germs into her room, he could not use traditional art materials to create for her a hand-made gift. He was able to use the iPad to draw a piece of art for her. The art therapist printed these for him, so that he could see his product, then gave another copy to the patient in the bone marrow transplant unit. The patient was very excited to have a gift made by her friend and fellow patient, and she hung it on her wall to remind her of that support (Figure 7.6). Digital media helped these young people to connect and support each other, while keeping infection control policies intact.

Malchiodi (2012) shares a different example of tablet technology with a pediatric patient. Josh, a 10-year-old boy, was admitted to a children's hospital for injuries from an all-terrain-vehicle (ATV) accident. Josh underwent several painful surgical procedures and had a difficult time adjusting to his hospital stay. On three occasions he was non-compliant with medical procedures and had to be restrained in order for nursing staff to administer medications and IVs. He did enjoy working with the art therapist and child life staff, and in particular liked using an iPad (a portable and compact computer device that can be used bedside) to make images.

To help Josh get settled down, the art therapist introduced apps called SpinArt Studio and Spawn Glow. Both apps are easy to use and involve making colorful designs through spinning virtual paint (SpinArt) or moving colorful lines around the screen using one's fingers. Josh often became so occupied with using the iPad to make designs that the nursing staff could more easily give injections or perform routine medical procedures, without Josh becoming anxious or complaining about pain.

After a few days, the art therapist taught Josh about another way to make art on the iPad through an app called Doodle Buddy, a program with numerous drawing tools (colored pencil and paintbrush lines) and special effects that only require the use of a finger on the screen, like the apps previously mentioned. It is a particularly good program for children, because they enjoy using these tools and effects, along with the stamps that allow them to add icons for animals, environmental elements, and other objects or

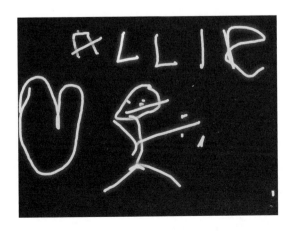

FIGURE 7.6. Digital artwork created by a friend for a patient at risk for infection.

emoticons (e.g., a "smiley face"). An audio feature can be selected so that each stamp makes its own sound when the artist places a stamp on the digital artwork. Making a piece of artwork only takes a few minutes. The child first selects a background (a color or environmental scene, such as a beach, mountains, or forest), and each artwork can be saved using a screenshot feature; artwork can then be printed or sent to other devices for viewing.

Josh used the Doodle Buddy over the course of several days to develop a story about one of the stamps, a sea turtle that he said had "superpowers." Superheroes are a common theme among children spending time in the hospital, and children in general, because they often are found in cartoons, digital games, and other media. At first Josh's sea turtle was surrounded by many threatening characters, including several ominous spiders that lived on a dangerous cliff by the ocean. He mentioned that his turtle was often afraid but learned how to make the spiders follow him into the ocean, where they eventually drowned. Eventually he found a special island, where he met a friendly lady-bug that helped him to feel less lonely while on the island and was "very nice to talk to." They played games on the beach during sunny days together; eventually the story ended with the sea turtle returning home to his own island of safety, where he lived with other turtles at his house.

From this brief vignette, it is not difficult to conclude that Josh at least partially used the story of the sea turtle (himself), dangerous elements and entities (the discomfort of the hospitalization and psychosocial struggles), and the ladybug (the therapist) to explore and communicate his feelings during his hospital stay and eventual recovery. While the art therapist could have also introduced drawing or sculpting materials bedside, digital media are an attractive alternative for younger clients like Josh, who are adept at learning how to use apps for self-expression.

Finally, tablet technology can also be used to reduce isolation by expanding a child's world when he or she is not able to leave the room. For example, we have used Skype on a laptop computer and Facetime on an iPad to allow children to participate in events that they could not attend in person, or to visit a friend in another room. This technology allowed these children to connect with others, an important element in maintaining wellness during a hospital stay.

ETHICAL AND LEGAL ISSUES IN DIGITAL ART THERAPY

The rapid emergence of digital technology is influencing how art therapy is practiced in all settings, including hospitals. Digital media have created possibilities for new ways to archive art expressions, communicate with patients, record data on patient progress, and interact with individuals living in remote or rural areas who are otherwise not easily served by medical staff. Tablet technology and other devices provide increased accessibility for some young patients whose physical challenges prevent them from using traditional pencils or paintbrushes. Despite these advantages, digital art therapy introduces new and emerging ethical dilemmas and, in some cases, legal concerns. Because this chapter cannot cover all possible ethical and legal aspects of digital art therapy, two areas of key importance to art therapy practice are briefly summarized: secure storage and confidentiality.

Secure Storage

Secure storage of images and patient data is an ongoing concern. With the advent of e-health procedures, physicians and other professionals now routinely use handheld computers to record patient data; these devices have software that encrypts data to provide safe storage of sensitive information. Encryption does not ultimately solve all problems of secure storage, because devices may be synchronized with other computers that must encrypt data as well (Plovnick, 2010).

For example, if a patient uses tablet technology, procedures and policies for secure storage must be made in advance. This may include backup on a remote site, hard drive, or CD or DVD or in the form of print images. Just like the accidental breakage of a clay sculpture, if a young patient damages a laptop computer or iPad, or if it malfunctions or "crashes," any artwork or confidential information may be permanently lost. A special casing for a tablet or laptop can prevent damage, but electronic loss of artwork or data may be impossible to recover.

Confidentiality

Confidentiality is a complex area for art therapists using any form of art expression during treatment, including digital technology. While there are many aspects to consider in working with pediatric patients, there are two major ones for practitioners using digital media in psychosocial care. One challenging aspect of using devices like iPads with multiple children involves protecting the confidentiality of previous users. In other words, when a child uses a computer or tablet to create an art expression, any images must be stored, so that the next patient does not have access to them. Because online sites are recorded as "history" on most devices, this is a complex issue; it may require the therapist constantly to delete logs or anything that can be used to track the activities of the previous user.

The second major aspect involves social networking sites and online platforms. While young clients may be encouraged to utilize social networking to enhance social support and share their stories (and art expressions) with others, participation in social media is difficult to monitor. It is challenging to advise children and adolescents about sharing information with other young patients, and when is helpful and when it may be counterproductive or compromising. The same holds true for display of digital photographs and films on sites such as Flickr or YouTube. Public display of these digital art forms can provide a sense of pride, mastery, and self-efficacy under certain circumstances; for a pediatric patient confined to bed at home or at a hospital, this type of self-expression can be critical to a sense of empowerment and connection. On the other hand, any public exhibition of art expressions by patients also brings up issues of boundaries, confidentiality and unpredictable adverse effects. Digital art expressions, photographs, and films, in contrast to traditional art expressions, can be transmitted easily and downloaded by others who can alter their content or post them to other sites. Rice (2009) notes that cyberspace does not "forget"; once something is uploaded to a site, downloaded, or viewed, a record of the event or image is always somewhere on the Internet. In contrast, tangible art expressions (drawings, paintings, collages, or sculptures) can be securely stored or even destroyed, if necessary (for a more complete discussion of exhibition of patient artwork, please see Chapter 23).

CONCLUSION

Digital art therapy is, at best, a changing landscape; new technologies are emerging every month that improve technology or change the way technology is delivered to users. This chapter has summarized current practices and approaches to applying digital technology to art therapy with pediatric patients. For the foreseeable future, it seems that digital media are here to stay and not only are art forms preferred by young patients but also are accepted as a ubiquitous part of communication and social interaction among children and adolescents. As art therapists and others who address the psychosocial care of pediatric patients continue to explore digital media in their work, it is likely that new and exciting apps will emerge to help young clients use technology as a way to cope adaptively with the challenges of medical illnesses.

REFERENCES

Asawa, P. (2009). Art therapists' emotional reactions to the demands of technology. *Art Therapy: Journal of the American Art Therapy Association, 26*(2), 58–65.

Austin, B. (2009). Technology, art therapy, and psychodynamic theory: Computer animation with an adolescent in foster care. In C. Moon (Ed.), *Materials and media in art therapy* (pp. 199–213). New York: Routledge.

Canter, D. S. (1989). Art therapy and computers. In H. Wadeson, J. Durkin, & D. Perach (Eds.), *Advances in art therapy* (pp. 296–316). New York: Wiley.

Collie, K., & Cubranic, D. (1999). An art therapy solution to a telehealth problem. *Art Therapy: Journal of the American Art Therapy Association, 16*(4), 186–193.

Collie, K., & Cubranic, D. (2002). Computer-supported distance art therapy: A focus on traumatic illness. *Journal of Technology in Human Services, 20*(1–2), 155–171.

Collie, K., Cubranic, D., & Long, B. (2002). Audiographic communication for distance counseling: A feasibility study. *British Journal of Guidance and Counseling, 30*(3), 269–284.

Collie, K., Kreshka, M. A., Ferrier, S., Parsons, R., Graddy, K., Avram, S., et al. (2007). Videoconferencing for delivery of breast cancer support groups to women living in rural communities: A pilot study. *Psycho-Oncology, 16*, 1–5.

Davis, A. (2011). What about digital toys? *Play Therapy, 6*(4), 18–21.

Hoffman, H. (2004). Virtual-reality therapy. *Scientific American, 291*(2), 58–65.

Klorer, P. G. (2009). The effects of technological overload on children: An art therapist's perspective. *Art Therapy: Journal of the American Art Therapy Association, 26*(2), 80–82.

Lenhart, A., Madden, M., Macgill, A. R., & Smith, A. (2007). *Teens and social media: The use of social media gains a greater foothold in teen life as they embrace the conversational nature of interactive online media.* Washington, DC: Pew Internet and American Life Project.

Macedonia, M. (2009). Virtual worlds: A new reality for treating posttraumatic stress disorder. *IEEE Computer Graphics and Applications, 29*(1), 86–88.

Malchiodi, C. A. (2000). *Art therapy and computer technology: A virtual studio of possibilities.* London: Jessica Kingsley.

Malchiodi, C. A, (2009). Art therapy meets digital art and social multimedia. Retrieved from *www.psychologytoday.com/print/34389.*

Malchiodi, C. A. (2012). Art therapy materials, media, and methods. In C. A. Malchiodi (Ed.), *Handbook of art therapy* (2nd ed., pp. 27–41). New York: Guilford Press.

Peterson, B., Stovall, K., & Elkins, D. (2005). Art therapists and computer technology. *Art Therapy: Journal of the American Art Therapy Association, 22*(3), 139–149.

Plovnick, R. M. (2010). The progression of electronic health records and implications for psychiatry. *American Journal of Psychiatry, 167*(5), 498–500.

Project Spectrum. (2011). Project spectrum—strengths of autism shine through 3D. Retrieved November 15, 2011, from *http://sketchup.google.com/intl/en/spectrum.html.*

Reger, G., Holloway, K., Candy, C., Rothbaum, B., Difede, J., Rizzo, A., et al. (2011). Effectiveness of virtual reality exposure therapy for active duty soldiers in a military mental health clinic. *Journal of Traumatic Stress, 24*(1), 93–96.

Reid, D. T. (2002). Benefits of a virtual play rehabilitation environment for children with cerebral palsy on perceptions of self-efficacy: A pilot study. *Pediatric Rehabilitation, 5*(3), 141–148.

Reid, D. (2005). Correlation of pediatric volitional questionnaire with the test of playfulness in a virtual environment: The power of engagement. *Early Child Development and Care, 175*(2), 153–164.

Rice, J. (2009). *The church of Facebook: How the hyperconnected are redefining community.* Colorado Springs, CO: David C. Cook.

Seiden, D. (2001). *Mind over matter: The uses of materials in art, education and therapy.* Chicago: Magnolia Street.

Seymour, J. (2011). Digital dilemma: Play therapy and online social networking. *Play Therapy, 6*(1), 16–19,

Starlight Foundation. (2011). *Starbright World.* Retrieved December 1, 2011, from *www.starlight.org/starbrightworld.*

Thong, S. A. (2007). Redefining the tools of art therapy. *Art Therapy: Journal of the American Art Therapy Association, 24*(2), 52–58.

Weinberg, D. J. (1985). The potential of rehabilitative computer art therapy for the quadriplegic, cerebral vascular accident and brain trauma patient. *Art Therapy: Journal of the American Art Therapy Association, 3*(2), 66–72.

Weiser, J. (1999). *PhotoTherapy techniques: Exploring the secrets of personal snapshots and family albums* (2nd ed.). Vancouver: PhotoTherapy Centre Press.

Weiser, J. (2010). Using photographs in art therapy practices around the world: PhotoTherapy, Photo-Art-Therapy, and Therapeutic Photography. *Fusion, 2*(3), 18–19.

Weiser, J. (2012, January 15). PhotoTherapy Centre homepage. Retrieved from *www.phototherapy-centre.com/home.htm.*

PART II

ART THERAPY
WITH ADULT PATIENTS

INTRODUCTION

British artist and author Adrian Hill is credited for coining the term "art therapy" in 1942 and recorded his ideas about the rehabilitative qualities of art in 1945 in *Art versus Illness*. His conceptualization of art therapy resulted from his own convalescence from tuberculosis at King Edward VII Sanatorium in 1938, where he passed long months of hospitalization by drawing and found the process helpful in his own recovery. In 1939, Hill was invited to teach art to other patients as part of an occupational therapy program at the sanatorium, including injured soldiers and civilian patients. Hogan (2001) noted that Hill felt art making was a way to take patients' minds off their illnesses and to release stress. In later years, he went on to become the president of the British Association of Art Therapists and was a proponent for art therapy becoming an integral part of the National Health Service in the United Kingdom (Waller, 1991). In brief, Hill's contribution became a milestone in the acceptance and implementation of art therapy as part of treatment for adult patients with medical illness or physical disabilities.

Today in the 21st century, there is growing evidence for the application of art therapy to work with adult patients, particularly those with cancer or chronic conditions, including those that involve pain and fatigue. Art therapy as an intervention for patients with breast cancer shows promise. In one study (Oster, Magnusson, Thyme, Lindh, & Astrom, 2007), a standard instrument used to measure coping resources, was used to identify the impact of art therapy on how patients viewed their illness. The results demonstrated a connection between art therapy and talking about protecting one's own boundaries, when compared to a control group. The researchers concluded that art therapy provided patients with a means to more accurately express their own interpretations and experience with cancer. In a second study (Svensk et al., 2009), art therapy was examined in relationship to the impact of diagnosis, treatment, and the experienced quality of life as measured by a standard instrument. It compared two groups of women undergoing radiotherapy treatment for breast cancer, one that received individual art therapy and one that did not. Those who received art therapy showed a significant increase in total health, total quality of life, physical health, and psychological health, as compared to the control group. A significant positive difference within the art therapy group was also seen, concerning future perspectives, body image, and systemic therapy side effects. These improvements were achieved in a relatively short time, underscoring that art therapy can be applied in the short-term and still demonstrate significant effects.

Pain and fatigue are two symptoms of many illnesses in adults and often come as unwelcome side effects of various medical treatments, including chemotherapy for cancer. Like many art therapists who work with individuals with chronic illness or physical disabilities, I ask clients about the degree of pain and fatigue they are experiencing so that we can co-create a plan to address these symptoms and quality of life. For example, Ana was in her late 40s when she was referred to me for art therapy and counseling when her rheumatoid arthritis (RA) became more severe. RA is an illness in which the body essentially attacks its own joints causing pain, swelling, and eventual loss of function, if not treated aggressively and consistently. Ana was first diagnosed with RA in her late 20s and had been prescribed many different medications including nonsteroidal anti-inflammatory drugs and injections. Her illness had progressed to the point where more powerful interventions were necessary, including Methotrexate, an immunosuppressant that inhibits inflammation and is also used to treat certain cancers. Ana was put on this drug because her RA was no longer responding to the first line of medical treatments.

Initially, Ana wanted to try art therapy as a form of relaxation and distraction and particularly as way to exercise her hands, increase flexibility, and maintain fine motor skills that were jeopardized by the inflammation in her joints. But we quickly found that when given meaningful and enjoyable ways to engage in self-expression, Ana also reported how much the pain throughout her entire body was reduced. In initial sessions, we began with some easy drawing, painting, and collage activities, using art expression as a physical intervention (fine motor exercise), stress reduction, and a form of communication about feelings and perceptions about chronic illness. Ana eventually became interested in creating detailed drawings and cut-paper designs of imaginary animals and birds (see Figure II.1); she enjoyed planning these images and how to use layers of colored papers and inks to express her ideas. Despite the difficulty and intricacy of cutting layer upon layer of paper and using fine-tipped pens, Ana found this art form self-soothing and as she said, a "way to make pain irrelevant." Once in awhile she would laugh and observe that her knuckle joints "squealed the next morning" after spending an hour or two designing, cutting, arranging, and layering colored papers and drawing. But she also observed that just imagining what her next design would look like would often take her mind off the pain, and she reported to her rheumatologist that she had less need for narcotic medications to ease any flares of inflammation or pain.

Some initial studies point to art therapy as an effective intervention in reducing perceptions of pain and fatigue. Nainis, Paice, and Ratner (2006) investigated the impact of art therapy sessions on oncology patients who were experiencing pain and tiredness.

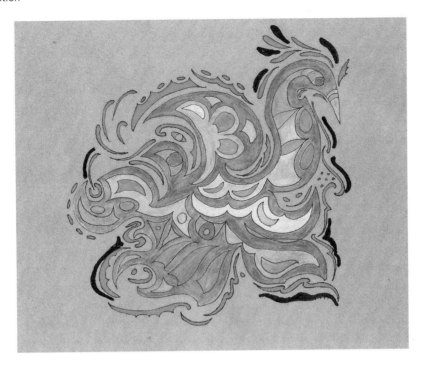

FIGURE II.1. Ana's cut paper image of a bird.

The specific goal of the study was to determine the effect of a 1-hour art therapy session on pain and other symptoms common to this patient population. Participants were given the opportunity to choose from a wide range of materials and projects, providing an individualized approach. For those patients who could not easily use their hands, the art therapist provided assistance and took directions from patients. In brief, the researchers found that there were statistically significant reductions in eight of the nine symptoms measured. Surprisingly, participants made numerous comments that art therapy energized them, underscoring that the process decreased perceptions of tiredness in the short-term.

Chapters in this part explain and illustrate the variety of ways that art therapy can make a difference in the lives of adults with cancer (Chapters 8, 10, and 11), physical trauma (Chapters 9, 16, and 17), chronic illnesses (Chapters 12, 13, 14, and 15), and Alzheimer's disease and dementia (Chapter 18). Each reflects the important role that art therapy has in helping individuals address the psychological and interpersonal consequences of life-threatening illnesses, such as cancer and HIV/AIDS and disability. Additionally, many of these chapters underscore the emerging knowledge that art expression complements somatic approaches, health psychology, and the neurobiology of how and why art therapy supports emotional and physical aspects of recovery. In all cases, the case material, interventions, and research presented in this part highlight the rapidly expanding "best practices" in work with adults in a variety of medical settings.

As described in the Introduction, oncology patient Michaela used art expression not only to explore her feelings about cancer but also as a way to summarize life experiences. It was her way to "reclaim personal power, to create a lasting visual legacy, and to say, therefore, 'I am' and 'I exist'" (Malchiodi, 1997, p. 51). Art is a form of visual narrative (Chapter 8) for people of all ages, but particularly for adults, who when confronted with serious illness or a life-changing condition, search for a sense of wholeness and a way to re-examine and reframe life stories.

REFERENCES

Hill, A. (1945). *Art versus illness*. London: Allen & Unwin.

Hogan, S. (2001). *Healing arts: The history of art therapy*. London: Jessica Kingsley.

Malchiodi, C. A. (1997). Invasive art: Art as empowerment for women with breast cancer. In S. Hogan (Ed.), *Feminist approaches to art therapy* (pp. 49–64). London: Routledge.

Nainis, N., Paice, J., & Ratner, J. (2006). Relieving symptoms in cancer: Innovative use of art therapy. *Journal of Pain and Symptom Management, 31*(2), 162–169.

Oster, I., Magnusson, E., Thyme, K., Lindh, J., & Astrom, S. (2007). Art therapy for women with breast cancer: The therapeutic consequences of boundary strengthening. *The Arts in Psychotherapy, 34,* 277–288.

Svensk, A. C., Öster, I., Thyme, K. E., Magnusson, E., Sjodin, M., Eissmann, M., et al. (2009). Art therapy improves experienced quality of life among women undergoing treatment for breast cancer: A randomized controlled study. *European Journal of Cancer Care, 18,* 69–77.

Waller, D. (1991). *Becoming a profession: The history of art therapy in Britain, 1940–1982*. London: Routledge.

CHAPTER 8

Art Therapy as a Form of Visual Narrative in Oncology Care

Jill V. McNutt

The experiences of a cancer patient can be turbulent and traumatic. Facing life after diagnosis and treatment for cancer has become a subject for research and growth in the medical literature. This chapter explores the cancer patient experience and explains some of the interfaces patients undergo within the medical system. With the assistance of the art therapist, patients are able to express themselves through visual images, reflect on life through imagery, and re-create life as cancer survivors.

DEFINING THE PATIENT EXPERIENCE

Perhaps the most popular frame through which the cancer experience is discussed is that of the seasons of survivorship defined originally by Mullan (1986), describing his journey through cancer as a physician and cancer survivor. The seasons begin as "acute survivorship" as patients undergo active cancer treatments and monitoring. The "transitional season" is defined as the time when the patient is transitioning from regular treatments to ongoing monitoring and/or maintenance treatments. The "extended season" includes three subsections: "maintained remission, cancer free, and living with cancer" (Miller, Merry, & Miller, 2008, p. 371). The final season, "permanent survivorship," is applicable to those who have reached the extended survivorship phase as cancer free. Those who develop cancer again reenter the acute season of survivorship.

Psychological health decreases rapidly following the shock of diagnosis with cancer (Andrykowski, Lykins, & Floyd, 2008; Clemmons, Knafl, Lev, & Mc Corkle, 2008; Reb, 2007). Physical health treatments take precedence over mental health or more holistic methods. Treatments such as surgery, chemotherapy, and radiation therapy fill the days, weeks, and months of nausea, loss of body image, inability to work, and changes in lifestyle. For those who do not succumb to cancer, the journey continues to provide challenges. Fears and need for coping resources include physical, behavioral, and personal life changes; fear of reoccurrence; emotional distress; loss of the safety net of health care; and difficulties returning to normal life (Allen, Savadatti, & Levy, 2009). Concerns for the patient in the re-entry phase include self-image, others' attitudes toward cancer, social narratives of survivorship, and re-adaptations to "normal" life (Heywood, 2003).

Andrykowski et al. (2008) charted four possible state paths for the cancer survivor: (1) continued deterioration, (2) continued impairment, (3) recovery and return to former life patterns, or (4) growth in light of the cancer experience. Continued deterioration is the path of survivor despair leading to continued loss of functioning and inability to return to a purposeful life. Continued impairment allows the survivor to regain some functioning, but not to the extent that he or she can return to life as it was precancer. Recovery and return to former life patterns restore the survivor's prediagnostic condition. Finally, growth in light of the cancer experience describes the survivors who find underlying value in the cancer experience.

In a series of interviews with U.S. cancer survivors, Kaiser (2008) learned that some women have rejected the survivor identity on the basis of (1) not being sick enough; (2) not wanting to be part of that group; (3) preferring to be identified beyond the illness; or (4) because they were still sick. Survivors may not express pain and fear disclosing the reality of breast cancer. Kaiser writes that some may prefer the labels of warriors or thrivers to being lumped in with the collective survivor identity. Svensk et al. (2009) add that medical discourse often makes women's own stories invisible. A balance in patient perception between subjective and objective, stress burden and coping resources, and perhaps global and personal aspects of survivorship define patient experience (Andrykowski et al., 2008).

PERCEPTIONS OF ILLNESS AND MENTAL HEALTH CONCERNS

Associated psychological conditions for some patients may meet diagnostic criteria for posttraumatic stress disorder (PTSD), depression, or other diagnoses (American Psychiatric Association, 2000). After cancer diagnosis there is a risk for increased anxiety and depression (Bush, 2009). There is, however, no indication that that degree of anxiety and depression impedes normal functioning. Many symptoms are associated with PTSD, but diagnosis with PTSD and/or major depression is rare (Andrykowski et al., 2008).

Mental health remains a concern, however, particularly when it impedes quality of life. Hoffman, McCarthy, Recklitis, and Ng (2009) using results from a national survey by the U.S. Census Bureau, compared psychological distress in 4,636 cancer survivors to 122,220 never-diagnosed individuals and found that a significantly larger percentage of survivors suffered psychological distress. Two-thirds of those with psychological distress had not met with mental health providers. Many of these survivors face emotional distress due to fear for the future, fear of cancer in general, poor perceived health, and poor coping skills.

CULTURAL VARIATION IN THE CANCER EXPERIENCE

The cancer experience is not independent of ethnicity. Although symptoms may be similar, global, cultural, and individual lenses, along with courses of treatment and stages of cancer diagnosis, all combine with other factors to create the patient-survivor experience. Efforts are being made internationally to address the needs of all patients (Thomas, Carlson, & Bultz, 2009).

Cultural identity is very important when considering the needs of the oncology patient. Economic, geographic, and racial disparities in cancer care are present throughout the United States. According to the American Cancer Society (2009), African Americans have higher rates of cancer diagnosis and higher percentages of mortality. Economic concerns and becoming dependent on oncology treatments are but two of the potential struggles of the underprivileged in the United States. Health disparities, health care inequities, and reduced access to health care translate into discrimination for high-risk populations (Barton-Burke, Barreto, & Archibald, 2008). Cultural identity must be considered during any meaning making and reidentification interventions.

Geography also has an impact on the survivor experience and narrative. For the cancer survivor living in rural areas, with large distances to travel for access to health care, remote access to information helps to ground the survivors' personal experience by offering access to oncology professionals and accurate information about cancer. Misconceptions about cancer and its treatment placed limits on the creative freedom of the survivor. Rural survivors were shown to have slower adjustment, lower vitality, and higher perceptions of stigmatization following cancer treatment (Bettencourt, Schlegel, Talley, & Molix, 2007).

VISUAL NARRATIVE, MEANING MAKING, AND IDENTITY INTEGRATION

Artwork created by patients can serve as a valuable "visual" narrative of the cancer experience. Generalized narratives help to transform individual experience by allowing the patient or survivor to feel supported and heard. Art making can help to ensure that individual identities are not lost in the context of the collective cancer survivor identity. Visual images help to make visible connections to individual experience (Radley & Bell, 2007). This occurs in many ways, including but not limited to the following:

1. *Maintenance of self-identity.* Maintenance of self-identity within the context of the collective is vital to the subjective experience of cancer treatment and the path to

survivorship. Reflecting on the cross-cultural experience in art therapy, McNiff (1984) found "interdependence between universal and particular forms of communication" (p. 126). McNiff explains that through creativity individuals can access, through the self, relationships to the universal. Preservation of the self within the cancer survivor identity requires a personal balance between one's individual identity and the collective model.

2. *Perceptions of illness.* Reynolds and Vivat (2010) investigated art making's influence on the perceptions and experiences of chronic illness. They interviewed 13 women with chronic illness and ongoing pain about their art-making practice. From their interviews, Reynolds and Vivat discerned two major ways of experiencing the illness. Some art makers were bound by their illness, while others were able to live beyond the illness through the art-making process. Art processes reported by participants who were bound by illness were defined by the limitations of pain accommodation within the illness. These participants did not identify themselves as artists. Those who were able to live beyond the illness often described themselves as growing artists, and their works were defined in possibility revealing the person as opposed to the illness.

3. *Meaning making.* For those who have experienced cancer, finding ways to integrate past events and cancer experiences into reformulated identities is necessary in order to be able to move beyond the illness. Andersen, Bowen, Morea, Stein, and Baker (2008) surveyed 636 breast cancer survivors and found two modes of meaning making. Survivors who made meaning of their experience either made sense of the situation or found benefit from the experience. The cancer patient must take inventory of her precancer identity and synthesize it with new notions of identity. This type of reconstruction is available through the art making and art therapy process (Reynolds & Prior, 2006). This process adds to potential optimism and advances the collective identity. The breast cancer survivor identity builds constructs by which individuals can begin to frame their experiences. Both positive and negative effects can be seen on the ability personally to create a postdiagnosis and posttreatment identity (Kaiser, 2008).

4. *Search for greater meaning.* Cancer diagnosis is traumatic for the patient (Geffen, 2000). But if the patient uses it to reflect on experiences and chooses to make new life connections rather than dispose of old ones, the illness experience can be transformative. Those who thrive posttreatment take cancer as a challenge that elicits a search for greater meaning. Expression through art has the potential to help make those connections (Dreifuss-Kattan, 1990). Dreifuss-Kattan notes about the cancer patient turned artist that "the artist's inside is no longer only an incubator for a malignant, cancerous process, but is a healthy soil for symbolism and form giving" (p. 133).

5. *Self-efficacy and locus of control.* Art making and thoughtful reflection are theorized to bring about a balance of internal and external locus of control, adding a sense of purpose to life (Malchiodi, 1998). This sense of purpose in turn provides motivation and a will to live, and feelings of satisfaction and completeness leading to the idea of accomplishment and integrity as opposed to despair (Erikson, 1978). From this creative

participation comes meaning making, reduced stress, reduced depression, increased coping strategy development, increased active engagement in health care, and increased self care (Heywood, 2003; Luzzatto & Gabriel, 2000; Monti et al., 2006; Svesnk et al., 2009). Art therapy has been noted to encourage active rather than passive participation in health care and oncology options, and positive coping and adjustment strategies, and it has been shown to stimulate catharsis and emotional balance (Heywood, 2003).

BENEFITS OF ART AND ART THERAPY

Engagement in creating art has been shown to have attributes of homeostatic motivation, cognitive orientation, and affect (Camic, 2008). "Homeostatic motivation" is described as a tension created by interaction between the individual's internal triggers and the artwork that is then integrated and released by the viewer (Dewey, 1934; Kreitler & Kreitler, 1972). "Cognitive orientation" occurs during the integration of stimulus into cognitive knowledge structure (Kreitler & Kreitler, 1972). The experience of art by the viewer involves a dialogue with the artwork. This dialogue challenges the cognitive structure of the viewer in such a way as to disrupt the homeostatic state. The viewer then integrates the art and experience in order to return to balance (Dewey, 1934). Through the process of creating and reflecting on personal visual narratives, the cancer survivor encounters these attributes and is able to integrate identities.

Sixty-three patients on 15-bed cancer unit participated in a nurse's investigation into the benefits of art making. Rockwood-Lane (2005) found that art narratives were created in a spiral growth process starting with physical or psychic pain. A shift often occurred during the art making or storytelling process in which themes of "emerging from darkness," "surrendering to the process," and "slipping through the veil" (p. 288), among others, emerged. Patients' internal self witnessed the art and helped them see the self as body energy, including feelings of compassion, oneness, and transcendence (Rockwood-Lane, 2005).

The use of art therapy in identity re-formation has been shown to help cancer survivors find and maintain individual identities within the context of the survivorship identity. Predeger (1996) worked with an art therapy breast cancer focus group through which a qualitative review of artwork, coresearchers' reflections on artwork, and group discussion formed the basis of feminist inquiry. Predeger was curious about the process of co-creating personal and collective meaning making. She found that art as a method of inquiry helped tap inner creativity, made notable progress in meaning making, provided connections and empowerment, and was a source for a way of knowing. Through the study of women attending art therapy groups, she found that the art therapy groups helped to actualize a need to express; lose and gain control; illuminate a changing perspective; transcend the experience, lead to braver perspectives; connect with others; fuel a creative spark; and celebrate the feminine (Predeger, 1996). The group created a safe place where cancer survivors could safely explore the situation in which they found themselves through diagnosis, treatment, and survivorship.

Collie, Bottorff, and Long (2006) interviewed 17 cancer survivors about their experience with art and art therapy. Of them, 10 reported experiencing "art as a harbor." Nine, who were participating in art therapy, used art to "get a clearer view"; 12 used art to "clear the way emotionally"; and 10 found that art "enhanced and enlivened the self" (p. 765). Art and art therapy were found to reduce the threat of annihilation of the self; to help women affirm and appreciate present existence; and to enhance the possibility of an ongoing self. Art and art therapy benefits listed in the survey of cancer survivors who had participated in the past were as follows: (1) promotes emotional expression; (2) permits trust in what has been expressed; (3) facilitates personalized expression and resistance to disempowering discourses; (4) brings a sense of personal worth; (5) provides intrinsic motivation through its aesthetic dimension; and (6) brings a feeling of connection with a larger whole (Collie et al., 2006).

CASE EXAMPLES

Each patient and/or survivor has his or her own experience in the process of creating and reflecting on art therapy visual narratives. The following two composite experiences help to demonstrate some of the elements. Gina came to art therapy 3 months after the completion of her chemotherapy treatments for breast cancer; Catherine had 4 years of posttreatment survivorship before beginning her art therapy visual narrative experience. Gina opted to participate in art therapy through a series of individual sessions, and Catherine joined a small group of five women who met weekly in the studio clinic.

Gina

During the first session, Gina was introduced to art therapy as a way of seeing the world and the cancer experience, and was initially given the opportunity to sort through art materials. Gina professed no art experience and was attracted to magazine images. Gina sifted through the magazines and removed images that both metaphorically and literally reflected her experience of cancer. The images were then sorted into a timeline and taken home between sessions.

Gina returned to the second session with the images sorted into treatment and posttreatment. Paint was selected as the medium through which Gina's visual narrative would be created. General painting instructions were provided by the art therapist. Gina positioned the magazine images revealing a two-sided canvas, with treatment depicted on the left side and posttreatment on the right. As the painting progressed, Gina began to question how the art therapist knew that shades were more intense closer in the foreground of the canvas and why water was drawn with horizontal lines. Through this painting instruction dialogue, Gina was motivated to notice subtleties in nature. During the fourth session, she noted that she had a new way of looking at the world.

As the painting process continued, Gina was encouraged to notice successes, struggles, and notable moments that arose during the session. The painting engaged her in dialogue and reflection. Gina noticed that some abstract shapes created in the negative spaces reminded her of the medical facilities where she received treatment and, subsequently, that the buildings were partially hidden by a haze. Further dialogue between Gina, the painting, and the art therapist led Gina to uncover some of the fears she had experienced during treatment. She also noticed that the colors around the treatment side reflected toxicity. The art therapist's validation helped to ground Gina's experience of treatment and encourage further discoveries. The art therapist kept field notes each week to keep a record of insights gleaned through this art process.

The validation and new vision Gina experienced gave her self-confidence and a voice. She became able to integrate the hope found on the posttreatment side of her painting into her health care decision-making process. The eighth session followed the completion of the painting and offered the opportunity for the creation of an artist statement and consent for display. Visual narrative participants are offered the opportunity to display their work to new patients in oncology clinics. Gina found new life in her visual narrative and was able to re-create hope for her future through the art therapy experience.

Catherine

Catherine was introduced to art therapy through a hospital-based open studio while recovering from surgery to remove tumors from her brain. She continued to attend open studio sessions periodically for the 4 years following her treatment. To begin her visual narrative participation, Catherine met with the art therapist to learn about the visual narrative process and opted to join a small group in which all members were creating visual narratives with the intent of displaying the finished products in a touring exhibit. Catherine came to the group with a three-dimensional diorama in mind. She looked through objects she found and fabrics to find materials to build a model of the hospital room she lived in during her treatment. Many of the objects she collected that day reminded Catherine of elements of her medical treatment.

While sharing her reflections during the group time, Catherine found camaraderie with other group members who acknowledged her experience. She became cognizant of how certain triggers of hope and fear emerged in her surroundings following diagnosis. Four years following her treatment, Catherine maintained detailed visual memories of the hospital room. As the diorama progressed, Catherine was able to revive and transform her memory of this significant moment in her life. She was validated and supported by the group and the art therapist. Through the experience of creating and reflecting on the diorama, Catherine was able to find an altruistic voice and exhibited a great deal of pride in sharing her work with new patients. Since participation in the visual narrative group, Catherine has found ways of supporting new patients. She discovered and articulated many of the positive elements provided her by medical staff and has chosen to give back by supporting new patients in many of the same ways.

CONCLUSION

This brief chapter underscores that art therapy in the form of visual narrative facilitates both metaphorical and tangible self-expression regarding the experience of cancer.

Seeing relationships and connections within the context of the art or visual narrative heightens the relationship between patients and their artwork. Art expression becomes a viable member of the triadic art therapy relationship, along with the patient and therapist. Through validation and witnessing the art process and product, the art therapist supports the development of the patient's strengths. These strengths add to the patient's voice and abilities to cope with treatment, and eventually to re-create life outside of cancer.

REFERENCES

Allen, J. D., Savadatti, S., & Levy, A. G. (2009). The transition from breast cancer patient to survivor. *Psycho-Oncology 18*, 71–78.

American Cancer Society. (2009). *Cancer facts and figures*. Atlanta: American Cancer Society.

American Psychiatric Association. (2000). *Diagnostic and statistical manual of mental disorders* (4th ed., text rev.). Washington, DC: Author.

Andersen, M. R., Bowen, D. J., Morea, J., Stein, K., & Baker, F. (2008). Frequent search for sense by long-term breast cancer survivors associated with reduced HRQOL. *Women and Health, 47*(4), 19–37.

Andrykowski, M. A., Lykins, E., & Floyd, A. (2008). Psychological health in cancer survivors. *Seminars in Oncology Nursing, 24*(3), 193–201.

Barton-Burke, M., Barreto, R. C., Jr., & Archibald, L. I. S. (2008). Suffering as a multicultural cancer experience. *Seminars in Oncology Nursing, 24*(4), 229–236.

Bettencourt, B. A., Schlegel, R. J., Talley, A. E., & Molix, L. A. (2007). The breast cancer experience of rural women: A literature review. *Psycho-Oncology, 16*, 875–887.

Bush, N. J. (2009). Post traumatic stress disorder related to the cancer experience. *Oncology Nursing Forum, 36*(4), 395–399.

Camic, P. M. (2008). Playing in the mud: Health psychology, the arts and creative approaches to health care. *Journal of Health Psychology, 13*(2), 287–298.

Clemmons, D. A., Knafl, K., Lev, E. L., & McCorkle, R. (2008). Cervical cancer: Patterns of long term survival. *Oncology Nursing Forum, 35*(6), 897–903.

Collie, K., Bottorff, J. L., & Long, B. C. (2006). A narrative view of art therapy and art making by women with breast cancer. *Journal of Health Psychology, 11*(5), 761–775.

Dewey, J. (1934). *Art as experience*. New York: Penguin.

Dreifuss-Kattan, E. (1990). *Cancer stories: Creativity and self-repair*. Hillsdale, NJ: Analytic Press.

Erikson, E. H. (1978). *Identity and the life cycle*. New York: Norton.

Geffen, J. R. (2000). *The journey through cancer: An oncologist's seven level program for healing and transforming the whole person*. New York: Crown.

Heywood, K. (2003). Introducing art therapy into the Christie Hospital, Manchester, UK, 2001–2002. *Complementary Therapies in Nursing and Midwifery, 9*, 125–132.

Hoffman, K. E., McCarthy, E. P., Recklitis, C. J., & Ng, A. K. (2009). Psychological distress in long-term survivors of adult onset cancer. *Archives of Internal Medicine, 169*(14), 1274–1281.

Kaiser, K. (2008). The meaning of survivor identity for women with breast cancer. *Social Science Medicine, 67*(1), 79–87.

Kreitler, H., & Kreitler, S. (1972). *Psychology of the arts*. Durham, NC: Duke University Press.

Luzzatto, P., & Gabriel, B. (1998). Art psychotherapy. In J. C. Holland (Ed.), *Psycho-oncology* (pp. 743–757). New York: Oxford University Press.

Luzzatto, P., & Gabriel, B. (2000). The creative journey: A model for short term group art therapy with post treatment cancer patients. *Art Therapy: Journal of the American Art Therapy Association, 17*(4), 265–269.

Malchiodi, C. (1998). *Medical art therapy with adults.* London: Jessica Kingsley.

McNiff, S. (1984). Cross-cultural psychology and art. *Art Therapy: Journal of the American Art Therapy Association, 1*(3), 125–131.

Miller, K., Merry, B., & Miller, J. (2008). Seasons of survivorship revisited. *Cancer Journal, 12*(6), 369–374.

Monti, D. A., Peterson, C., Shakin-Kunkel, E., Hauck, W. W., Pequignot, E., Rhodes, L., et al. (2006). A randomized controlled trial of mindfulness based art therapy (MBAT) for women with cancer. *Psycho-Oncology, 15*(5), 363–373.

Mullan, F. (1986). Seasons of survival: Reflections of a physician with cancer. *New England Journal of Medicine, 313*, 270–273.

Predeger, E. (1996). Womanspirit: A journey into healing through art in breast cancer. *Advances in Nursing Science, 18*(3), 48–58.

Radley, A., & Bell, S. E. (2007). Artworks, collective experience and claims for social justice: The case of women living with breast cancer. *Sociology of Health and Illness, 29*(3), 366–390.

Reb, A. (2007). Transforming the death sentence: Elements of hope in women with advanced ovarian cancer. *Oncology Nursing Forum, 34*(6), 70–81.

Reynolds, F., & Prior, S. (2006). The role of art making in identity maintenance: Case studies of people living with cancer. *European Journal of Cancer Care, 15*, 333–341.

Reynolds, F., & Vivat, B. (2010). Art making and identity work: A qualitative study of women living with chronic fatigue syndrome/myalgic encephalomyelitis (CFS/ME). *Arts and Health: An International Journal for Research, Policy and Practice, 2*(1), 67–80.

Rockwood-Lane, M. (2005). Spirit–body healing: A hermeneutic phenomenological study examining the lived experience of art and healing. *Cancer Nursing Journal, 28*(4), 285–291.

Svensk, A. C., Oster, L., Thyme, K. E., Magnusson, E., Sjodin, M., Eisemann, M., et al. (2009). Art therapy improves experienced quality of life among women undergoing treatment for breast cancer: A randomized controlled study. *European Journal of Cancer Care, 18*, 69–77.

Thomas, B. C., Carlson, L. G., & Bultz, B. D. (2009). Cancer patient ethnicity and associations with emotional distress—the 6th vital sign: A new look at defining patient ethnicity in a multi-cultural context. *Journal of Immigrant Health, 11*, 237–248.

CHAPTER 9

Using Imagery to Address Physical and Psychological Trauma

Ephrat Huss
Orly Sarid

In this chapter we present two interventions within health care settings using art therapy and guided imagery with accident-induced acute stress disorder (ASD). These cases both utilize images and are then compared. The analysis points to the importance of interactive shifts from physical to cognitive interventions that use images in both art therapy and guided imagery. We discussed differences between artwork and guided imagery, and their implications in health care with accident survivors.

Within today's complex and fast-moving reality, motor accidents are central reasons for clients to seek out therapeutic intervention in health care settings. Accidents often involve actual or threatened death, serious injury, or a threat to physical integrity of self or other, to which the individual's response involves intense fear, helplessness, or horror. As a traumatic event, an accident exacts a toll on body as well as mind, as described in the *Diagnostic and Statistical Manual of Mental Disorders* (DSM-IV-TR; American Psychiatric Association, 2000), and is thus a psychophysiological experience, even when the traumatic event causes no direct bodily harm. The challenge for therapists thus becomes how to address the interlocking physical and psychological characteristics of disturbing events, such as medical treatment and other potentially traumatic events, that demand both verbal and nonverbal interventions. Treatments such as the arts therapies and guided imagery, although they have different theoretical bases, integrate verbal and nonverbal elements. Both utilize recalled and restructured memories. The use of guided imagery in health settings is highly recommended as such a complementary therapy (Antall & Kresevic, 2004; Barnes, Powell-Griner, McFann, & Nahin, 2004).

Guided imagery has been shown to improve the postoperative course of adult and older adult surgical patients (Antall & Kresevic, 2004; Berger & Sarid, 2010; Fors,

Sexton, & Götestam, 2002). Guided imagery has been used successfully to significantly reduce children's pain associated with invasive procedures and improve selected medical conditions (Lambert, 1996). Guided imagery of an event such as an invasive, painful, and stressful medical procedure is often implemented as preparation for the event or afterward as a way of dealing with disturbing memories and physical symptoms (Antall & Kresevic, 2004; Lambert, 1996; Fors et al., 2002).

Art therapy is also used to relieve physical and emotional symptoms within health care settings. As a clinical intervention it is based on the belief that the creative process involved in the making of art is healing and life enhancing. The literature points to its use with patients or their families to cope with symptoms, and to adapt to stressful and traumatic experiences (Hughes & Mann da Silva, 2011; Nainis et al., 2006)

Our aim in this chapter is to examine these interventions comparatively, so as to learn more about the use of images in treating patients within health care settings and providing focused interventions to ease their symptoms.

ACUTE STRESS DISORDER

A diagnosis of ASD regards traumatized people within a time span of 2 to 4 weeks after the occurrence of the trauma (Bryant & Harvey, 1997). The symptoms of ASD include a combination of one or more dissociative and anxiety-related symptoms, and avoidance of reminders of the traumatic event. Examples of dissociative symptoms experienced in ASD are emotional detachment, temporary loss of memory, depersonalization, and derealization (Isserlin, Zerach, & Solomon, 2008).

Previous studies have regarded the period of ASD as especially significant for intervention in order to prevent long-term posttraumatic stress disorder (PTSD; for a review on the neurobiological aspects of stress, see Yehuda, McFarlane, & Shalev, 1998; Elzinga & Bremner, 2002). Between 63 and 80% of patients with ASD suffer PTSD 2 years posttrauma if not treated soon after the traumatic event (Bryant, Moulds, & Nixon, 2003; Harvey & Bryant, 1999, 2000). Thus, an early intervention in ASD may contribute to the overall prevention and treatment of future PTSD.

The scientific literature proposes a distinction between ordinary memories that have a clear structure, are easy to remember, and tend to be voluntary and conscious, and memories of traumatic experiences (Sotgiu & Moromont, 2008; Van der Kolk & Fisler 1995). A "traumatic memory" is as a special kind of memory that is experienced in the form of vivid fragments of images, sounds, smells, and bodily sensations (Ogden, Minton & Pain, 2006; Sotgiu & Mormont, 2008; Van der Kolk, Hopper, & Osterman, 2001; Whitfield, 1995). McCleery and Harvey (2004) suggest that the physiological overexcitation of the senses may initiate the repetition of traumatic memories that creates a continuous stress response (McNally, 2003, 2006; Peace & Porter, 2004). Thus, memory distortions caused by trauma can cause a loss of control and lack of coherent narrative relative to the traumatic event (McNally, 2003; 2006; Van der Kolk et al., 2001). This points to the need to address both physical stress and the specific memories that cause the stress. Indeed, several researchers have proposed that the detrimental effects of stress on the brain's memory systems can be reversed or blocked in the immediate aftermath of trauma, before memories become stabilized through a time-dependent process (Alberini, Milekic, & Tronel, 2006; Bremner, 2006).

Thus, the underlying principle in favor of the immediacy of intervention in the ASD period is the possibility of monitoring physiological responses and modulating traumatic memories, so that retrieved traumatic memories will be experienced less intensively and cause fewer symptoms.

ART THERAPY

Art therapy incorporates different levels of intervention in treating clients suffering from potentially traumatic experiences such as accidents, illnesses, and medical procedures (Hass-Cohen, 2003; Hass-Cohen & Carr, 2008; Klingman, Koenigsfield, & Markman, 1987; Mallay, 2002). It engages the senses through observing, touching, and manipulating art materials, while relating to the specific sensory characteristic of the materials chosen. The art therapy process and products become not only the symbolic manifestation of traumatic memories but also a hermeneutic zone for more positive reinterpretations of memories and perceptions of the traumatic events. Art therapy accesses and modulates traumatic memories through the personal symbolic meanings the client attributes to shapes, textures and colors. Client and therapist together, through elaboration, repetition, and reframing of the art product, create a more coherent narrative of the traumatic memories and meanings of symbols (Appleton, 2001; Hass-Cohen, 2008; Perry Pollard, Blakely, Baker, & Vigilante, 1995). Pifalo (2002) noted a significant reduction in trauma symptoms in sexually abused children after art therapy.

Art therapy however, is an emerging field, and while much practice-based anecdotal and theoretical research supports the relevance of art therapy for trauma and ASD intervention, and it is widely used in natural disaster and war trauma situations, (Chapman, Morabito, Ladakakos, Schreier, & Knudson, 2001; Talwar, 2007) there is little empirical research on art therapy in general as a pioneering field of therapy (Mollica et al., 2004).

GUIDED IMAGERY

Within guided imagery the individual is asked to recall and to imagine an image of an illness, accident, medical intervention, or other trauma, while being guided by techniques that include modifying shapes, colors, textures, and distancing images (Bryant & Harvey, 1997, 1998; Bryant, Sackville, Dang, Moulds, & Guthrie, 1999). Thus the client undergoes exposure to the potentially traumatic memories by working with images, in order to achieve emotional regulation.

Guided imagery integrates both physical and perceptual elements as it focuses on images of the traumatic memories, providing modulation and a restructuring of the negative image into a less intense and more integrated memory. The physical elements include relaxation through breathing exercises, autogenic training, and/or progressive muscle training. The aim is to modify psychophysiological reactions in the body and thus to reduce the excitatory effect of implicit traumatic memories (Davis, McKay, & Eshelman, 2000; Norris & Fahrion, 1993). Another component of guided imagery focuses on cognitive elements, such as learning rational self-talk to manage anxiety-producing situations and using cognitive restructuring techniques to reinterpret autobiographical traumatic memories (Hickling, Blanchard, & Kuhn, 2005; Meichenbaum, 1985).

CASE EXAMPLES

In this section we demonstrate the previously discussed interventions of art therapy and guided imagery in two case studies of trauma due to car accidents. The two cases are adapted from our extensive field work and supervision. (One of us [O. S.] teaches and supervises cognitive-behavioral intervention, while the other [E. H.] teaches and supervises art therapy.) We have the consent of the clients, and all identifying features of the cases have been changed.

Art Therapy Intervention

A 48-year-old woman was referred to a community medical clinic after a car accident. Her main complaints were sleep problems and overwhelming anxiety, accompanied by rapid heart palpitations. She described repeated, vivid visual memories of the motorbike driver she had injured in the accident. She recalled her two children standing and crying in the rain by the ruined car late at night. These visual memories were accompanied by a sense of deep guilt and fear. She repeatedly stated that she was a "bad person" who drove carelessly and exposed her children and the motorbiker to an accident situation. The intervention included four meetings that took place in the ASD period about 3 weeks after the accident.

In the first session, the art therapist heard the preceding description and encouraged the client to make a visual representation of any feelings or memories related to the accident. The client chose a large sheet of paper and drew a lump in the middle of the road, using intense back and forth movements with black oil pastel. After observing her picture, she added two additional shadowy figures and black paint drops to the whole picture. She explained, "The most disturbing image is the motorcyclist lying as if dead. This is the largest central lump. My two children are the shadowy figures, and the splashed water paint is their tears and the rain." The therapist reframed the flooding of stimuli experienced by the client by pointing out how organized the picture in fact was in terms of composition. The client agreed and continued her narrative. "Once we approached the motorcyclist he talked to us and said that his ankle hurt but that he was okay. I feel terrible that in addition to hurting the driver I exposed my children to such a traumatic experience." The therapist suggested drawing a strong contour line around the children to protect them. After making this change in the picture, the woman said, *"Actually, the children were okay; they hugged each other and consoled the motorcyclist."*

In the next session, the client stated that her concern was with her intense guilt over being the reason for the accident. "I'm a 'speedy' person. I don't slow down. I keep thinking that this was the reason for the accident." The therapist asked her to draw this sensation, and she rapidly drew a green spiral utilizing felt-tip pens that move quickly over the page. The therapist remarked that even when she was "speedy" she was in fact in control and kept the spiral's dimensions equal and within the page limit. The woman nodded in surprise, saying, "I never thought about it. It is true. In fact, I called for help so quickly because I am so 'speedy' so it also helped."

The therapist suggested that she add an image to contain the green spiral, and the client drew a purple box around the spiral. In the following sessions the purple box with its green spiral became a concrete container for additional art symbols of memories from the accident.

We see in this art therapy case study, that first, the physical agitation of the client was modulated through the manipulation of different art materials and their different sensations. Second, the experience of chaos expressed in the narrative was given control through its organization and symbolization on the page. Third, the art product gained new meanings as verbalized by the therapist and the client, who together modified or corrected disturbing memories. For example, the children were protected by drawing "coats." Fourth, the problem (e.g., being "speedy"), was symbolized, then integrated into an enabling narrative.

We see that physical art making, symbolization, and interpretation were utilized simultaneously or separately to reintegrate the sensory and emotional, as well as cognitive, levels of reaction to trauma (Hass-Cohen, 2008; Talwar, 2007). This enabled the client to rearrange both the sensory and the cognitive overexcitation of the traumatic memories, and to gain distance by placing them on the page, thus re-creating a coherent narrative and sense of control (Hass-Cohen, 2008; Kozlowska & Hanney, 2001; Rankin & Taucher, 2003).

Guided Imagery

An 18-year-old girl was referred to a community medical clinic after a car accident. She was injured in the accident and had undergone surgery in which her spleen was removed; one leg was in a cast due to shin bone fractures. The intervention included four sessions within the ASD period about 3 weeks after the accident. Her main complaint and reason for referral was a feeling of agitation, distress, and recurrent vivid images of the accident itself.

The therapist asked the girl to prioritize the most acutely disturbing memories. She stated, "I am floating in the air and viewing myself from above. It is very scary to see yourself from above. I feel I can't breath and my heart pounds when I remember this." The therapist taught her deep and slow breathing techniques and autogenic training (Norris & Fahrion, 1993). The relaxation was practiced throughout the whole intervention at the beginning of each session. The therapist then suggested that the girl make the first memory-image more comfortable, by moving physically closer to and embracing her wounded self on the road, rather than looking on from above. The client closed her eyes and described herself in this position, verbally comforting her wounded self. She was asked to repeat this image several times in order to construct a new, comforting memory. When asked by the therapist how she felt, the client stated that she felt consoled for now.

The client's next disturbing memory was being afraid of burning (the accident occurred in the desert on a summer afternoon). She kept repeating "I could have been burned." The therapist reminded her that in reality she didn't acquire any burns, and they adjusted the image with elements of coolness and comfort: The client imagined herself on the road in a lukewarm bath in which the water is very gentle and protective. On being prompted by the therapist as to what she would tell herself to deepen her sense of comfort she replied, "Everything is all right, I am comfortable, I am clean, and everything is taken care of."

In the next image, the client recalled the transition from the silence of being alone with the driver to the screams of the people around, the ambulances siren, and her uncle shouting, "I killed Lili!" The client identified her uncle screaming that she was dead as the most disturbing part of this image. The therapist and the client adjusted this memory by modifying the screams on the auditory level, and also by submerging the client's ears in the bath water of the previous image, to muffle the screams. She also added self-talk such as "The sounds are becoming quiet and distant."

The final disturbing image was a visual image of her injuries: "I remember myself on the road, my stomach was bleeding and my leg was in a very strange angle. I don't want to have this memory anymore." The therapist suggested restructuring this memory image by imagining a short movie of the process of being healed, with all her organs in their proper place, and the scars mending, renewing and regenerating. In the last two meetings, all of these techniques were further practiced, until the client reported control of these techniques and the ability to self-modify her disturbing memories and thoughts. A follow-up after half a year indicated that she was asymptomatic.

We see that this case study includes physical muscle relaxation and the adjustment of visual, tactile, and auditory images of the traumatic event. This involved a modification of all the senses within the recalled images. By describing sensations of movements, warmth, textures, specific colors, shades, smells and auditory elements, the therapist helped the client to change the traumatic memories. This was paired with comforting and positive "self-talk" to intensify the cognitive reframing of the painful memories. The restructuring of these trauma-related images and the new "self-talk" regarding the event altered the client's autobiographical memories.

In summary, the case study reiterates data in the literature review, showing how guided imagery integrates both sensory and perceptual elements as it focuses on the traumatic memories and psychophysiological responses of the client. The behavioral interventions relax the physical excitation, while the imaginable exposure modulates and restructures negative images.

DISCUSSION

Comparing art therapy and guided imagery in relation to ASD highlights the operative commonalities of two seemingly different theoretical and clinical methods commonly used in health care settings. From a theoretical perspective, both therapies intervene on the psychophysiological level of excitation. Art therapy starts from actual sensory experiences based on the visual and tactile characteristics of art materials that enable physical expression of body muscles and postures, and the involvement of the senses in the here and now. Guided imagery also focuses on modifying excitatory reactions by shifting excessive arousal to regulatory processes, through shifting images.

Both therapies relate to perceptual processes. For example, the art therapy intervention organized the traumatic experience on the cognitive level through symbolization. The client reported repeated flashbacks of the injured motorcyclist lying on the road in the rain, and how this image flooded her with guilt and distress. This image was drawn in a symbolic way, then reframed by noticing that the injured shape was organized and the injury was in fact very moderate. The client treated with guided imagery saw herself from above, looking down at her wounded self, which aroused agitation. She modified these disturbing memories by a deliberate mental process that involved visually adjusting the image by shifting the relative size, composition, and content of the image. Most important, and common to both interventions, are the constant and recurring shifts from physical overexcitation to physical relaxation, and from disturbing perceptions to modified, enabling perceptions (Tronel, Mikelic, & Alberini, 2005; Whitfield, 1995).

Thus, both art therapy and guided imagery modulate recalled images and challenge explicit traumatic memories and negative "self-talk" by stimulation of subsequent cognitive processing of existing images and symbols. From a biological perspective, this process enables the modification of implicit and explicit memories by initiating an inhibitory process (Cohen et al., 2006; Radley, Williams, & Sawchenko, 2009).

The differences between these two interventions, as can be seen in the case examples, are that the cognitive component of guided imagery does not create a concrete product from the image. The therapist helps to modulate disturbing memories as soon as the client describes them. Metaphorically, the client redraws her image, but in her mind rather than on a page. Art therapy on the other hand, externalizes the image into a concrete art product that is then physically adjusted and symbolized, as a result of a subsequent cognitive process. In art therapy the image modulation involves distinct stages of drawing, observing, and adjusting the art product or understanding of the art. Both of these interventions can be technically employed with relative ease in health care settings, although guided imagery may be easier to implement when patients are physically debilitated.

CONCLUSION

This chapter has shown how in health care settings art therapy and guided imagery work with images of accidents. We have pointed to the potential of creating new connections and pathways among the physical, emotional, and cognitive components of traumatic memory that is common to both art therapy and guided imagery. This is very important for professionals in health care settings, as these connections regulate and integrate the very components that become deregulated following the traumatic experience.

REFERENCES

Alberini, C. M., Milekic, M. H., & Tronel, S. (2006). Mechanisms of memory stabilization and de-stabilization. *Cellular and Molecular Life Sciences, 63*(9), 999–1008.

Antall, G. F., & Kresevic, D. (2004). The use of guided imagery to manage pain in an elderly orthopaedic population. *Orthopaedic Nursing, 23*(5), 335–340.

American Psychiatric Association. (2000). *Diagnostic and statistical manual of mental disorders* (4th ed., text rev.). Washington, DC: Author.

Appleton, V. (2001). Avenues of hope: Art therapy and the resolution of trauma. *Art Therapy, 18*(1), 6–13.

Barnes, M. P., Powell-Griner, E., McFann, K., & Nahin, R. L. (2004). Complementary and alternative medicine use among adults: United States. *Seminars in Integrative Medicine, 2*(2), 54–71.

Berger, R., & Sarid, O. (2010). Introducing the use of brief cognitive-behavioral intervention for treating acute episodes of migraine in emergency room. *Internet Journal of Allied Health Sciences and Practice, 8*(3), 1–5.

Bremner, J. D. (2006). Stress and brain atrophy. *CNS and Neurological Disorders—Drug Targets, 5*(5), 503–512.

Bryant, R. A., & Harvey, A. G. (1997). Acute stress disorder: A critical review of diagnostic issues. *Clinical Psychology Review, 17,* 757–773.

Bryant, R. A., & Harvey, A. G. (1998). Relationship of acute stress disorder and posttraumatic stress disorder following mild traumatic brain injury. *American Journal of Psychiatry, 155,* 625–629.

Bryant, R. A., Moulds, M. L., & Nixon, R. V. (2003). Cognitive behavior therapy of acute stress disorder: A four-year follow-up. *Behaviour Research and Therapy, 41*(4), 489–494.

Bryant, R. A., Sackville, T., Dang, S. T., Moulds, M., & Guthrie, R. (1999). Treating acute stress disorder: An evaluation of cognitive behavior therapy and supportive counseling techniques. *American Journal of Psychiatry, 156,* 1780–1786.

Chapman, L. M., Morabito, D., Ladakakos, C., Schreier, H., & Knudson, M. (2001). The effectiveness of art therapy interventions in reducing post traumatic stress disorder (PTSD) symptoms in pediatric trauma patients. *Art Therapy, 18*(2), 100–104.

Cohen, H., Zohar, J., Gidron, Y., Matar, M. A., Belkind, D., Loewenthal, U., et al. (2006). Blunted HPA axis response to stress influences susceptibility to posttraumatic stress response in rats. *Biological Psychiatry, 59*(12), 1208–1218.

Davis, M., McKay, M., & Eshelman, R. E. (2000). *The relaxation and stress reduction workbook.* Oakland, CA: New Harbinger.

Elzinga, B. M., & Bremner, J. D. (2002). Are the neural substrates of memory the final common pathway in posttraumatic stress disorder? *Journal of Affective Disorders, 70*(1), 1–17.

Fors, E. A., Sexton, H., & Götestam, K. G. (2002). The effect of guided imagery and amitriptyline on daily fibromyalgia pain: A prospective, randomized, controlled trial. *Journal of Psychiatric Research, 36*(3), 179–187.

Harvey, A. G., & Bryant, R. A. (1998). Relationship of acute stress disorder and posttraumatic stress disorder following motor vehicle accidents. *Journal of Consulting and Clinical Psychology, 66,* 507–512.

Harvey, A. G., & Bryant, R. A. (1999). The relationship between acute stress disorder and post-traumatic stress disorder: A two-year prospective evaluation. *Journal of Consulting and Clinical Psychology, 67,* 985–988.

Harvey, A. G., & Bryant, R. A. (2000). Two-year prospective evaluation of the relationship between acute stress disorder and posttraumatic stress disorder following mild traumatic brain injury. *American Journal of Psychiatry, 157,* 626–628.

Hass-Cohen, N. (2003). Art therapy mind body approaches. *Progress: Family Systems Research and Therapy, 12,* 24–38.

Hass-Cohen, N., & Carr, R. (2008). *Art therapy and clinical neuroscience.* London: Jessica Kingsley.

Hickling, E. J., Blanchard, E. B., & Kuhn, E. (2005). Brief, early treatment for ASD/PTSD following motor vehicle accidents. *Cognitive and Behavioral Practice, 12*(4), 461–467.

Hughes, E. G., & Mann da Silva, A. (2011). A pilot study assessing art therapy as a mental health intervention for subfertile women. *Human Reproduction, 26*(3), 611–615.

Isserlin, L., Zerach, G., & Solomon, Z. (2008). Acute stress responses: A review and synthesis of ASD, ASR, and CSR. *American Journal of Orthopsychiatry, 78*(4), 423–429.

Klingman, A., Koenigsfield, E., & Markman, D. (1987). Art activity with children following disaster: A preventative-oriented crisis intervention modality. *The Arts in Psychotherapy, 14,* 153–166.

Kozlowska, K., & Hanney, L. (2001). An art therapy group for children traumatized by parental violence and separation. *Clinical Child Psychology and Psychiatry, 6*(1), 49–78.

Norris, P. A., & Fahrion, S. L. (1993). Autogenic biofeedback in psycho physiological therapy and stress managemmnet. In P. M. Lehrer & R. L. Woolfolk (Eds.), *Principles and practice of stress management.* New York: Guilford Press.

Lambert, S. A. (1996). The effects of hypnosis/guided imagery on the postoperative course of children. *Journal of Developmental and Behavioral Pediatrics, 17*(5), 307–310.

Mallay, J. N. (2002). Art therapy, an effective outreach intervention with traumatized children with suspected acquired brain injury, *The Arts in Psychotherapy, 29*(3), 159–172.

McCleery, J. M., & Harvey, A. G. (2004). Integration of psychological and biological approaches to trauma memory: Implications for pharmacological prevention of PTSD. *Journal of Traumatic Stress, 17*(6), 485–496.

McNally, R. J. (2003). *Remembering trauma.* Cambridge, MA: Harvard University Press.

McNally, R. J. (2006). Cognitive abnormalities in post-traumatic stress disorder. *Trends in Cognitive Sciences, 10*(6), 271–277.

Meichenbaum, D. (1985). *Stress inoculation training.* New York: Pergamon Press.

Mollica, R. F., Lopes Cardozo, B., Osofsky, H. J., Raphael, B., Ager, A., & Salama, P. (2004). Mental health in complex emergencies, *Lancet, 364*(9450), 2058–2067.

Nainis, N., Paice, J. A., Ratner, J., Wirth, J. H., Lai, J., & Shott, S. (2006). Relieving symptoms in cancer: Innovative use of art therapy. *Journal of Pain and Symptom Management, 31*(2), 162–169.

Norris, P. A., & Fahrion, S. L. (1993). Autogenic biofeedback in psychophysiological therapy and stress management. In P. M. Lehrer & R. L. Woolfolk (Eds.), *Principles and practice of stress management.* New York: Guilford Press.

Ogden, P., Minton, K., & Pain, C. (2006). *Trauma and the body: A sensorimotor approach to psychotherapy.* New York: Norton.

Perry, B., Pollard, R., Blakely, T., Baker, W., & Vigilante, D. (1995). Childhood trauma, the neurobiology of adaptation, and "use-dependent" development of the brain: How "states become traits." *Infant Mental Health Journal, 16*(4), 271–291.

Pifalo, T. (2002). Pulling out the thorns: Art therapy with sexually abused children and adolescents. *Art Therapy, 19,* 12–22.

Radley, J. J., Williams, B., & Sawchenko, P. E. (2009). Noradrenergic innervations of the dorsal medial prefrontal cortex modulates hypothalamo–pituitary–adrenal responses to acute emotional stress. *Journal of Neuroscience, 28*(22), 5806 –5816.

Rankin, A. B., & Taucher, L. C. (2003). A task-oriented approach to art therapy in trauma treatment. *Art Therapy, 20*(3), 138–147.

Sotgiu, I., & Mormont, C. (2008). Similarities and differences between traumatic and emotional memories: Review and directions for future research. *Journal of Psychology, 142*(5), 449–469.

Talwar, S. (2007). Accessing traumatic memory through art making: An art therapy trauma protocol (ATTP). *The Arts in Psychotherapy, 34*(1), 22–35.

Tronel, S., Milekic, M. H., & Alberini, C. M. (2005). Linking new information to a reactivated memory requires consolidation and not reconsolidation mechanisms. *PLoS Biology, 3*(9), e293.

Van der Kolk, B. A., & Fisler, R. (1995). Dissociation and the fragmentary nature of traumatic memories: Overview and exploratory study. *Journal of Traumatic Stress, 8,* 505–525.

Van der Kolk, B. A., Hopper, J., & Osterman, J. (2001). Exploring the nature of traumatic memories: Combining clinical knowledge with laboratory methods. *Journal of Aggression, Maltreatment, and Trauma, 4*(2), 9–31.

Whitfield, C. L. (1995). The forgotten difference: Ordinary memory versus traumatic memory. *Consciousness and Cognition, 4*(1), 88–94.

Yehuda, R., McFarlane, A. C., & Shalev, A. Y. (1998). Predicting the development of posttraumatic stress disorder from the acute response to a traumatic event. *Biological Psychiatry, 44*(12), 1305–1313.

CHAPTER 10

Expressive Arts and Breast Cancer
Restoring Femininity

Fiona Chang

Breast cancer has ranked as the number one cancer among women in Hong Kong since the early 1990s. It accounts for one-fifth of all new cancers in women (Centre for Health Protection, 2011). In 2008 there were 2,633 new cases of female breast cancer (Hong Kong Cancer Registry, 2010). According to the Hospital Authority (2011), the number of inpatient episodes of breast cancer was 17,278 in the year 2010. There is a significant demand for psychosocial support for women with breast cancer.

There are several organizations providing holistic care, cancer education, and self-empowerment. The Cancer Patient Resources Centres in hospitals, CancerLink Support Centres in communities, Hong Kong Breast Cancer Foundation, and other self-help organizations all provide arts-related services. These include Chinese painting, calligraphy classes, arts-and-crafts classes, and art therapy groups and workshops on "Use of Arts for Recovery."

Breast cancer treatment may not only removes a body part but it may also take away self-confidence, feminine identity, sexuality, and faith in life. Women experience complicated emotions and seek ways to transform fear, despair, anger, and bewilderment into positive healing energy. They need a safe platform to talk about the taboo of sexuality and loss of feminine attractiveness. All these issues and more are heard through the voices of women with breast cancer and revealed through the creative process.

Drawing, images, and visualization can be powerful tools to help deal with important issues in our lives (Siegel, 1990). Expressive arts are considered safe alternatives to authentic expression for connecting our inner and outer reality, and our body, mind, and spirit (Rogers, 1993). This chapter begins with the courageous journey of Chung to demonstrate the needs of a woman coping with breast cancer and how arts healed her body–mind–spirit. It also presents the examples of women's strength and recovery of femininity through expressive arts therapy groups. Through empathetic witnessing and loving companionship, therapists can facilitate a unique experience for women with breast cancer and apply arts for their well-being.

WHEN CHUNG MET BREAST CANCER

Chung was diagnosed with breast cancer in 1995, at the age of 47. She was distressed by the loss of her breast and the axillary lymph nodes. She was single and longed for a family, and she felt she was not a "real" woman with only one breast. While still struggling with her body image, she also had to go through radiotherapy and chemotherapy. It never occurred to her that she would have the full course of treatment. On the surface, she seemed calm, because she was a "happy peanut" (happy person) in the eyes of her friends. Deep down she was frustrated and depressed. Like many cancer patients, she found it hard to express her bodily experiences in words (Oster, Magnusson, Thyme, Lindh, & Astrom, 2007).

Physically Chung suffered from pain around the wound and the side effects of treatment. She had pain and dryness in her vagina, and she lost her sexual desire. From her body portrait, we can better understand both the changes in her body and how the physical illness impacted her psychological well-being. She painted one arm in black to symbolize the lymphedema (swelling of her arm); her red fragile heart was surrounded by dark dots representing her worry about relapse, suffering, and death. It was entangled with grief, anger and intense fear common in breast cancer patients (Schover, 1991). These emotions affected her daily life and weakened her immune system. Chung could not sleep well at night. She also tried to hide the fact that she was a breast cancer patient and felt embarrassed when people stared at her breast. She was puzzled by the way God arranged these misfortunes for her, but at the same time she felt guilty thinking this way.

Chung's "happy face" did not take away her pain and anxiety. She could feel the deep resentment and shame inside. She rarely verbalized her feelings and thoughts. When the emotions were running high, she tried to suppress her feelings. She realized the need for an alternative and cathartic language to ventilate. When she lost her temper with the medical staff in the clinic, her oncologist advised her to seek professional help. However, because she found the verbal therapy unhelpful, she turned to art workshops and expressive arts groups.

I met Chung at an open art studio. She did not have any prior art experience, but she was open-minded to receive help. Although she had difficulty raising the affected arm, she insisted on coming to the studio because she enjoyed the freedom of playing with the art materials. Her first work was a piece of A3-size paper covered totally and thickly by black oil pastel; Chung expressed her anger by rubbing the pastel with all her might onto the paper. At the end she used up three regular black pastel sticks. There were still tiny white spots on the paper. She understood that it was impossible to cover all the emotions. She learned to accept the shadow parts in life.

In the creative exploratory expression, Chung's body and mind were relieved as she let go of the resentment in each moment of making art. She felt a "lighter" sense of self and a refreshed spirit. She described feeling like a shrinking balloon with more room for creativity after the well-hidden anger came out of her tummy. She began to pursue art for healing in her daily life. Chung's overall experience demonstrated the effects of the arts in improving quality of life, increasing self-understanding, enhancing feelings of health, and reducing anxiety and depression (Chang, 2011; Chang & Ho, 2000; Malchiodi, 1999; Oster et al., 2007).

Chung finally completed all the treatment and moved toward recovery. To celebrate the new lives of those with chronic illness, we organized an art exhibition called "Tears, Smiles, and Creation," with 50 pieces of precious artwork by participants. Art is a public platform between the artists and the visitors, and participants shared illness and life and death through their art. The viewers who attended the exhibition wrote down their own aesthetic responses to each piece of work as an exchange. Having taken part in organizing the exhibition, the creators/patients felt empowered. They even received donations for more arts programs. They had strong support from the community.

The cancer journey of Chung was not a smooth ride at all. She was saddened and felt helpless when her peers had relapses of cancer. Yet she, too, had a relapse in 2009. She began to have turbulent thoughts and emotions all over again. Because emotion is the source of creativity (Rogers, 1993), Chung came back to the expressive arts group again. She put black tempera paints on her palm and hit them strongly on paper. Each palm print was her statement of disappointment. After this cathartic expression, she gently added lively yellow and orange colors to the black prints to transform the negative feelings into positive healing energy for herself. During a music improvisation, she had fun listening to the tiny sounds made by popping bubble wrap and imagined her obsessive thoughts vanishing with each burst bubble. Chung found her true voice through singing, and she used dance to understand mind and body. She also made a magazine collage of different images of women's faces to explore different roles and identities. This was a gift to herself as a real woman, with many strengths and resources from within.

Sadly, Chung's cancer progressed, and she passed away in 2010. Before she died, I visited her once every 2 weeks. Her last drawing was made when she was unable to speak. She used her fragile hand to draw a heart slowly on my palm. I held it tightly, with tears and deep gratitude. I suggested bringing her more material next time so that she could transfer the heart into a visual image. Two weeks later, she was very much weaker and her breath was short. She would still try to draw a heart. No one could "see" it but I clearly saw it in my heart.

EXPRESSIVE ARTS PRACTICE

Chung's story illustrates how the arts can be used therapeutically to help women with breast cancer during diagnosis, treatment, rehabilitation and palliative stages. It demonstrates the effects of arts on soul-soothing, self-healing, and personal transformation. Chung embraced peace in the sacred space of the arts up to the end. She wanted me to disseminate these experiences to the world. I kept my promise and shared our experience here.

The story of Chung inspired me to include femininity by forming an expressive arts group called "Unlock your Knots and Unleash your Feminine Side," designed for women with breast cancer. It included both hospital and community venues. Some participants preferred to stay away from the hospital to enhance a true sense of recovery and being closer to normal life. Others trusted a group organized by the hospital. Although the group did not have a proper art studio, we used our creativity to make a comfortable group environment. This set a good example of how to make "something out of nothing."

The integrated use of the multimodal expressive arts process, the belief in self-actualization, and the empathetic and nonjudgmental environment of a person-centered expressive arts approach shaped the group plan (Rogers, 2011). A person-centered expressive arts therapist believes that everyone has the innate ability to create, and that the creative process is healing. The role of the therapist is to co-create with the group members a safe and supportive environment. Participants can use the arts freely for self-expression, self-awareness, and personal transformation. They are encouraged to support and learn from each other.

Objectives

The arts have helped women with breast cancer to understand their losses, bodily changes, and relationships affecting their identities (Halprin, 2002; Malchiodi, 1997). Therefore, the group's objectives for participants were as follows:

1. To understand the impact of breast cancer through the arts in a safe and supportive group environment.
2. To enhance self-awareness of the inner strength and the beauty of femininity in the Creative Connection® process.[1]
3. To actualize hidden creativity and self-healing capacity.
4. To promote mutual support, respect, and appreciation among the participants.

Group Structure

The group met once a week for 6 weeks. Each session lasted 2½ hours, and participants were encouraged to attend all the sessions. Each group recruited 10 women. To give them a sense of safety and to understand the group flow, a clear structure, developed for each session, included the following:

1. Welcome and Warm-up
2. Core Arts Activities
3. Exploration and Witnessing
4. Sharing and Feedback
5. Closing Ritual

---

[1] The process of Creative Connection through integrative creative art modalities addresses the body, mind, emotion, and spirit (Chang, 2012; Rogers, 1993, 2011).

Session Plans

Weekly session themes and experiences are summarized in Table 10.1.

Preparation

To build rapport, we met each participant in person or by phone 2 weeks before the beginning of the group. A brief interview was conducted, including the following areas:

1. Introduce the group content and schedule.
2. Understand each participant's arts background.
3. Identify any special needs.
4. Note whether a participant is currently in psychotherapy.
5. Offer recommendations for comfortable and suitable clothing for participation.
6. Encourage participants to bring a journal and a camera to record their work.
7. Explain confidentiality, including consent needed to record, film, or photograph others' creative work during the group.

Unfolding the Group Process

This section describes the activities and participants' responses to creative work; pseudonyms are used to protect the identity and confidentiality of participants.

Session 1: "My Hands"

As a welcome ritual, each participant drew her intentions on a white paper cup. Yi drew a happy face to symbolize her search for happiness. Mei Ling drew a beach "for

TABLE 10.1. Group Session Plan

Session	Theme	Art modality
1	"My Hands"	• Exploration of hands • Hands drawing
2	"Femininity, Sexuality, and Beauty"	• Guided imagery exploration • Body awareness exercise • Body portrait painting
3	"Who Am I?"	• Authentic movement • Writing
4	"My Home and Relationships"	• Miniatures • Three-dimensional (3-D) creation
5	"My Dream Sculpture"	• Clay sculpturing • Museum pose
6	"Our Gift for the Future"	• Reflective writing/storytelling • Closing ritual

a comfortable life." Some drew trees and flowers to show the vitality of nature. We put jasmine green tea in the cups and engaged in a tea meditation. We slowed down our breathing, concentrated on the steam, the aroma and warmth. When we were enjoying each sip mindfully, we connected our inner experience with the image of our intention.

To introduce the group content and ground rules in a stimulating way, we used different pictures to depict respect for emotions (tears), nonjudgmental attitude, confidentiality, mutual respect, and empathetic listening. I prepared a script (see Table 10.2) to facilitate participants' exploration of their hands. It was about understanding ourselves by reading the stories invisibly printed on our hands. The script is supposed to be only an outline; any facilitator has to be fully present to each woman's unique gestures, facial expression, and emotional responses.

Mei Ling used different colors to represent different stages of her hands (Figure 10.1). The green hand on the left was her hand when she was a child.[2] It was full of fun and happiness. The blue hand was the swollen hand after surgery; she wished to keep it healthy inside the "safe box." The group members empathetically listened and visualized how restricted the hand was inside the small box. They encouraged her to take it out of the box and be free.

This session ended up with a simple breathing and giving ritual. We stood in a circle and put all our hands in the center. We looked at our hands. We expressed our gratitude to each other and to our hands. When we exhaled, we imagined our burdens leaving our hands. When we inhaled, we imagined receiving support from the group and giving our love to each other.

TABLE 10.2. Script for the Guided Exploration of Hands

Be curious about your hands, explore them without any judgment.

Just being with them, breathing in . . . breathing out . . .

Quietly look at your hands deeply with your breathing . . .

Follow your tempo . . . tenderly . . . bring your awareness to the hands . . .

Try to make friend with them . . . feel and touch them . . .

Give full attention to each small part of the hands . . . the wrinkle lines, the texture, the colors, any special marks, special memories . . .

Listen to your sensations about each spot . . .

How do they feel? What is their thought?

Let your hands speak to you . . . try to listen to them at this present moment . . .

You may know more about it gradually and follow your pace without a hurry . . .

You are invited to take a few minutes for free and spontaneous exploration . . .

If you want to stay a little bit longer, we certainly respect your need.

If you are ready, you can start the hands creation or write about this process.

---

[2] The original artwork for this chapter was in color. It is reproduced here in black and white.

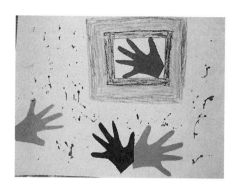

FIGURE 10.1. "Reaching Out of the Box!" Copyright 2012 by Fiona Chang.

Session 2: "Woman, Sexuality, and Beauty"

This session started with making a body from Sculptina (a form of clay) to introduce ourselves. I then facilitated a short body exploration as a warm-up for the body portrait drawing (see Table 10.3).

Most enjoyed the joy and freedom of the movement with their eyes closed. It was full of feminine beauty, the tender touch of the body and expression of sexual energy. Some were embarrassed at the beginning and held a scarf for confidence. But eventually each woman experienced the process of liberation and felt good about her body. The women were invited to transfer the movement experience into a life-sized portrait. Siu Fung drew her deformed body (see Figure 10.2); she was shy to show her "ugly and deformed body." But her body spoke to her, saying "Never give up!" She felt her inner strength and realized the importance of accepting her body and being who she was; she added a sun to her portrait to symbolize hope.

Yee created a blue and green running figure (Figure 10.3). Her head was filled with worries. She felt empty, having lost her breast. She drew a feminine body to show the beauty of being a woman and added in strokes of motions and hair blowing in the wind to make it even more lively. The creative process was a delight to her, because she strived for freedom and experienced it through art making.

Each portrait was unique. It reminded us of our own physiological, psychological, social, and spiritual aspects. The ending ritual was to say thanks to the portrait and tell what we have learned from it in one sentence.

Session 3: "Who Am I?"

For deeper exploration we hung our portraits on the wall and used authentic movement (an expressive, improvisational movement practice) to give them life. The room suddenly turned into an art-based dance studio. Getting our body–mind–spirit ready, we did arm movement to prevent lymphedema in a symbolic way. We imagined our shoulders, our elbows, and our arms as paintbrushes to draw imaginary circles of different sizes and colors. I played a song called "The Dreaming" to express our Yang-masculine energy.

TABLE 10.3. Script for Guided Body Exploration: "Our Femininity"

Move around this room . . . slow down your movement and breathing . . .

Find a comfortable space in your own dancing hall . . .

Relax your body and listen to the rhythm of your body . . .

Gently move your body in response to your own rhythm . . .

Close your eyes . . . follow your pace . . .

Listen to your beat and move in your own way . . .

Just follow your body to move . . . follow your senses to express . . .

There is no right or wrong . . . just experience and stay open . . .

Allow your body to lead your movement . . .

Dance freely . . . be mindful of your moving . . .

Be curious on your body, listen to it . . .

Feel it and explore it without any judgment . . .

Just be with your body . . . move freely to express your female energy . . .

Feel the feminine force inside you . . . your woman power . . .

Be aware of the feelings inside your body . . .

Dance spontaneously in response to your feelings . . . resonance to your body . . .

Express your true beauty . . . your unique exotic energy . . .

Explore and feel your sexual resources . . .

Just be open . . . grasp this precious opportunity to discover your sexual body parts . . .

Be curious about them . . . be friendly with them . . . let them be liberating . . .

Pay attention to your sensations . . . follow your pace without a hurry . . .

Prepare to close your movement with an ending pose . . .

When you are ready, gradually bring your attention back to this room.

You are invited to do some writing or start the portrait painting.

This was followed by "The Thread" to connect with our Yin-feminine energy. Several dyads that formed to start the movement-based exploration took turns being the mover and the witness. The movers talked about their art first, followed by movement to express how the portrait would dance. The witnesses provided a supportive and safe space for the mover to dance freely and remained fully present to the moving process without judgment. After each dance, the mover shared first and the witness followed. The witnesses could share what they saw, how they felt, and how they experienced the process.

The engagement in an external activity provides a "distancing" that can help us gain a new perspective that may help to resolve the struggle (Liebmann, 1996). In some cases, I suggested that participants experienced their creative work from a different orientation. For example, the portrait by Yuen Kwan was in a vertical, resting posture. She turned it by 90° (Figure 10.4) and realized that the portrait became an exhausted person who was trying to stand up. The figure could not even raise her head and was in an inferior position. Yuen observed that she could do much better than this and should open up more to others.

Art making, along with dialogue, is a helpful way to explore the motivations and needs underlying struggles (Kaplan, 2007). I always invited the participants to write

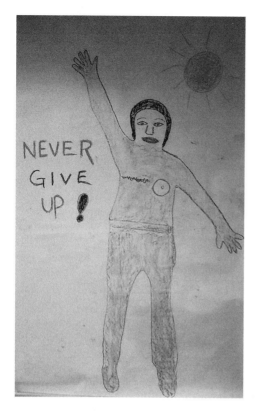

FIGURE 10.2. "Never Give Up!" Copyright 2012 by Fiona Chang.

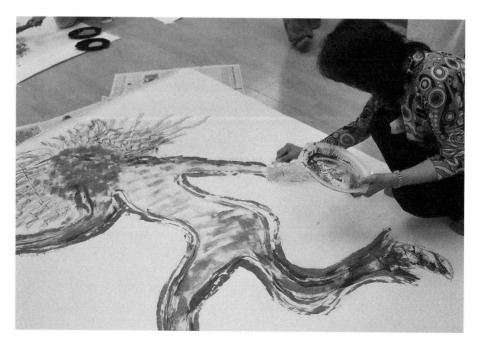

FIGURE 10.3. "From Emptiness to Energizing Body." Copyright 2012 by Fiona Chang.

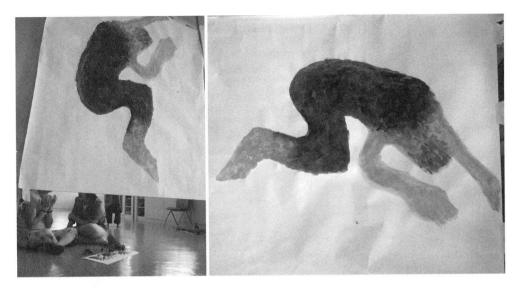

FIGURE 10.4. "Lying Down and Reaching Out." Copyright 2012 by Fiona Chang.

about their dialogue with the art and movement. In my invitation I asked each woman to describe her art, to let it speak to her, and to listen to the wisdom from within. Yuen Kwan rarely expressed herself in words. She was amazed at how the magic of arts helped her to organize her thoughts and articulate her suppressed feelings. The ending ritual for this session was for each woman to create a body from Sculptina to state her needs.

Session 4: "My Home and Relationships"

Breast cancer strains relationships. It is helpful to understand how it affects the family relationship and to explore how to improve it. In the fourth session, we began with an ice-breaking encounter involving nonverbal clues and mindful listening to the sounds around us and in various environments. The members enjoyed discovering the "new" sounds in the room, in the hospital, in their homes, then back to the room, as well as sounds inside their bodies. They then used miniatures and art materials to explore their close relationships and to create images of "home."

In the process of creating, arranging, and fixing, Carmen selected an orange bear to represent her. She was carrying a dinosaur; a lizard and a cat piggyback style (Figure 10.5). She visualized that she was carrying so much of the burden of her sons and husband. There was an old Chinese saying, "The tortoise is good at nurturing energy, so it can survive a century without food" (Dreher, 2000, p. 42). From her artwork, Carmen visualized her family interaction and learned that a quality connection with all needs met is created through compassionate giving and receiving (Rosenberg, 2000). Therefore, she transformed her work and learned to be a relaxed bear, and let her family share her duties. She then could finally enjoy more relaxation with her family to restore her own energy. She affirmed her need to respect, love and nurture herself.

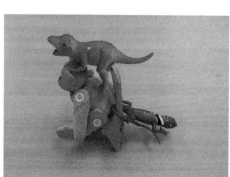
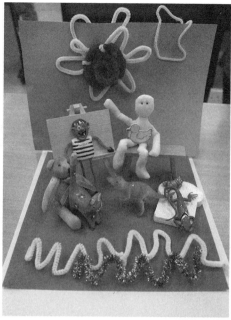

FIGURE 10.5. "Burdens on the Shoulder." Copyright 2012 by Fiona Chang.

We visited each "home" and explored changes for the better in the family relationship. The women in the group discovered new abilities to take action, to make their situation clearer for themselves and establish a comfortable boundary for their own space in the creative healing process (Oster et al., 2007). Once participants were able to clarify conflicts in family relationships, they could begin see new possibilities and share solutions (Dreher, 2000). The closure for this session included a dyadic ritual to share love and support with each other.

The depth of sharing in any group of this nature depends on the concerns, the ability to be open, and the readiness of the group. Sometimes they felt shy and, at times, ashamed to share the difficulties in their sexual relationships. Sex and intimacy are still taboo. It was easier to use metaphoric language to symbolize their distant relationships with their partners. The artwork often subtly shared the negative feelings caused by body mutilation and the adjustment in the marital relationship. The therapist's sensitivity and openness played an important part in nurturing a safe and accepting atmosphere.

Session 5: "My Dream Sculpture"

In this session, participants were invited to use ceramic clay to sculpt a pose representing "my ideal self." Group members used their senses to connect with the clay by beating, squeezing, modeling, and putting their feelings into the clay. Then they resculpted and transformed the clay into their ideal selves; many different expressions resulted from this process. Yuen Kwan made a sculpture of rowing a boat with her husband. Oi Lee created four smiling faces of her family. Carmen weaved a delicate basket to collect her strength and beauty. Yuk Ling crafted a meditating self to remind herself to have a mindful heart and peaceful mind (Figure 10.6). They also wrote poems to express the content of their art expressions.

Siu Fung created a dancing girl to embrace hope. She wrote the following poem about her sculpture:

Never give up!
Never give up! Never give up!
I hear the cheers in my mind.
I am tired. I am tired.
I hear the voices in my body.
I can do it. I can do it.
I hear the clapping within my heart.
Never give up! Never give up!
I realize the need to rest.
I see a green light of hope.
I feel the love from others.
I sense the power of autonomy.
I know I will stay alive.
I know I will live even better.

The group members took turns sharing their poems. At the end of the session, they paired up and with their hands sent healing energy to their partner. It was a miraclous moment of giving and receiving.

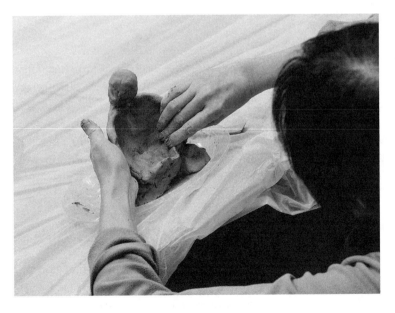

FIGURE 10.6. "Meditating Self." Copyright 2012 by Fiona Chang.

Session 6: "Our Gift for the Future"

Telling one's story can be a tool for making sense of life (Mathieson & Stam, 1995). In the final session, members were invited to display their artwork and revisit their creative journey. Some wrote stories; others used dance and song to share their gain from the group. Combining arts and group process provides a creative and supportive group environment for sharing common concerns (Rogers, 2011). The women observed that art could more easily facilitate self-expression and communication than words alone. Art is a natural form of communication for women with breast cancer that offers an alternative way to express feelings and thoughts in a manner that is less threatening than strictly verbal means (Malchiodi, 2006). In using art, verbalization is often not necessary. Individuals can communicate creatively and naturally through movement, colors, images, singing, sounds, and journal writing. The integrated use of the arts can make use of women's senses as they become aware of themselves and their inner healing resources in a holistic way.

Art therapy has been found to be helpful in reducing cancer symptoms such as pain, fatigue, fear, and anxiety (Nainis et al., 2006). This was true for Po Lin. She found it hard to express herself, was always under stress, and was bound by rules and social values. Before participating in group activity, she hid all her emotions and suffered from insomnia. Through the arts, like others who are struggling with illness, she could accept her pain and suffering (Levine & Levine, 2000). She learned to handle her negative feelings and understand her challenge from different perspectives. Now she could go to sleep quickly and with a calm mind. The entire group was touched while witnessing her changes. We ended the session in a circle holding hands and felt the healing energy and love circulating among us.

What Was Learned

The previous section illustrates a kind of art-based observation that reveals the effect of the arts in helping women with breast cancer. Apart from qualitative understanding of the expressive arts process, we also looked for empirical data. From the pre–post self-rating scores of the group members (see Table 10.4), we discovered that arts were effective in relaxing their bodies (94.4%), staying open (83.3%), increasing creativity (83.3%), and facilitating family communication (83.3%). More than three-quarters of the group improved in self-image and positive thinking.

DISCUSSION

As a therapist, I constantly learn from my "clients." I hesitate to name my group "clients," because they were wonderful creators, artists, and teachers. When I start with a new group of women, I first perform a comprehensive needs assessment. I look on the Internet for images created by others who underwent similar medical challenges. It is a kind

TABLE 10.4. Pre–Post Self-Rating Scores of the Group Members

Personal growth	Pre–post difference of the group members			
	Negative difference (regression)	Positive difference (progress)	No difference (no change)	p value
Self-understanding	1 (5.6%)	11 (61.1%)	6 (33.3%)	.006
Expression of feelings	0 (0%)	13 (72.2%)	5 (27.8%)	.000
Communication with others	2 (11.1%)	11 (61.1%)	5 (27.8%)	.022
Creativity	3 (16.7%)	15 (83.3%)	0 (0%)	.008
Openness	0 (0%)	15 (83.3%)	3 (16.7%)	.000
Trust others	1 (5.6%)	13 (72.2%)	4 (22.2%)	.002
Self-image	0 (0%)	14 (77.8%)	4 (22.2%)	.000
Ventilation of emotion	1 (5.6%)	13 (72.2%)	4 (22.2%)	.002
Self-confidence	0 (0%)	12 (66.7%)	6 (33.3%)	.000
Relaxation of body	0 (0%)	17 (94.4%)	1 (5.6%)	.000
Family communication	1 (5.6%)	15 (83.3%)	2 (11.1%)	.001
Positive thinking	2 (11.1%)	14 (77.8%)	2 (11.1%)	.004

of art-based needs assessment to imagine the possible creative expression of the target group. Moreover, we could share with them these images in postcard size to stimulate creativity. This can also convey mutual understanding and connection.

The major challenge of working with cancer patients is their unstable health condition. We have to be sensitive to their needs and accept their limitations. Sometimes women dropped out because of unexpected physical deterioration. The group was for the members a life laboratory on coping with impermanence in life. Fortunately, we could use art to demonstrate these uncertainties in life and visually transform them. I was always touched by the members who strived to participate in the group even though they were in great pain. Each time they would feel much better at the end, because the arts had energized their bodies and diminished their sense of suffering. As shared by Anna Halprin (2002), a person with a cancer may not be cured, but she can always be healed. Our group members told us that they could feel a state of physical, psychological, and spiritual well-being when engaging in the arts.

Body is the foundation of all expression (Levine, 1996, cited in Levine & Levine, 2000, p. 32). This was especially true for these group members, who were facing many bodily changes; they enjoyed the process of drawing body portraits and moving their bodies. Moving brought them to deeper feelings (Halprin, 2003) and facilitated the understanding of their art as well. I also integrated lymphedema exercises in the warm-up exercises for the dance and movement part: for example, drawing imaginary, many-colored circles that became bigger and bigger in the air.

Sometimes people were tempted to interpret the art. Being a person-centered therapist, I kept myself mindful of staying open and listening to each person's story. I treasured the equal and respectful time with each woman with whom I was working. With empathetic listening and unconditional positive regard, members felt support and sense of safety. Through their hands-on experience in the Creative Connection process (Rogers, 1993), each found her unique way in coping with cancer. They were truly empowered by the arts.

CONCLUSION

Expressive arts therapy may not be the prevailing means of individual and group counseling in health care. Yet it is an effective means to connect with and release our deep emotions. Unlike conventional cancer treatment, the arts do little harm and carry no side effects. The symbolic and metaphoric nature of the arts provides a safe space for women with breast cancer to explore the taboo of sexuality and sensitive issues of feminine identity and couple relationship (Ertl, 1999; Malchiodi, 1997; Oster, Astrom, Lindh, & Magnusson, 2009; Rogers, 1993). Cancer patients can choose their favorite art modalities to actualize their latent creativity and bring out the underlying potential for self-healing. Art can inspire energy and creativity during the journey through cancer.

The interplay of art, music, writing, and movement not only healed our bodies, but it also helped us to channel our emotions and enhance our self-confidence. We found a new sense of self with feminine power and infinite creativity. We let go of the suppressed emotions from within. We experienced the sacred space in the arts to transform our negative emotions into healthy and liberating energy. In the person-centered expressive arts process, we enjoyed a safe platform in the group. Through deep listening to our art, music, movement, and poetry, we allowed ourselves to express and regain our "woman power." We found our true beauty and exotic energy in the arts. These are the true voices of the women with breast cancer participating in an expressive arts therapy group.

REFERENCES

Centre for Health Protection. (2011). Breast cancer. Retrieved October 13, 2011, from *www.chp.gov.hk/en/content/9/25/53.html.*

Chang, F. (2011). Using person-centered expressive arts therapy for advancing group development. *Social work group case book* (pp. 157–193). Hong Kong: Riding Word Press.

Chang, F. (2012). Integrating person-centered expressive arts with Chinese metaphors. In D. L. Kalmanowitz, J. S. Potash, & S. M. Chan (Eds.), *Art therapy in Asia* (pp. 253–266). London: Jessica Kingsley.

Chang, F., & Ho, S. (2000). From expression to empowerment: Using creative arts as self-healing media for cancer patients. In R. Fielding & C. L. W. Chan (Eds.), *Psychosocial oncology and palliative care in Hong Kong: The first decade* (pp. 189–211). Hong Kong: Hong Kong University Press.

Dreher, D. (2000). *The tao of inner peace.* New York: Penguin.

Ertl, M. (1999). Art in Vienna's hospitals: Decoration or challenge? In D. Haldane & S. Loppert (Eds.), *The arts in health care: Learning from experience* (pp. 47–57). London: King's Fund.

Halprin, A. (2002). *Returning to health with dance, movement and imagery.* Mendocino, CA: Life Rhythm.

Halprin, D. (2003). *The expressive body in life, art and therapy: Working with movement, metaphor and meaning.* London: Jessica Kingsley.

Hong Kong Cancer Registry. (2010). Summary of cancer statistics in Hong Kong in 2008. Retrieved October 13, 2011, from *www3.ha.org.hk/cancereg/summary%20of%20canstat%20 2008.pdf.*

Hospital Authority. (2011). *Hospital Authority statistical report 2009–2010.* Hong Kong: Statistics and Workforce Planning Department, Strategy and Planning Division, Hospital Authority.

Kaplan, F. F. (2007). Art and conflict resolution. In F. F. Kaplan (Ed.), *Art therapy and social action* (pp. 89–102). London: Jessica Kingsley.

Levine, S., & Levine, E. (2000). *Foundations of expressive arts therapy: Theoretical and clinical perspectives.* London: Jessica Kingsley.

Liebmann, M. (Ed.). (1996). *Arts approaches to conflict.* London: Jessica Kingsley.

Malchiodi, C. A. (1997). Invasive art: Art as empowerment for women with breast cancer. In S. Hogan (Ed.), *Feminist approaches to art therapy* (1st ed., pp. 49–64). London: Routledge.

Malchiodi, C. A. (Ed.). (1999). *Medical art therapy with adults.* London: Jessica Kingsley.

Malchiodi, C. A. (2006). *The art therapy sourcebook.* Los Angeles: Lowell House.

Mathieson, C. M., & Stam, H. J. (1995). Renegotiating identity: Cancer narratives. *Society of Health and Illness, 17*(3), 283–306.

Nainis, N., Paice, J. A., Ratner, J., Wirth, J. H., Lai, J., & Shott, S. (2006). Relieving symptoms in cancer: Innovative use of art therapy. *Journal of Pain and Symptom Management, 31*(2), 162–169.

Oster, I., Astrom, S., Lindh, J., & Magnusson, E. (2009). Women with breast cancer and gendered limits and boundaries: Art therapy as a "safe space" for enacting alternative subject positions. *The Arts in Pscyhotherapy, 36,* 29–38.

Oster, I., Magnusson, E., Thyme, K. E., Lindh, J., & Astrom, S. (2007). Art therapy for women with breast cancer: The therapeutic consequences of boundary strengthening. *The Arts in Psychotherapy, 34,* 277–288.

Rogers, N. (1993). *The Creative Connection: Expressive arts as healing.* Palo Alto, CA: Science & Behavior Books.

Rogers, N. (2011). *The Creative Connection for groups: Person-centered expressive arts for healing and social change.* Palo Alto, CA: Science & Behavior Books.

Rosenberg, M. B. (2000). *Non-violent communication: A language of compassion.* Encinitas, CA: Puddle Dancer Press.

Schover, L. R. (1991). The impact of breast cancer on sexuality, body image, and intimate relationships. *CA: A Cancer Journal for Clinicians, 41*(2), 112–120.

Siegel, B. S. (1990). *Peace, love and healing: Bodymind communication and the path to self-healing: An exploration.* New York: Harper Perennial.

CHAPTER 11

Healing across Cultures

Arts in Health Care with American Indian and Alaska Native Cancer Survivors

Elizabeth Warson

"Art is healing." This is a phrase that I had to retrain myself to say after 2 years of graduate art therapy training. *How* does art heal? That was always the question. Intuitively, many of us can say art is healing because of our own experience with the art-making process. I know this from a cultural lens as well, one that is grounded in the holistic perspective of indigenous people. This chapter considers wellness from a Native American perspective; art is part of this framework, as it is an integral part of life. It draws upon my personal experience within the Native American culture, including personal life, clinical art therapy practice with Indigenous Peoples, and collaborative research with American Indian cancer survivors and their family members, to present how arts in health care is considered a culturally respectful healing practice.

ART IS A UNIVERSAL LANGUAGE

"Art is a universal language" is an assumption shared by many expressive arts practitioners and often used as a rationale for arts-based therapies being inherently culturally respectful. Within the field of art therapy, the notion of art as a universal language has been inextricably intertwined with art as a healing practice. References to art making as a healing practice abound from the American Art Therapy Association's definition of art therapy as "healing and life enhancing" (McNiff, 2004) and contemporary media sources, such as *A Universal Language for Healing* (Rubin, 2011). At face value, these sources naively suggest that art making transcends cultural differences, reinforcing a more global perspective of art therapy.

Not all theorists are in agreement though, Bruce Moon (2009) states, "I do not believe art is a universal language" (p. 154), adding that he is aware in his own work of "cultural truisms" (p. 154) from Western culture, reflecting a more contextualized viewpoint. Similarly, Cathy Moon (2002) articulates a more postmodern philosophy stating that a "universal quality of art as a mode of expression" (p. 255) is reflective of the individual's life experience and cultural background. McNiff (2004) deconstructs the romanticized notion of art as a healing practice, reaffirming the "universal healing qualities of art by people inside and outside therapy" (p. 6). However, the *how* aspect is not well defined in terms of culture-bound meaning, reinforcing a vague notice of a universality. Arts-related anthropologist Ellen Dissanayake (1992) presents a different stance on meaning making through the arts, referring to this process as "making oneself special" (p. xi), further intimating an innate tendency to make art within a culture-bound context. In this respect art making is situated within both a cultural context and biologically driven tendency.

CULTURAL RELEVANCY

Cultural relevancy is often an applied concept resulting from an attempt to modify a directive, intervention, or task related to a broad aspect of the culture, or even a related culture. It is more a complex process not only involving collaboration but also establishing relationships with stakeholders; assembling advisory committees; interviewing community members; assessing relevancy of art materials processes; piloting art interventions; co-creating curriculum; and being involved with the community. This involves a degree of reciprocity: "*How* do you intend to give back to the community?" In essence, one is practicing in what Hays (2008) refers to as a culturally responsive approach. More specifically, she recommends that practitioners and researchers develop an understanding of indigenous, religious, and traditional practices to devise and implement culturally relevant arts-based therapies. This understanding follows an ongoing process of self-assessment through the ADDRESSING framework, which "begins with an emphasis on understanding the effect of diverse cultural influences on therapists' worldviews" (p. 6). This framework that comprises categories ranging from age-related generational experiences to ethnic and racial identity, maps out one's worldview, as well as the role of privilege. This self-awareness is crucial in terms of conceptualizing the ADDRESSING framework or worldview of others.

To be culturally responsive in health care requires an understanding of the notion of worldview. A person's worldview is defined by aspects such as cultural upbringing, values systems, and life experiences, which have a profound influence on how we think, interact with one another, and make decisions (Sue & Sue, 2008). Self-assessment is the first step in being able to experience divergent worldviews (Hays, 2001). Without this awareness, "cultural oppression" (p. 293) may result unknowingly because of a lack of understanding. "It has become increasing clear that many diverse groups hold worldviews that differ from members of the dominant culture and their practicing therapists.

In a broader sense, worldviews determine how people perceive their relationship to the world (nature, institutions, other people, etc.)" (Sue & Sue, 2008, pp. 293–294).

Although it is well known that divergent worldviews exist between Western and Native American thought, especially in relation to illness and wellness, Duran (2006) underscores the need for culturally relevant approaches that extend beyond the *application* of Native practices to that of an *understanding* of Native concepts of healing and illness. Duran refers to this understanding as the "Native epistemological root metaphor" (p. 10) or *knowing* Native ways of existing in the world as they relate to multiple worlds (e.g., spiritual, physical, and psychological). This concept of Native epistemology is especially salient in working with American Indians/Alaska Natives (AI/AN), as holistic approaches in Western medicine, comprising alternative and complementary therapies, are gaining recognition (Office of Cancer Complementary and Alternative Medicine [OCCAM], n.d.).

COMMUNITY-DRIVEN AND PARTICIPATORY APPROACHES

Developing a sense of Native epistemology lays the groundwork for co-creating community-driven projects. A community-driven focus is often confused with community-based participatory models, when in actuality this is more of a continuum. The community-based approach to research and program development is one for which Native communities have a stated preference because of the degree of shared decision making and collaboration between the research team and community (Boyer et al., 2005). This collaboration, one that is formed in the beginning stages of the project, is geared toward providing an effective model or program that can be integrated or sustained within these communities. An important component of this approach is a Community Board or Advisory Committee, comprising a diverse group of community members to oversee the development and outcome of the study. The community-driven approach can develop into community-based participatory research involving more of an active partnership approach geared toward implementing sustainable practices.

NATIVE CONCEPTS OF HEALTH AND ILLNESS

Clements's *Primitive Concepts of Disease* (1932) provided one of the earliest ethnographic studies among Indigenous Peoples throughout the world. His study provided a description and classification of disease concepts from traditional practices. Duran (2006) made reference to Clements's five main types as a foundation for understanding Native concepts of healing and illness, providing a bridge between Western and non-Western perspectives. Clements's concepts were broadly defined into three categories: natural causes (modern medicine), human agency (sorcery), and supernatural agency (supernatural factors). His study extended these three categories into five main types: sorcery (human infliction), breech of taboo (guilt), disease-object intrusion (object removal), spirit intrusion (outside entity intruding), and soul loss (loss of soul). Variants of these concepts continue to represent the worldview that many Indigenous Peoples maintain, and perceptions of illness and wellness.

Broadly stated, Native Americans view wellness and illness as an interrelated system. As such, illness is caused by an imbalance or disharmony in one's life (Sue & Sue, 2008). This notion may sound simple but the belief systems, traditions, and value systems vary tremendously between tribal cultures, and are seemingly affected by degrees of acculturation. Romanticized notions of shamanic practices and traditional healers in the dominant society have seemingly clouded the importance of these concepts and their meaning. Much of what is practiced in Western society is due in part to the influence of "Indian medicine," primarily botanical preparations and natural remedies (Vogel, 1970)."The meaning of the term medicine to an Indian was quite different from that which is ordinarily held in white society. To most Indians, medicine signified an array of ideas and concepts rather than remedies and treatment alone" (pp. 24–25). In more recent times, efforts to reintegrate traditional medicine with Western practices have been in the forefront of health care reform for AI/AN. In spite of this integration, concepts of wellness and illness differ considerably between Native Americans and non-Natives.

In spite of these holistic efforts in Western medicine, the Native American perspective on wellness is largely misunderstood (Hodge, Limb, & Cross, 2009). Wellness from a Native or Indigenous perspective is more "relationally based" (p. 213), focusing on the interrelated concepts of mind, body, spirit, and context. This approach differs substantially from more westernized linear concepts of mind–body interaction in that spirituality is central to understanding the mind–body connection and that *mind* extends beyond cognition to include emotional well-being (Cross, 1997). The notion of *context* is unique to Native people, emphasizing a collectivist worldview that Native people share; that is, a person is understood in relation to his or her family, tribal community, history, culture, environment, work, and so on (Cross, 1997). This worldview counters the rugged individualism observed in Western secular culture, which places importance on autonomy and the belief that an individual can control his or her environment (Sue & Sue, 2008). As such, wellness from a more holistic Native American perspective addresses quality-of-life factors by achieving balance and harmony through the reciprocal relationship among mind, body, spirit, and context (Cross, 2001).

CANCER INCIDENCE AND SURVIVORSHIP AMONG AMERICAN INDIANS AND ALASKA NATIVES

Modern medicine has benefited from, and continues to rely on, traditional American Indian medicine. By contrast, the Native people of today are the most medically underserved racial group in the Western world. This seems to be an unfortunate juxtaposition when one considers the advancements and progress in Western medicine and the poor survival rates for medically ill Native Americans (Pfefferbaum, Pfefferbaum, Rhoades,

& Strickland, 1997). Reports of acute and chronic illness among Native Americans continue to rise, with diseases of the heart and stroke as the leading cause of death (American Heart Association, 2007, Statistical Fact Sheet, para. 1) and cancer as the second leading cause of AI/AN deaths of persons 45 years and older (Association of American Indian Physicians, [AAIP], n.d., Cancer Statistics para. 1). With respect to cancer survival rates, AI/AN have the highest mortality rates for "all cancers combined" (Intercultural Cancer Council [ICC], n.d., para. 4). These mortality rates reflect the current disparities in the AI/AN health status, including access and quality of health care (Roubideaux & Dixon, 2001).

Although research studies on cancer incidence among Native Americans have reported lower rates among AI/AN than among white Americans (Centers for Disease Control and Prevention [CDC], 2003; Espey et al., 2007), this discrepancy is partly attributed to racial misclassification (Frost, Taylor, & Fries, 1992; ICC, n.d.). For the vast majority of Americans, cancer rates are declining for the first time in 70 years (American Cancer Society [ACS], 2007), and according to the National Cancer Institute (NCI, 2007), the number of survivors from 1971 to 2002 has more than doubled to 10 million survivors. These gains have seemingly clouded higher rates of cancer for the medically underserved, including people of color, lower socioeconomic status, and non-English-speaking people (Intercultural Cancer Council, 2012). The ICC was charged with the task to oversee racial and ethnic disparities in health care delivery, identifying five different criteria for cancer care: Available, Accessible, Acceptable, Affordable, and Accountable (p. 2). The ICC's mission is "to promote policies, programs, partnerships, and research to eliminate the unequal burden of cancer among racial and ethnic minorities and medically underserved populations" (p. 1). Their 2006 Survivorship Report details the impact of poverty and lack of insurance as a primary reason for poor survival rates for the medically underserved populations.

The statistics on cancer incidence and mortality rates are neither reliable nor are they representative of the overall AI/AN population, because there is no single database for tracking incidence and survivor rates. In addition to racial misclassification, occurrences of underreporting are widespread due to barriers in data collection efforts (ICC, 2012). AI/AN cancer data are often clustered with other racial/ethnic minority groups under the "other" data category. The appearance of less cancer in AI/AN communities is partially attributed to the younger AI/AN median age reported in 2000 by the U.S. Census Bureau (2001), when in fact cancer is more prevalent in the older adult population (ICC, 2012). Cancer rates overall continue to be reportedly lower for AI/AN by database sources from Surveillance, Epidemiology and End Results (SEER; Clegg, Frederick, Hankey, Chu, & Edwards, 2002), the ACS (2007), CDC (2003), and the U.S. Department of Health and Human Service's Office of Minority Health (AI/AN Profile, n.d.). Conversely, available cancer data through organizations such as the ICC (American Indian/Alaska Natives and Cancer, n.d.), indicate that AI/AN cancer has been increasing the past 20 years. Moreover, cancer is the second leading cause of death for AI/AN persons over age 45. AI/AN people also have the poorest survival rate from all cancers combined of any racial/ethnic minority group.

ART THERAPY WITH CANCER SURVIVORS

Art therapy considers the mind–body interaction for healing, personal growth, and an enhanced quality of life. Art therapy is practiced in different settings with diverse populations, using traditional and nontraditional art processes, nonverbal and verbal approaches, and an array of formats, ranging from open studios and workshops to independent practice. Specialized approaches, such as medical art therapy, have led to the development of art-based psychosocial interventions for individuals experiencing acute and chronic illness. The efficacy of art therapy with the medically ill has been a focus in art therapy research, concentrating on variables such as pain management, increased self-expression, stress management, and enhanced quality of life (Nainis et al., 2006). Art therapy is rooted in many ancient traditions, and the use of art and medicine is no exception. As a complementary form of therapy, medical art therapy has demonstrated significantly lower ratings of depression, anxiety, and somatic symptoms with breast cancer survivors (Egberg Thyme et al., 2009). Many novel approaches within the field of medical art therapy have surfaced for cancer survivors, focusing on wellness-based models (Malchioidi, 1999) and symptom management (Nainis et al., 2006). Innovative approaches such as mindfulness-based art therapy (MBAT) successfully integrate mindfulness-based stress reduction with visual forms of self-expression for cancer survivors (Monti et al., 2006). Art-based interventions in cancer research often consider the mandala, an Eastern-based form of meditation incorporating circular symmetry, as a model for stress reduction. Quasi-experimental studies have suggested that coloring a predesigned mandala can reduce self-report measures of stress (Curry & Kasser, 1999; Lorance, Warson, & Rosencrans, 2008). Mandala imagery has also served as an assessment tool to convey perceptions of breast cancer treatment (Elkis-Abuhoff, Gaydos, Goldblatt, Chen, & Rose, 2009).

ART THERAPY WITH AMERICAN INDIANS AND ALASKA NATIVES

Grounded in Native epistemology, complementary therapies such as art therapy could provide a more culturally responsive, holistic approach for addressing psychosocial factors in health care for Native Americans. The creative arts, including art therapy, have been beneficial in attending to concepts related to Native wellness (Herring, 1997): "The expressive arts represent avenues of emotional, religious, and artistic expression that remain an essential part of the life of most Native people" (p. 106). To Native people, the creative arts provide a nonverbal outlet for expression of feeling, allowing disclosure to occur without the need for verbalization; this nonverbal outlet is significant when one considers that Native people use silence as a form of respect, especially toward authority figures and elders. From a Native perspective, art is a form of life and ritual, and one that is rich in metaphor, symbolism, and meaning; this is reflective of a Native way of being in the world (Herring, 1997).

There is a paucity of literature focusing on art therapy with AI/AN. The majority of these publications have focused on anecdotal evidence to support art therapy as a culturally relevant approach (Bien, 2005; Moody, 1995). American Indian art therapist Phoebe Dufrene was the first academic to articulate the interrelationship between art therapy practice and American Indian methods of healing (Dufrene, n.d.; Dufrene, Coleman, & Gainor, 1992). Her collaborative work with American Indian psychologist Herring (1997) outlined culturally respective approaches in art therapy. Presently, there are only two art therapists conducting research in Indian country: Dr. Cueva, a registered nurse and cancer educator, who has been researching culturally relevant art-based interventions as part of her ACS-funded Arts-Based Cancer Education with Alaska Native People and the Community Health Representatives (CHR) Cancer Education Module (Cueva, Kuhnley, Stueckemann, Lanier, & McMahon, 2010). I also focus on cultural relevancy in devising and implementing art-based psychosocial interventions specific to stress and pain management (Basto, Warson, & Barbour, 2012; Warson, 2009, 2012). Both Dr. Cueva and I consider a relationally based Native perspective of wellness comprising the interrelationship among mind, body, spirit, and context in our approach (Cross, 2001; Hodge et al., 2009).

HEALING PATHWAYS: PILOT STUDY

Method

The Healing Pathways pilot project was developed in 2006 and implemented through funding from the Johnson & Johnson Foundation through the Society for the Arts in Health care and in partnership with the North Carolina Commission of Indian Affairs. The aim of this mixed-methods community-driven project was to develop a culturally relevant art therapy workshop as a means of stress reduction for American Indian cancer survivors and their family members in North Carolina. During this 1-year grant period, three workshops were conducted for two settlements of the Coharie and one urban intertribal center in Cumberland County. A total of 46 participants attended the three workshops. No specific criteria were indicated with respect to cancer site, gender, current medical treatment, or duration of time as a survivor. As a community-driven workshop, all generations were included whether they were cancer survivors or a family member directly affected by cancer. A culturally relevant format for conducting the art therapy workshops was one of the outcomes of this study. This feasibility study incorporated an emergent design allowing the Advisory Committee, comprising seven tribal members from the Coharie community, to provide constant feedback and recommendations that were incorporated immediately following each workshop.

In collaboration with the North Carolina Commission of Indian Affairs, the investigator was introduced to the commission members representing the nine tribes within North Carolina through a letter drafted by the Executive Director Greg Richardson. In addition, the investigator attended a Commission meeting to introduce herself in person and discuss the details of the study. Through these preliminary meetings with the Commission, an Advisory Committee was formed; a Commission member Sadie Barbour from the Coharie tribe was designated to assist with the workshops. Prior to forming the Advisory Committee, the investigator piloted her art interventions with Ms. Barbour to obtain feedback about the cultural appropriateness of the art directives for the community workshops. This meeting led to the formation of an Advisory Committee from the Coharie tribe comprising seven members who were either cancer survivors or family members.

The Advisory Committee members participated in a workshop prior to implementing the protocol in the tribal communities. Based on this workshop, three art interventions and a warm-up exercise were agreed upon for the first community workshop. Committee members made additional recommendations to provide the art therapy workshops with a more culturally relevant format for the Coharie elder community, consisting of a kinesthetic warm-up "clearing the air" with a feather; a gestural drawing on large sheets of paper; a guided visualization drawing; for stress and/or pain management; a "response" piece to the visualization drawing; and an open-ended "closing" piece. The inclusion of pain management in the protocol was the most significant modification to attend the beliefs of the elders within this community. Additional recommendations included limiting the amount of art supplies made available, the inclusion of an opening and closing prayer, and an altar with ceremonial pieces specific to the tribal community.

To measure the effectiveness of these interventions on stress reduction, a 40-item self-report inventory, the State–Trait Anxiety Inventory (STAI; Spielberger, 1983) was included as a pretest and posttest measure. There was some initial hesitation from the Advisory Committee and the North Carolina Commission of Indian Affairs about using this inventory, because the length and wording of the questions was not culturally specific for American Indians. A suggestion was made to reduce the number of questions by half from the original 40-item self-report inventory and a modified STAI, referred to as the State–Trait Personality Inventory (STPI; Spielberger, 1986), was acquired from the publisher.

Research Design

The mixed-methods design incorporated a single group pretest–posttest with a qualitative content analysis of the artwork. Three separate workshops (3 hours/workshop) were held within two settlements of the Coharie tribe, in addition to an intertribal urban site in Cumberland County. The workshops were announced to the community at tribal meetings and culturally relevant flyers approved by the Institutional Review Board (IRB) were posted throughout the tribal center with the PI's contact information. The 3-hour workshops at the tribal centers were followed by a healthy lunch and a raffle. The participants were apprised of the study individually and consented as a group, using a 5-page IRB document. The pretest STPI was administered prior to the implementation of the art intervention, and the posttest STPI, at the conclusion of the workshop. The tribal representatives, who were trained by the PI to administer the tool, assisted with this process by reading the questions aloud and assisting with their self-report scores based on a 4-point Likert scale.

This study incorporated an emergent design enabling the PI to modify the art interventions throughout the study, based on feedback from the Advisory Committee. The first workshop with the Coharie tribe provided the environment to explore a range of art materials and directed art tasks. The resulting art interventions were modified for the second workshop and replicated again in the third workshop. A follow-up member check was conducted to discuss the impact of the workshop.

Data Collection

Workshop 1

The Coharie tribe assembled the group of 28 older adult women who had overlapping health conditions (diabetes) or stress-related problems due to cancer. Formatting of the workshop was based on the feedback from the Advisory Committee, which included "clearing the air" with a feather; kinesthetic drawing; visualization and corresponding depiction of stress or pain; and a response piece (medium of choice). The third open-ended task was not completed because of time constraints. The women were provided with a package of Model Magic (a self-hardening molding material) to experiment on their own, in addition to a visual journaling kit that included watercolor pencils, watercolor paper, eraser, and a paintbrush.

Prior to the workshop, in the middle of the room, Ms. Barbour created an altar with a lit candle to recognize those from the tribe who had passed on from cancer. The oldest woman in the room gave the prayer. The protocol for this workshop included a warm-up of "clearing the air" with a white feather. This ritual was developed by the Advisory Committee and was culturally specific to the Coharie. Each participant in a circle passed around a feather and drew in the air. This warm-up was followed-up with a gestural drawing on 18″ × 24″ sheet of grey paper tape on the wall. Participants were encouraged to make gestural marks in the air first (circle, up and down, and back and forth) before reproducing these marks on the paper. Participants sat down at a grouping of tables to participate in a guided visualization drawing focused on the depiction of stress or pain. Participants depicted their stress or "pain" using lines, shapes, and color in the center of the circle. (Prior to this implementation, we used an Eastern-based mandala as a stimulus to work from, then modified this circular configuration to a "healing circle" [a term coined by Linda Burhanisstipanov] to make this drawing task culturally relevant.) They were encouraged to participate in breathing exercises to reflect on this image, then rated their level of stress or pain on a 1- to 10-point scale (10 = highest level). Continuing with the breathing exercises, they visualized a lesser degree of pain or stress and were encouraged to depict this in consecutive stages. Once participants had reached their lowest level, they verbally processed their responses to this exercise. After they had identified an area in their circle with which they connected, they were encouraged to create a "response" piece using a medium of choice. The STPI posttest was completed prior to breaking for lunch, again with the assistance of the tribal representatives. In addition to a raffle, the PI provided a gift of a visual journaling set and a visual example and brief introduction to visual journaling, along with written guidelines. Participants were encouraged to draw, paint, or collage in their journals for at least 5 minutes a day as a means of reducing stress.

Workshops 2 and 3

Prior to the second workshop, I reviewed the audio- and videotapes to modify the format. The Advisory Committee reviewed these modifications and supported the revised format for the second workshop with another settlement of the Coharie tribe. The modifications included fewer choices regarding art media and the "clearing the air" warm-up, without a follow-up gestural drawing, because it was not perceived as being purposeful enough. Grey paper was used for all drawing tasks, as many of the participants displayed a preference for white media; white pastels, for example, cannot be seen on a white paper or background. The healing circle intervention remained unchanged with the exception of the inclusion of grey paper. The response intervention to the healing circle exercise was narrowed down to a predrawn circle on watercolor paper with a watercolor set vs. a broad range of art materials. The Model Magic self-hardening clay was used as a closing intervention, in lieu of an open-ended task. The second workshop consisted of 10 Coharie elder women and men. The modified protocol was piloted with this community, which with the feedback from the Advisory Committee, decided that the format was culturally relevant and acceptable to replicate. The third workshop at an intertribal site included eight female cancer survivors and family members from the Lumbee, Cherokee, Waccamau Siouan, and Coharie tribes. The protocol from the second workshop was replicated in a standardized manner: an initial workshop that included a "clearing the air" warm-up exercise, healing circle drawing, "response" painting, and an introduction to visual journaling; and a follow-up workshop that included a "clearing the air" warm-up exercise, review of visual journal, creation of a cover for the visual journal, and a "response" clay task.

Data Analysis

The STAI (Spielberger, 1983) is an inventory that has high validity in studies with medically ill patients. This inventory was reviewed and modified three times to provide more culturally appropriate wording. I consulted with the publisher to obtain guidance during this modification process. The final condensed version referred to as the STPI (Spielberger, 1986) comprised 17 questions, as opposed to 40 questions with the STAI. The final modification resulted in omitting two questions that participants perceived to be duplications and an easier-to-read format. In spite of the modifications, the scoring system (4-point Likert scale) presented a challenge, because most participants were completing the inventory as a dichotomous rating system and inadvertently reversed the numbers to reflect the opposite of their intention. Participants from all three groups stated that the wording was confusing and were not receptive to completing the postassessment as a result. The inventories were neither rated nor considered in a more formal analysis because of the degree of difficulty in completing them. The Advisory Committee also expressed concern that the STPI was biased, and that the analysis from the inventories could be misleading.

Qualitative Analysis

The artwork of the 46 participants from three community workshops was analyzed with an inductive approach to open coding from grounded theory (Creswell, 2007) and mapping techniques from situational analysis (Clarke, 2005). The open coping was conducted by creating lists of words describing formal art qualities, symbolic content, and narrative themes that emerged from the artwork. The mapping technique was a second level of coding, clustering observations in radial maps, "situating" the dominant themes in context to the participants' worldviews. Three dominant themes resulted from the two levels of coding: an emphasis on pain management; narrative depictions of nature and human figures; and a personal, symbolic approach to color use. The Advisory Committee reviewed the findings from each workshop and gave additional feedback to provide more of a context.

The emphasis on pain in the healing circle intervention was observed in 87% of the art productions. This focus on pain and stress levels was indicated by the Advisory Committee, which made the recommendation to include the option of pain. The color associated with pain was red or black for all of the pain-related healing circles. A target configuration, created using concentric layers of color, was the most common design for the healing circle (Figure 11.1). The color associated with less pain or stress was consistently white or a lighter hue of color; 100% of the healing circles incorporated five or more colors, resulting in a vibrant effect.[1]

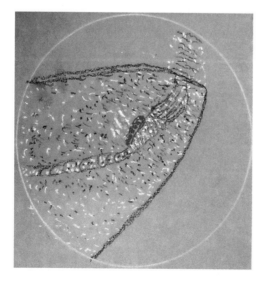

FIGURE 11.1. Healing circle drawing.

---

[1] Original artwork for this chapter was in color. It is reproduced here in black and white.

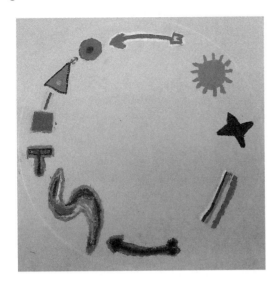

FIGURE 11.2. Healing circle "response" painting.

The narrative depiction of nature and human figures surfaced in the "response" painting (Figure 11.2). Participants were asked to look at a section of their healing circle and create a "response" painting. Approximately 30% of the participants opted to continue to focus on pain, observed in the depiction of red monochromatic human figures, with emphasized interiors (layered paint) suggestive of the source of pain (Figures 11.3 and 11.4). The narrative themes corresponded with the storying process and stories of cancer survival and events from everyday life were indicated symbolically through the painting and clay process. Cultural images reminiscent of dreamcatchers surfaced during the painting process and served as a metaphor for weaving together parts of participants' lives (Figures 11.5 and 11.6).

Consistent personal and symbolic use of color was evident in all the art-based interventions. The use of color became a dominant theme, because the majority of the art productions included a full range of primary and secondary colors. The symbolic meaning of color was explored in terms of collective meaning (e.g., white representing

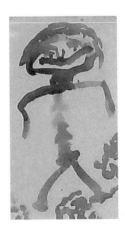

FIGURE 11.3. Response painting: Pain.

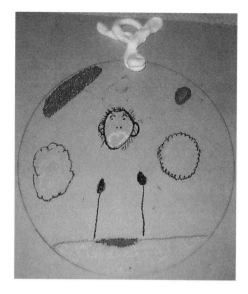

FIGURE 11.4. Response drawing: Pain.

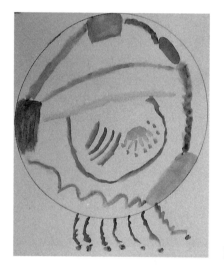

FIGURE 11.5. Dreamcatcher.

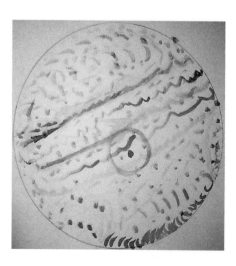

FIGURE 11.6. Dreamcatcher.

"purity"), as well as personal meaning (e.g., one participant's depiction of a yellow cancer cell; Figure 11.7). Most often observed was the vibrancy of colors reinforced through repetitious marks and dashes reflective of patterns of beading and stitching from quilting (Figures 11.8 and 11.9). Color also served as a catalyst for the storying process; participants were literally "speaking" through color to tell their stories.

Follow-Up Interviews

Two separate interviews were conducted as a form of a member check with a mother–daughter pair that had participated in the Coharie workshops. The mother was a cancer survivor and the daughter, her caregiver. They requested that I join them for lunch at their family farm to discuss their visual journals presented to them at the end of the workshop. Over the course of several months, these women had been maintaining a daily visual journal, recording thoughts, observations, and feelings. Both reported that visual journaling gave them an opportunity to spend time to themselves, away from other responsibilities. This "member check," along with other reports from tribal representatives, and requests from the communities for additional "books," suggested that visual journaling was becoming an accepted practice within this tribal community.

Discussion

The aim of this mixed-methods study was to provide a culturally relevant art therapy workshop to promote stress reduction for cancer survivors and their family members. Statistical significance was not achieved based on the pretest and posttest STPI, because as the study progressed, it became apparent that the inventory was not transferable to southeastern American Indian tribes. Moreover, the North Carolina Commission of Indian Affairs, as well as the Advisory Committee, had concerns from the beginning about the use of this instrument within their tribal communities. The qualitative analysis was limited with respect to evaluating the research question, and it is not known to what extent the interventions had an effect on stress reduction. What resulted from this study was a culturally relevant workshop format that could be replicated in a larger study. Using an emergent design and community-driven approach, this format was modified to embrace the mind, body, spirit, and context associated with Native American wellness by embracing the importance of prayer, art making, storying, and community (Cross, 1997). The results of this study reinforced a Native American concept of wellness-based mind, body, spirit, and context, evident in the three domains from the coding analyses. More specifically, the emphasis on pain reflected a body-based awareness. Originally, this pain emphasis was presumed to be connected with the Christian beliefs associated with this particular community, in that once a person has given his or her life to Christ, there are no worries (S. Barbour, personal communication, June 1, 2006). The concentration on pain during the healing circle exercise, as well as the continuation of the pain theme in the "response" painting, also seemed to indicate a highly interrelated mind–body connection: Thoughts, feelings, perceptions, and somatic sensations are simultaneously

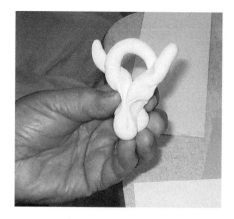

FIGURE 11.7. Cancer cell.

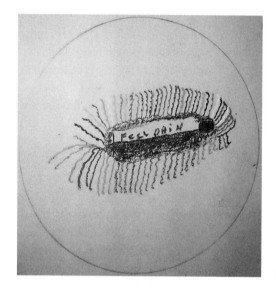

FIGURE 11.8. Healing circle drawing: Patterning.

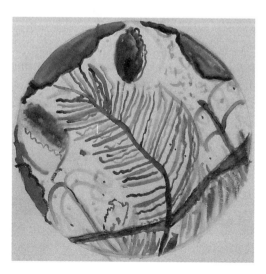

FIGURE 11.9. Response painting: Patterning.

experienced rather than compartmentalized as stemming from one's mind or body. This concept warrants further research, as it seems to counter a more Western secular perspective that somatic experiences can be pathological in nature. Little is known about the implications of an interrelated concept of wellness based on mind, body, spirit, and context in Western medicine (Cross, 1997).

The storying process elicited through the art process seemed to string together mind, body, spirit, and context; without storying, many of these images would have been reduced to colorful decorative patterns, devoid of meaning. Storytelling is central to indigenous cultures as part of an oral tradition of teaching and sharing tribal knowledge, as well as a source of entertainment and inspiration. The storying process in qualitative research—specifically, narrative inquiry—is a method of exploring the deeper layers of meaning making. Although this was not a narrative inquiry, the storying process was a central yet a separate aspect of the study that could neither be observed in the context of the artwork nor recorded in a self-report inventory. In addition to the storying process, another unanticipated outcome was the self-guided visual journaling that was sustained after completion of the workshops. The impact of this intervention—that was intended more as a gift than a formal intervention—in addition to the storying process became a primary consideration in a follow-up study.

HEALING PATHWAYS STUDY

An expanded study was supported by an Institutional Research Grant (IRG-08-091-01) from the ACS, to The George Washington University Cancer Institute and a community grant from the Mayo Cancer Clinic's Spirit of EAGLES program. The workshop format stemming from the Healing Pathways pilot study is currently being replicated in tribal communities throughout North Carolina. The aim of this project was broadened to provide a culturally relevant art therapy intervention as a means to promote a sense of wellness (through stress reduction), thus affecting quality-of-life factors for American Indian cancer survivors from North Carolina tribes. The study is currently being conducted throughout North Carolina, and modifications to the research design and an overview of the standardized format for the workshops are discussed in the next section.

Methods

This replication was expanded to include a total of 14 art therapy workshops (seven initial and seven follow-up) for approximately 300 American Indian cancer survivors and their family members (average of 21 participants per workshop) from five rural and urban North Carolina tribal communities: Coharie (two settlements), Waccamau Siouan (two settlements), Occaneechi Band of the Saponi Nation, and Cumberland County Indian Association (an urban intertribal center). American Indian cancer survivors and their family members from North Carolina will be included in this study, including children, adolescents, adults, and older adults as part of the community-driven focus. A waiver of documentation was approved for this study because of the difficulty in obtaining participants' consent during the pilot using a 5-page consent form.

Modifications to the Research Design

A grounded theory approach from qualitative research replaced the mixed-methods design because of the storying emphasis from the pilot, as well as limitations experienced with the self-report measure. The workshop format was expanded to include a follow-up workshop incorporating visual journaling exercises and clay work. Visual journaling was also included as a self-guided intervention between the two workshops, spaced approximately 4 weeks apart. A clay intervention using red ceramic clay rather than self-hardening clay was added as the final art intervention, based on the recommendation from the pilot study Advisory Committee. The replicated design also considered a more thorough rationale for each of art-based intervention. As part of the community-driven approach, a five-member Advisory Committee was assembled, including providers, professionals, and scholars from the Lumbee Nation and Coharie tribe.

Data Collection

Preliminary Workshop

As a warm-up activity for the first intervention, participants were asked to "clear the air" with a white turkey feather. Within the North Carolina tribes, white signifies "purity" and was an acceptable choice for this purpose. This process entails moving a feather in a circular manner, up and down, and back and forth, first with the dominant hand, then with the nondominant hand. This exercise was an outcome from the pilot study and in combination with a traditional prayer ceremony, is how we center participants in body, mind, spirit, and context before our workshops begin.

The focal part of this workshop was the guided visualization and depiction of stress or pain. This form of visualized was devised from similar psychoneuroimmunologal (PNI) interventions; PNI focuses on the relationship between psychological processes and the immune system (Kiecolt-Glaser, McGuire, Robles, & Glaser, 2002). Visualization is one technique that PNI specialists use to help reduce perceptions of pain and levels of stress. The inclusion of art with this technique was meant to enhance the effects through experiential means. Participants depicted their stress or pain using lines, shapes, and color in the center of the circle. They were encouraged to participate in breathing exercises to reflect on this image, rating their level of perceived stress or pain on a 1- to 10-point scale (10 = highest level). Continuing with the breathing exercises, they were prompted to visualize a lesser degree of pain or stress, depicting these responses in consecutive stages or layers moving toward the outside of the circle. Once they had reached their lowest level, participants verbally processed their responses with the group. The breathing exercises were included in the protocol based on the effectiveness of mindful breathing from the MBAT study (Monti et al., 2006). I also completed training in mindfulness meditation to integrate this practice fully.

Although they are related experiences, the rationale for focusing on both stress and pain stemmed from the pilot study, because of the interrelationship among mind, body, spirit, and context (Cross, 1997). After they had identified an area in their healing circle with which they felt connected, participants were directed to create a watercolor painting within a predrawn circle (same size as circle used in guided visualization). In art therapy this is referred to as "response" painting; that is, one is literally responding metaphorically to a visual image or stimulus to deepen the experience. Ideally, the participant elaborates on his or her experience with stress or pain while the fluidity of the watercolor painting induces a state of flow (Csikszentmihalyi, 1992). Flow experiences are intrinsically motivated and imply such a deep level of concentration that the stressors of everyday life are not in one's conscious mind. Our aim was to elicit this state of flow through the soothing quality of watercolor painting and allow participants to experience a self-induced state of relaxation.

At the end of the first workshop, a brief introduction to visual journaling was provided along with a handout of basic guidelines. Participants were encouraged to work in their journals (both artwork and written reflection) for up to 5 minutes a day until the follow-up workshop. Visual journaling was an unexpected outcome from the pilot study. Originally, we handed out visual journals at the end of the study to encourage personal art making. Small-scale journals (5" × 7") were provided to encourage participants to make brief entries rather than feel the need to use up all of the paper. Because of this, we decided to focus on visual journaling in both workshops and as a self-guided process between workshops. Specific art directives were not provided, so that we could track the themes that emerged from this process.

Follow-Up Workshop

This workshop began with the same warm-up of "clearing the air" and saying a prayer for those whose lives have been affected by cancer. Again, this set the stage for the focus of the group. I facilitated discussion of the visual journals and encouraged participants to discuss specific entries and to identify themes or patterns that were apparent to the group. Once themes or patterns were identified, the participants were encouraged to create covers for their journals using natural materials. Supplemental journals were provided to encourage participants to continue this process. The clay task was introduced as a final intervention. We used red clay, per the request of tribal members, as it resembles the natural clay from this community. My co-facilitator Sadie Barbour recommended clay as a final intervention based on the receptiveness of this medium in a needs assessment we conducted with the youth from her community (Basto et al., 2012). Participants were asked to reflect on a theme from either the workshop or visual journaling on which to elaborate throughout the clay process. Art supplies were provided at the end of both workshops to encourage ongoing personal art making as a form of self-care.

Method of Analysis

The artwork and audio recordings from the workshops will be analyzed with the qualitative coding software program NVivo*9© (QSR International, n.d.; findings will be made available in 2012 when the study is completed). This qualitative coding program will enable the researcher to cross-reference the descriptive memos and content tally from the artwork with the transcriptions created from the audio-recorded workshops. This approach was considered in lieu of statistical analysis based on the emphasis on the storying process observed during the pilot study. The coding software will assist in providing more of context for the relationship between the art making and storying process. The expected outcome of the coding analysis is twofold: to understand the interplay between Native American wellness and quality-of-life factors, and to develop a hypothesis that can be tested in a larger efficacy study.

CONCLUSION

Developing partnerships to foster a collaborative relationship is key to any study conducted with diverse groups of people. This was certainly my experience during the inception of the feasibility study. Because I am an American Indian researcher, this does not grant me automatic access to tribal communities; relationships must be nurtured and sustained over time to conduct meaningful research. Moreover, knowing the Native epistemology of a particular tribe is vital to developing sustainable practices. Cultural relevancy is just one aspect of a study that cannot be applied, and what is required in cancer care is development of an understanding of the complexity of Native American wellness.

REFERENCES

American Cancer Society (ACS). (2007). *Cancer facts and figures 2007.* Atlanta: Author.

American Heart Association. (2007). Statistical fact sheet—2007 update: American Indians/ Alaska Natives and cardiovascular disease. Retrieved July 11, 2008, from *www.American heart.org/downloadable/heart/1046238734663fs02Am03.PDF.*

Association of American Indian Physicians. (n.d.). American Indian/Alaskan Native cancer statistics. Retrieved March 24, 2008, from *www.aaip.com/resources/cancer.html.*

Basto, E., Warson, E. A., & Barbour, S. (2012). Exploring American Indian adolescents' needs through a community-driven study. *The Arts in Psychotherapy, 39,* 134–142.

Bien, M. B. (2005). Art therapy as emotional and spiritual medicine for Native Americans living with HIV/AIDS. *Journal of Psychoactive Drugs, 37*(3), 281–292.

Boyer, B. B., Mohatt, G. V., Lardon, C., Plaetke, R., Luick, B. R., Hutchinson, S. H., et al. (2005). Building a community-based participatory research center to investigate obesity and diabetes in Alaska Natives. *International Journal of Circumpolar Health, 64*(3), 281–290.

Centers for Disease Control and Prevention. (2003, August 1). Cancer mortality among

American Indians and Alaska Natives—United States, 1994–1998. *Morbidity and Mortality Weekly Report,* pp. 704–707.

Clarke, A. E. (2005). *Situational analysis: Grounded theory after the postmodern turn.* San Francisco: Sage.

Clegg, L. X., Frederick, P., Hankey, B. F., Chu, K., & Edwards, B. K. (2002). Cancer survival among US Whites and minorities: A SEER (Surveillance, Epidemiology, and End Results) program population-based study [Electronic version]. *Archives of Internal Medicine, 162,* 185–1993.

Clements, F. E. (1932). *Primitive concepts of disease.* Berkeley: University of California Press.

Creswell, J. W. (2007). *Qualitative inquiry and research design: Choosing among the five traditions.* Thousand Oaks, CA: Sage.

Cross, T. (1997). Understanding the relational worldview in Indian families [Part I]. Retrieved January 5, 2011, from *www.nicwa.org/relational_worldview.*

Cross, T. (2001). Spirituality and mental health: A Native American perspective. *Focal Point, 15,* 37–38.

Csikszentmihalyi, M. (Ed.). (1992). *Optimal experience: Psychological studies of flow in consciousness.* Cambridge, UK: Cambridge University Press.

Cueva, M., Kuhnley, R., Stueckermann, C., Lanier, A. P., & McMahon, P. (2010). *Understanding cancer: Cancer education module.* Anchorage, AK: Indian Health Service. Retrieved from *www.ihs.gov/nonmedicalprograms/chr/docs/chrnewcancermanualbinder82710.pdf.*

Curry, N. A., & Kasser, T. (2005). Can coloring mandalas reduce anxiety? *Art Therapy: Journal of the American Art Therapy Association, 22*(2), 81–85.

Dissanayake, E. (1992). *Homo aestheticus: Where art comes from and why.* New York: Free Press.

Dufrene, P. M. (n.d.). *Utilizing the arts for healing from a Native American perspective: Implications for creative arts therapies.* Unpublished manuscript, Purdue University, West Lafayette, IN.

Dufrene, P. M., Coleman, V. D., & Gainor, K. A. (1992). Counseling Native Americans: Guidelines for group process. *Journal for Specialists in Group Work, 17*(4), 229–234.

Duran, E. (2006). *Healing the soul wound: Counseling with American Indians and other Native Peoples.* New York: Teachers College Press.

Egberg Thyme, K., Sundin, E. C., Wiberg, B., Oster, I., Astrom, S., & Lindh, J. (2009). Individual brief art therapy can be helpful for women with breast cancer: A randomized controlled clinical study. *Palliative and Supportive Care, 7*(1), 87–95.

Elkis-Abuhoff, D., Gaydos, M., Goldblatt, R., Chen, M., & Rose, S. (2009). Mandala drawings as an assessment tool for women with breast cancer. *The Arts in Psychotherapy, 36*(4), 231–238.

Espey, D. K., Wu, X. C., Swan, J., Wiggins, C., Jim, M. A., Ward, E., et al. (2007). Annual report to the nation on the status of cancer, 1975–2004, featuring cancer in American Indians and Alaska Natives [Electronic version]. *Cancer, 110*(10), 2119–2152.

Frost, F., Taylor, V., & Fries, E. (1992). Racial misclassification of Native Americans in a surveillance, epidemiology and end results registry. *Journal of National Cancer Institute, 84,* 957–962.

Hays, P. A. (2001). *Addressing cultural complexities in practice: A framework for clinicians and counselors.* Washington, DC: American Psychological Association.

Hays, P. A. (2008). *Addressing cultural complexities in practice: Assessment, diagnosis, and therapy* (2nd ed.). Washington, DC: American Psychological Association.

Herring, R. D. (1997). The creative arts: An avenue to wellness among Native American Indians. *Journal of Humanistic Education and Development, 36*(2), 105–113.

Hodge, D. R., Limb, G. E., & Cross, T. L. (2009). Moving from colonization toward balance and harmony: A Native American perspective on wellness. *Social Work, 54,* 211–219.

Intercultural Cancer Council (ICC). (2012). Cancer fact sheet. Retrieved January 10, 2012, from *iccnetwork.org/cancerfacts/index.html.*

Intercultural Cancer Council. (n.d.). American Indian/Alaska Natives and cancer. Retrieved March 24, 2008, from *www.iccnetwork.org/cancerfacts/icc-cfs2.pdf.*

Kiecolt-Glaser, J. K., McGuire, L., Robles, T. F., & Glaser, R. (2002). Psychoneuroimmunology: Psychological influences on immune function and health. *Journal of Consulting and Clinical Psychology, 70,* 537–547.

Lorance, J. D., Warson, E., & Rosecranz, D. (2008). *Prostate cancer survivors response to coloring a mandala or completing a maze puzzle.* Unpublished Master's thesis. Eastern Virginia Medical School, Norfolk, VA.

Malchiodi, C. A. (1999). *Medical art therapy with adults.* Philadelphia: Jessica Kingsley.

McNiff, S. (2004). *Art heals: How creativity cures the soul.* Boston: Shambhala.

Monti, D. A., Peterson, C., Shakin-Kunkel, E. J., Hauck, W. W., Pequignot, E., Rhodes, L., et al. (2006). A randomized, controlled trial of mindfulness-based art therapy (MBAT) for women with cancer. *Psycho-Oncology, 15,* 363–373.

Moody, J. (1995). Art therapy: Bridging barriers with Native American clients. *Art Therapy: Journal of the American Art Therapy Association, 12*(4), 220–226.

Moon, B. L. (2009). *Existential art therapy: The canvas mirror* (3rd ed.). Springfield, IL: Thomas.

Moon, C. H. (2002). *Studio art therapy: Cultivating the artist identity in the art therapist.* Philadelphia: Jessica Kingsley.

Nainis, N., Paice, J. A., Ratner, J., Wirth, J. H., Lai, J., & Shott, S. (2006). Relieving symptoms in cancer: Innovative use of art therapy. *Journal of Pain and Symptom Management, 31*(2), 162–169.

National Cancer Institute (NCI). (2007). Cancer survivorship research: Estimated U.S. Cancer Prevalence. Retrieved July 14, 2008, from *http://dccps.nci.nih.gov/ocs/prevalence/prevalence.html.*

Office of Cancer Complementary and Alternative Medicine (OCCAM). (n.d.). Retrieved January 6, 2007, from *www.cancer.gov/cam.*

Pfefferbaum, R. L., Pfefferbaum, B., Rhoades, E. R., & Strickland, R. J. (1997). Providing for the health care needs of Native Americans: Policy, programs, procedures, and practices. *American Indian Law Review, 21,* 211–258.

QSR International. (n.d.). NVivo*9. Retrieved February 9, 2011, from *www.qsrinternational.com/products_nvivo.aspx.*

Roubideaux, Y., & Dixon, M. (2001). Health surveillance, research, and information. In M. Dixon & Y. Roubideaux (Eds.), *Promises to keep: Public health policy for American Indians and Alaska Natives in the 21st century* (pp. 253–274). Washington, DC: American Public Health Association.

Rubin, J. A. (2001). *A universal language for healing* [DVD]. Available from *www.expressivemedia.org/f10.html.*

Spielberger, C. D. (1983). *Manual for the State–Trait Anxiety Inventory (STAI).* Palo Alto, CA: Consulting Psychologists Press.

Spielberger, C. D. (1986). *State–Trait Personality Inventory (STPI).* Palo Alto, CA: Consulting Psychologists Press.

Sue, D. W., & Sue, D. (2008). *Counseling the culturally different: Theory and practice* (5th ed.). Hoboken, NJ: Wiley.

U.S. Census Bureau. (2001). The American Indian and Alaska Native population: 2000. Retrieved January 4, 2007, from *www.census.gov/prod/2002pubs/c2kbr01–15.pdf.*

U.S. Department of Health and Human Service's Office of Minority Health. (n.d.). American Indian/Alaska Native profile. Retrieved September 23, 2008, from *www.omhrc.gov/templates/browse.aspx?lvl=3&lvlid=26.*

Vogel, V. J. (1970). *American Indian medicine.* New York: Ballantine Books.

Warson, E. A. (2009). Art-based narrative inquiry with American Indian breast cancer survivors. *Dissertation Abstracts International A: Humanities and Social Sciences, 70*(2), 487.

Warson, E. A. (2012). Healing pathways: Art therapy for American Indian cancer survivors and their family members. *Journal of Cancer Education, 27*(1), 47–56.

CHAPTER 12

In Body and Soul

Art Therapy with Socially Excluded People Living with HIV and AIDS

Marta Tagarro
Susana Catarino

This chapter presents two different art therapy interventions in Lisbon, Portugal, for socially excluded people (e.g., drug addicts, prostitutes, the homeless), including people with HIV and those in terminal stages of AIDS. It also explores the advantages of using art therapy with people living with HIV/AIDS and explains a model used in Portugal and theoretical concepts behind interventions. A psychoeducational semi-open-group intervention and an open-group intervention with terminal patients with AIDS using an art therapy approach are described, and examples are presented to illustrate "AIDS in the Soul." Finally, the chapter concludes with reflections on how creativity and art therapy are important with this population, and why holistic interventions are richer because they reach the physical, psychological, and social aspects of the individual.

HIV/AIDS AND BIOPSYCHOSOCIAL IMPLICATIONS

The news of testing positive for HIV triggers a profound alteration in the world of an individual, the guarantee of a healthy future disappears and the disease remains as background in the life of that person (Field & Kruger, 2008). Although in the initial phase the disease can be latent, with an absence of symptoms, after some time the manifestation of symptoms of fatigue, pain, peripheral nerve dysfunction, nausea, loss of appetite, headaches, among others, begins (Car & Cooper, 2000, cited in Rao et al., 2009). Later, chronic infections, opportunist infections, and serious neoplasms take place and culminate in the individual's death (André, 2005).

Receiving an HIV-positive diagnosis can therefore cause very stressful reactions and involve radical changes in the way subjects see themselves and their lives (Merz, 2007). Not only does the person receive the news that a disease can cause his or her death but the stigmatizing social representations associated with the disease are also realized (Thery, 1998, cited in André, 2005). The stigma and isolation provided by the socio-cultural environment may trigger psychopathological symptoms. Reis (2008) points out that after one gains knowledge of the infection, one experiences discrimination and obstacles to the accessibility of social and health services. People with HIV also have difficulties related to family environments, social relationships, job accessibility, housing, their financial system, and education. Managing the secret of the disease invariably affects relationships the individual establishes in the work environment, becoming an added source of stress.

Changes in routines and body image also occur. The regular intake of antiretroviral therapy (ART) or highly active antiretroviral therapy (HAART) medication brings the first sensation of being sick to an individual who previously may not have had symptoms of the disease (Berg, Michelson, & Safren, 2007, cited in Merz, 2007). One's professional life may also be affected due to the decrease of resistance and excessive fatigue. Side effects of the medication also become extremely stressful (Reid & Courtney, 2007, cited in Merz, 2007). A lipodystrophy syndrome, a frequent side effect, affects the metabolism and brings some physical changes that have negative consequences for the subject. Body image is altered, the subject becomes less attractive, and the physical aspect may even betray the HIV-positive state due to facial alterations, since there is a loss or gain of fat below the cheekbones (Behrens & Schmidt, 2006, cited in Merz, 2007).

The way individuals face these vast changes greatly influences their psychological and physical state. Olley et al. (2004, cited in Field & Kruger, 2008) state that people who believe their behavior directly influences the realization of their objectives have internal control of their actions, whereas people who believe that their behavior does not influence personal realization of their objectives are externally controlled, which contributes to feelings of depression and helplessness.

It is possible that people who believe that their personal actualization does not depend on themselves, but on some external control, develop a greater spiritual side. There is a necessity to believe in something superior that can bring hope to the subject and explain the reason for becoming sick. Kremer, Ironson, and Kaplan (2009) realized that discovering oneself to be a carrier of the virus becomes a turning point in one's life, providing a shift in priorities, an increase in altruism, greater care for relationships with others, and a healthier lifestyle. After becoming aware of the diagnosis there is a tendency in some individuals toward increased spirituality and a belief that one has been chosen to have the disease by a superior power.

Therefore, there are many factors at play following the subject's HIV-positive diagnosis. After the initial phase of shock, alterations in the subject's routines occur, and corporal symptoms and even physical alterations begin to appear. The social stigma weighs on one greatly, deeply affecting one's psychological state. The isolation, depression, and helplessness are symptoms that often cause individuals to resort to technical or spiritual help to deal better with the pain. It is important for helping professionals to be conscious of the multiplicity of problematic factors in order to give adequate interdisciplinary responses.

ART THERAPY AND HIV/AIDS

Stuckey and Nobel (2010) conducted a literature review in an attempt to understand the connection between artistic creation and health. Based on several studies, they concluded that creative involvement contributes to the improvement of a variety of physiological and psychological aspects in sick individuals, improving their state of health. Through creativity and imagination, individuals are able to concentrate their identity and strength toward finding a cure. Sometimes the disease itself can have a fundamental role in the search for a creative activity. Rao et al. (2009) noted that the physical and psychological symptoms of patients improved after art therapy sessions. The results suggest that art therapy can improve people's capacity to deal with the disease, and that physical symptoms may be more sensitive to change than psychological symptoms.

   Therefore, we infer that a creative therapeutic approach develops creative potential that in turn allows for change and the creation of new perspectives. The psychological effects of creative expression are manifested in positive moods, feelings of confidence and self-sufficiency, greater capacity for problem solving, less anxiety, and the capacity to adapt actively to the surrounding world (Field & Kruger, 2008). Creative individuals often seem to possess the necessary resources that allow feelings and internal experiences to come in contact with external reality, and enable the responses to be flexible and suitable to the situations. When the response to the situation is less rigid, there is greater and more satisfactory adaptation to reality (King & Pope, 1999, cited in Field & Kruger, 2008). Creative activity allows the modification of emotions and contributes to positive moods, feelings of confidence and self-sufficiency, and cognitive development, which in turn allows for greater problem-solving capacity that results from convergent thinking (Averill, 1999; Isen & Daubman, 1984; and Montgomery & Hodges, 2004, all cited in Field & Kruger, 2008). These benefits apply to the various facets of a person's life, including perception of his or her body and physical well-being, as well as the ways of handling the disease.

   From a psychodynamic point of view, material from the primary process may be examined, experienced, and transformed in order to permit new insights and new forms of connecting to the world. By express feelings and fantasies and containing the tension that results from some creations, individuals gain confidence to reformulate their positions in regard to the reality in which they live. This requires the capacity to portray the experience in images and words, and to give voice to not only the internal but also the external world (Holm-Hadulla, 1996, cited in Field & Kruger, 2008).

   Bien (2005) realized that art therapy is beneficial to the people suffering from HIV/AIDS who have difficulty in not only managing their emotions but also speaking about them. Also Borgman (2002, cited in Stuckey & Nobel, 2010) affirmed that art helps people express experiences that are too difficult to verbalize. Merz (2007) noted that art therapy can be conducted in a crisis intervention context, immediately after a positive diagnosis of HIV. In our experience, it can also be used as a long-term intervention, with the objective of improving the quality of individuals' lives. More importantly, art therapy is oriented toward action, which means that patients have an active role in the sessions. This approach helps them search for internal resources and gain the strength not only to accept and deal with the disease but also to discover vital new sources of energy and power.

THE POLYMORPHIC MODEL

Ruy de Carvalho (2001) conceptualized the "polymorphic model" as a multidimensional approach to how therapists decide what type of intervention is more appropriate. It involves focus on one or more therapeutic aspects of art: (1) creation (experimental art therapy); (2) learning (psychoeducational or thematic art therapy); (3) expression (integrative art therapy); and/or (4) attribution of deeper meaning (analytic–expressive art therapy). For example, psychoeducational or thematic art therapy is a semidirective or structured directive approach surrounding a theme, in which the art therapist establishes a work plan based on thematic workshops (Carvalho, 2009). It is intended to help individuals acquire certain skills through artistic techniques and resources. This type of approach is group-based and presupposes psychotherapy in which the art therapist assumes the role of leader in order to promote relationships among the individuals of the group. In contrast, experiential art therapy emphasizes creative expression as primal, and attention is given to the potential of the techniques. This facilitates communication and patients' discovery of their internal worlds through imagination and creative development (Carvalho, 2009). Therapists may use various strategies to promote communication among the members (verbal and nonverbal communication) in the group dynamic.

HIV IN THE BODY: ART THERAPY WITH PEOPLE LIVING WITH HIV

After we conducted a needs assessment in a day care center for people living with HIV, we determined that psychoeducational or thematic art therapy would be the most pertinent approach to take with this target audience. The members of this group participated in an interview and were asked to make a free drawing. We explained to each individual that he or she was free to be part of the group, but that the rules, such as confidentiality, would have to be respected. A questionnaire in the second meeting evaluated clients' quality of life, self-esteem, conceptions about HIV, and social and affective skills.

Through these interviews we realized that these individuals also had various problems with social exclusion. Many were separated from their families for a variety of reasons: family abandonment after knowing of the disease, history of prostitution, homelessness or drug addiction. Some of these individuals never had a family or were abandoned by their family in their childhood. We also noticed that their abilities to have insights were reduced, because most presented with poor skills in elaborating feelings and thoughts. Therefore, it appeared to us that the psychoeducational or thematic approach focusing on skills training would be best for the intervention with this population.

A semistructured group was organized, and intervention objectives that would respond to the previously discussed necessities were defined. The general objective of this project was to enhance psychosocial skills. For this objective, various skills were defined. We present the specific objectives and the skills in Table 12.1.

As an example, two of the various sessions where Objective 2 was central are presented. When we speak about corporality of an HIV patient, we refer to something that raises a variety of feelings. Reflections about a body that betrayed the person are painful. A previously full-functioning body that now has limitations brings on a time of mourning for what used to be and attempts to deal with the new (physical) body psychologically. Also, the psychological being in the body has been altered. Body-related feelings must be addressed, and the opportunity to work on self-image through reparation processes through creative expression must be provided.

In order to illustrate this idea, we describe two sessions in which clay was offered because of its potentialities to deal with body issues. Sholt and Gavron (2006) observe that working with clay relates to primary ways of communication and expression and at times raises memories connected to touch and movement. Thus, working with clay can function as a central window to unconscious, nonverbal representations and be used as a facilitating element for people who have difficulty expressing themselves verbally.

We developed the following themes for the group: "What do I value in my body?" and "What can I do to value it more?" The group sessions began with welcoming clients and allowing group members to share current concerns and emergent topics. The theme of the session was then presented (in this case, "What Do I Value in My Body?) and each participant was given time to speak about personal objectives and expectations regarding that theme. The first practical exercise followed: body expression with free

TABLE 12.1. Specific Objectives and Skills Development

Objectives	Skills
Specific Objective 1: To promote personal value and organization	• Check one's self-esteem • Ability to deal with stress factors and go beyond autonomy limitations • Ability to establish significant social and affective relationships
Specific Objective 2: To develop consciousness and acceptance of the disease	• Increase body consciousness and relaxation • Value the body • Deal with the disease • Lead a healthy life
Specific Objective 3: To promote skills for the elaboration of adaptation and life-planning strategies	• Develop a personal organization program

movements to the sound of music and interaction with other members of the group. We chose this technique to start since body expression and music can create a sense of body relaxation and flexibility. The participants had an opportunity to relax, respond to the sound of the music, and gain a greater consciousness of their bodies.

Following this experience, we suggested exercises to help them get used to the clay—kneading, feeling the clay's texture, touching the clay with their eyes closed, and touching it with different pressures. This technique enabled them to relieve unconscious tensions; various sensations may surface when contact is made with this material, and use of clay is also a form of stimulating the senses. Heimlich and Mark (1990, cited in Sholt & Gavron, 2006) referred to the importance of touching the clay, because the physical impressions left in the material generate greater involvement between subject and piece. These marks can be interpreted as the marks the person leaves in the real world.

Following this activity, we suggested that the participants model that which they valued in their body. Giving form to the clay helped to promote a sense of empowerment and self-worth in the participants as they examined more closely aspects of their bodies. This experience calls forth individuals' reflections about their bodies and themselves through modeling with their own hands. Last was verbal sharing of what was created, and we requested that each person speak about what the image meant to him or her, as well as feelings and insights related to the theme. For example, 38-years-old N. stated, "The brain of my figure doesn't work, nothing in him works," projecting his feelings regarding himself to what he had created. Sixty-three-year-old R. valued the hands, saying that they are very useful in her daily life, underlining her capacity to create and be proactive in life.

The next session began with the usual welcoming conversation, followed by a presentation of the work theme for that day: "What can I do to value my body more?" The members of the group reflected about the previous session's theme and how, they found their creations had changed since the last meeting (due to the properties of the clay, which is damaged when it dries if the pieces are not baked). N.'s creation became headless; it did not stay together. N. was disappointed and stated: "Headless. I never saw anyone headless. It does not look like a person, it looks like an astronaut." R.'s creation, which had been valued for its hands, had in fact lost its hands.

This confrontation with the clay pieces created the previous week allowed each person to face his or her own personal fragility. Experiencing reparation using the same matter (clay) enabled participants to transform the figures into something more consistent with themselves and to access their own capacity for internal reparation. For example, in the previous session, 33-years-old C. characterized his creation as "a humped back doll, all crooked. It doesn't have arms and it has a wide back. It is tired." During this session, C., the only person who found his piece still intact, stated: "Mine was the only one that did not break. It was mocked but it held up." Sholt and Gavron (2006) state that working with clay allows individuals to find both self-constructive and destructive aspects in psychological change and identity formation processes. N., who "lost his head," said, "I went to the dollar store and bought a head" (Figure 12.1). This affirmation indicated some depreciation of N.'s belief in his cognitive and intellectual capacities, as well as his capacity to believe in his potential for effective and gratifying internal reparation.

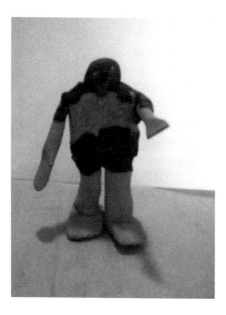

FIGURE 12.1. N.'s creation.

After repair of the clay objects', participants were asked to add plasticine [a form of malleable clay that comes in several colors] and glitter to them. Plasticine is very flexible and does not harden; it allows the individual to create freely and transform the object during the process. There is the possibility to mix colors, to put them together and to separate them. Glitter, with all its colors and sparkles, fortifies the life attributed to the object, thus reflecting one's interior sparkle. Participants reported: "An A. with greater value, a more colorful life" (55-year-old A.) and "I made a scarf and a necklace in order to feel prettier" (see R.'s clay object in Figure 12.2). Collie, Bottorff, and Long (2006, cited in Stuckey & Nobel, 2010) state that art can be a refuge for intense emotions related to

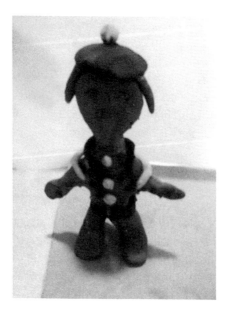

FIGURE 12.2. R.'s creation.

the disease. Imagination has no limits when creative forms to express pain are found. Working with clay in particular can be a powerful method to help people though tactile involvement with the object, and can facilitate verbal communication and cathartic release, revealing unconscious material and symbols that cannot be expressed through words. A. noticed in the end, "I did not remember to make the eyes or a mouth," and looking at the structure he created, said: "It is very fragile, just as I am."

Many emotions related to living with HIV can be difficult to verbalize. The expression though other mediums can be the solution to liberating internal tensions, sharing feelings, and discovering issues that were previously unknown. In addition to this, the very process of creation can create a sense of relief, and the final product can help the subject confront issues relating to the disease. C. stated, "I also didn't want to make the face because of the AIDS. Because the blood is everywhere and in the head as well."

AIDS AND THE SOUL: EXPERIENTIAL ART THERAPY

This section emphasizes the importance of creating art therapy groups of an experiential nature for institutionalized people living with AIDS. The open groups that we describe began in 2007, in a residence for people living with AIDS. The first art therapy groups with people living with AIDS in Portugal were implemented in this residence in Lisbon, and provided the development of internships in the following years. Some of the diagnoses that characterize this population include chronic hepatitis C infection, secondary epilepsy, thrombocytopenia, encephalopathy, hemophilia A, ganglion tuberculosis with aftereffects (memory alterations and left hemiparesis), cerebral toxoplasmosis, pneumocystosis, stroke with aftereffects, deep vein thrombosis of the left inferior member, HIV-2 infection (C3-CDC stage), and melanoderma. In the session described nine people between 35 and 73 years old (six males and three females) participated.

The sessions took place in the residence's garden, which was wheelchair-accessible and more compatible for art therapy groups. The exterior space allowed physical distance from the residence, because it placed individuals in contact with nature and gave them a feeling of greater freedom. It simultaneously permitted privacy because it allowed distance from others. It allowed other adult day care center helpers at the residence to see the creative capacity of the patients, because the helpers were often not present during patients' sharing. It also helped to educate day care center helpers about the need for an appropriate and confidential space for patients to engage in creative work and share feelings about their illness through art.

Finally, while the garden was not a traditional space for art therapy, it was a positive space for participants to reflect and share personal discoveries, and to strengthen connections with the center's staff. The helpers were able to see the capabilities of the participants and their personal efforts to create ("Look what they can do; they do in fact surprise us"). They were at times invited to join in a musical moment at the end of a session, providing agreeable moments with the patients, and beneficial reinforcement of their relationship, which usually was characterized only by moments of pain, grief, suffering, anguish, loneliness, and isolation.

Example of Group Session

Sitting around a table in the residence's garden and listening to Feng Shui music, we suggested that participants close their eyes, listen to the music, feel the breeze, let themselves be taken/transported anyplace they wanted, and let go and enjoy the experience. We encouraged a moment of silence and asked participants to keep their eyes closed, to leave everything behind and "dive" into another space, leaving the mind to wander. They were told to leave that location and to bring what they found significant with them, to gradually return to the garden and slowly open their eyes. With their eyes open and with paper and pastel pencils in front of them, we suggested that participants freely express what they would like to share about where they had been in their imaginations.

After the drawing experience was completed, participants were asked to talk about the places they drew. For example, L. wanted to talk about his old house, where he used to work, and the happy memories he has, not wanting to refer to anything else. Showing great tension, what he remembers from this space he swore never to talk about it again. He mentions after a brief pause that it was in this place that his wife and 7-year-old son died in a fire, while he was working close by. All the people in the group verbalized phrases of encouragement, of friendship and understanding in response to L.'s story. C. talked about his drawing: "a multimillionaire in front of a cemetery," having written "the hour of truth, Amen" (Figure 12.3), and asking, "What happens after you die?"

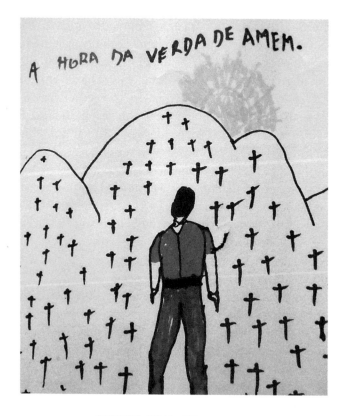

FIGURE 12.3. C.'s creation.

Following the sharing session, one of the patients expressed discontentment about the negativity in the group. He spoke of Jesus of Nazareth, because he had just lost a friend and was not ready to explore the death theme, challenging the group to be positive and to live their lives with hope. F. shared her drawing about the circus with joy, making a connection with her daughters, who were clowns. J. talked about his paradise, a place of peace and kindness. N. spoke about ocean and mountain sights that transmit hope and well-being. L. drew a big heart on the wallpaper and enunciated the names he wanted to place inside, as if fixing the internal pain he initially described and curing it with new affections, new friendships, and a new family. One of the patients wanted to sing a song with the following lyrics: "Let your life be painted by all colors. Let it be painted, let yourself be taken." Everyone then reached for available musical instruments—various types of maracas and tambourines—to celebrate the unity of the group (Figure 12.4).

At the end of the session participants said the following:

"L., you will forget the past and live the present in the company of your friends."
"Unity and Team Spirit, whether we like it or not, it is our family."
"Happiness is being loved and loving others."
"Unity, fraternity. Awesome."
"I wish good health to all."
"God exists."
"Willpower to reach our goals."

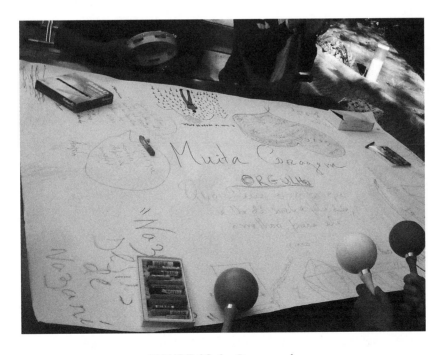

FIGURE 12.4. Group work.

"Friendship for all."
"Love for your neighbor and for yourself."

Guided fantasy, also called "guided imagery," can be a helpful intervention for people living with AIDS, because it allows a feeling of freedom from the physical body that imprisons them through pain and other symptoms. The use of guided fantasy helps to access imagination, memories, and forgotten or negated feelings. For example, L. shared that the music and imagery took him to the place where his wife and 7-year-old son died in a household fire. Previously, this was an experience he had refused to talk about or share, a secret that he always kept to himself.

In using music for guided imagery, it is essential to choose it carefully, keeping in mind the characteristics of the music and the target population. This particular application of music and imagery encouraged body relaxation, access to memories, and rejuvenation. Materials are also important. Pastel pencils are easily used by people with manual dexterity and movement challenges because of their fluidity and ease of control. They help simultaneously to reinforce the creative capacity and the potential for self-realization. Expression on the large paper occupying the entire surface of the table encourages participation on a "common ground." In other words, it reinforces intergroup sharing while facilitating individual expression. For example, other people expressed their support of L. by asking to write phrases such as "lots of courage" and "God bless him and give him luck and happiness; the best for him."

These art therapy groups with people living with AIDS have revealed important developments at different levels: increasing connections between staff and patients; promoting friendship and closer relationships; and motivating participation in visits to museums, shows, and summer camp. Participants became more conscientiousness and educated about taking responsibility for the rigorous administration of antiretroviral drugs and thus experienced a better quality of life, and social and spiritual well-being. Individually and collectively they became more self-confident and learned to share more deeply their emotions, and religious and spiritual beliefs.

CONCLUSION

HIV/AIDS is not limited to the physical disease, it also involves a holistic perspective that includes multidisciplinary interventions with this population. Weiser (1996) underscores the fundamental link between body and mind, and the strong connection between the emotional state and the immunological system in fighting the infection. In order to be effective, the therapeutic interventions must take into account the specificities of this population. Both medical intervention and nonpharmacological intervention are of extreme importance, so that the individual can maintain and/or regain emotional or social equilibrium. Art therapy is increasingly being accepted as complementary to medical intervention in the relief and treatment of symptoms associated with HIV/AIDS, as well as other illnesses (Nainis et al., 2006, cited in Rao et al., 2009). We believe that art therapy is indispensable as a complement to traditional antiretrovirals and other pharmaceutical treatments.

Art therapy for people living with HIV/AIDS is emerging as an approach that is able to free patients from the anguish, fears, and emotional trauma associated with the disease, and that enhances personal discovery and interpersonal learning. It is a potent weapon in both the psychosocial treatment of infection, and the stigmatization and social exclusion often found in HIV/AIDS patients. Creativity and empowerment are ultimately antidotes to physical, mental, and social devastation.

REFERENCES

André, M. (2005). *Adesão à terapêutica em pessoas infectadas pelo VIH/SIDA* [Adherence to therapy in people living with HIV/AIDS]. Lisboa: Stória Editores.

Bien, M. B. (2005). Art therapy as emotional and spiritual medicine for Native Americans living with HIV/AIDS. *Journal of Psychoactive Drugs, 37*(3), 281–292.

Carvalho, R. (2001). A arte de sonhar ser [The art of dreaming to be]. *Colecção Imagens da Transformação, 8.*

Carvalho, R. (2009). Art therapy/psychotherapy: The Portuguese perspective: From institutions to private practice. In SIPE (Ed.), *Jubilé de la SIPE (1959–2009): From yesterday to now* (pp. 121–129). Paris: Société Internationale de Psychopathologie de l'Expression et d'Art-Thérapie.

Field, W., & Kruger, C. (2008). The effect of na art psychotherapy intervention on levels of depression and health locus of control orientations experienced by black women living with HIV. *South African Journal of Psychology, 38*(3), 467–478.

Kremer, H., Ironson, G., & Kaplan, L. (2009). The fork in the road: HIV as a potential positive turning point and the role of spirituality. *AIDS Care, 21*(3), 368–377.

Merz, R. (2007). Art therapy and AIDS. *Music Therapy Today, 8*(3), 446–461.

Rao, D., Nainis, N., Williams, L., Langner, D., Eisin, A., & Paice, J. (2009). Art therapy for relief of symptoms associated with HIV/AIDS. *AIDS Care, 21*(1), 64–69.

Reis, A. (2008). Sida, pobreza e desenvolvimento humano [AIDS, poverty, and human development]. *Cidade Solidária, 20,* 52–55.

Reynolds, F. (2003). Conversations about creativity and chronic illness: I. Textile artists coping with long-term health problems reflect on the origins of their interest in art. *Creativity Research Journal, 4,* 393–407.

Sholt, M., & Gravon, T. (2006). Therapeutic qualities of clay-work in art therapy and psychotherapy: A review. *Journal of the American Art Therapy Association, 23*(2), 66–72.

Stuckey, H. L., & Nobel, J. (2010). The connection between art, healing, and public health: A review of current literature. *Framing Health Matters, 100*(2), 254–263.

Weiser, J. (1996). Psychosocial consequences of living with HIV/AIDS. *Social Worker, 64*(4), 18–33.

CHAPTER 13

Art Therapy
with HIV-Positive/AIDS Patients

Luis Formaiano

Setting up an art therapy workshop for HIV-positive/AIDS patients proved to be no easy task. My interest in the subject began when two HIV-positive/AIDS patients came to my practice for psychotherapy within a few days of each other. After a few sessions I began to realize that behind the medical aspects of the disease lay a complex thread of psychosocial, cultural, and ethical issues, making it a challenging subject to be addressed through art therapy. While it is comparatively easy to identify a wide variety of target groups for an art therapy project, one of the most serious problems I encountered was a perceived lack of visibility of the HIV-positive/AIDS population. This could be attributed to the very negative impact that the infection has had in society ever since its appearance, leading most importantly to stigmatization and discrimination.

In Argentina, as in most other countries in the world, no HIV-positive/AIDS patient is obliged to disclose his or her serological status. Thus, from the outset I understood that it would be quite a challenge to contact potential clients and get the project off the ground. The first art therapy meeting finally took place in July 2004. As news of the workshop began to circulate in specific peer Internet networks, and those who attended the first sessions began to recommend it and inform their doctors, the workshop attracted increasing attention. My work with various nongovernmental organizations (NGOs) that dealt with prevention, testing, and treatment for the virus also contributed to this, placing the focus on the innovative way in which art therapy could contribute to dealing with such a delicate subject.

Despite all the advances made in treating the disease, which have undoubtedly improved quality of life, stigmatization still remains, as do the psychological effects of the disease. This is why I believed that art therapy for PLWHA (people living with HIV-positive/AIDS) would prove to be an effective tool in addressing such a sensitive and complex issue. This chapter includes a description of the theoretical framework on which the project is based, a review of previous experiences worldwide, and the general characteristics of this particular project. This is followed by a short case study and the final conclusions.

THEORETICAL FRAMEWORK

The main goals of the art therapy project focus on the following points:

1. *Exploring healthy behaviors and self-care.* The perception of risk is a central characteristic here (Fernandez, Castro, & Pérez, 2002). With an already infected population, secondary prevention must be strengthened in order to avoid possible infection with a different strain of the virus, which might prove to be drug resistant and lead to failure of the treatment. A further issue is adherence to the treatment, that is, each patient's degree of compliance and commitment to the treatment is a suitable topic to be addressed by art therapy, since various external obstacles demotivate a patient and could cause abandonment of the treatment.

2. *Reinforcing self-esteem.* In the case of newly infected clients a positive diagnosis may provoke a decrease in their own self-worth and make them generally feel guilt-ridden and angry. Self-esteem is considered to be the immune system of the conscience (Branden, 1995). Thus, rebuilding self-esteem is an ongoing task with a PLWHA, since daily interactions put it to the test, especially when beginning a new relationship (how and when to address the subject), or when applying for a new job, with the fear of an HIV-positive result being revealed in the medical examinations for the post.

3. *Developing a sense of play.* For Winnicott (2005), creativity in a child or adult is freely expressed at play. Exploring the use of different art materials in order to create their own images allows PLWHA to experiment with different viewpoints in the safe environment of the art therapy room, without fear of being judged. In many cases, valuable childhood memories are recovered in the process and can be helpful in counteracting any painful memories associated with the time of infection. For PLWHA, there is generally a *before* and an *after* infection when the vision such clients had of their own lives changes dramatically, and they are able to incorporate new values and search for a deeper spiritual connection with life. Therefore, stimulation of potentialities would facilitate spontaneity and creativity, establishing the grounds for art therapy activities.

4. *Feeling dignified and becoming empowered.* Artwork created by PLWHA can produce a greater sense of dignity. Depending on the stage of the infection, different emotions prevail, and since art has the power to help clients gain a greater insight into themselves (Malchiodi, 1998), levels of self-satisfaction vary and prompt the search for new patterns of behavior that can be safely experienced in the process of art making.

5. *Managing psychological symptoms.* Other aspects considered central to art therapy exploration include two specific psychic symptoms suffered by most PLWHA: dealing with feelings of anxiety and mood disorders, particularly depression. Anxiety can

originate in the uncertainty associated with living with a virus in the body and the now improbable, thanks to current HAART (highly active antiretroviral treatment), progress of the infection to AIDS and the possibility of death. The future always poses a threat, and for some clients it is still very difficult to see light at the end of the tunnel, especially for those who regard the infection as a punishment.

Depression, on the other hand, appears as a desire to escape from the world, as alterations in mood, feelings of emptiness and a loss of self-esteem, sexual inhibition, a lack of interest in the performance of daily activities, and strong feelings of guilt. It is usually reinforced by a refusal to accept a positive diagnosis and a low CD4 count result (immune system markers) (Petrak & Miller, 2002).

CHALLENGES FOR ART THERAPISTS WORKING WITH PLWHA

Art therapists and others working with this population must continually update their knowledge of the subject, since great advances have been made in the 30 years since the epidemic first appeared. It is advisable to be accurately informed on the forms of transmission of the virus and to become familiar with certain medical terms, since during the activity clients tend to interact and share information that could prove valuable to the therapist in preparing future art therapy activities. It is essential for art therapists constantly to reexamine the ways in which they relate to clients. This is especially true in the case of recent infections, when some individuals who tend to be in a state of shock or emotional confusion experience guilt and shame, and might be in need of contention.

Consideration should also be given to those HIV-positive clients with an undetectable viral load who have been co-infected with the hepatitis C virus. Research into the latter has failed to keep pace with the advances made in treating HIV infection. Available hepatitis C treatments have had little or no success, meaning that many clients might experience complications. This is a further variable to be considered in art therapy activities, because, in these cases, this virus can prove to be as destructive as the HIV virus itself.

One of the key aspects of working with this population is handling countertransference. Art therapists must examine their own fears regarding the infection. However, an understanding of the ways of transmission does not guarantee that they will be able to act appropriately with their clients. Therapists' own prejudices must also be examined, since they might be working with a population that comprises mostly, but not exclusively, homosexual men, drug users, sexual workers, and so forth. Practitioners must also consider their reactions (based on religious beliefs and moral values, for instance) to the practices involved in the transmission of the virus, of which unsafe sex and drug abuse are the most common.

Other factors, such as the reassurance of confidentiality (Liebmann, 2004), are also of vital importance. Over time, and as a result of working on particular themes, some patients might offer information on their personal experiences from the time of infection, thus reinforcing key moments in their life histories.

HISTORY OF ART THERAPY AND HIV-POSITIVE/AIDS PATIENTS

Art therapy interventions on this subject can be traced as far back as the 1980s, a few years after the onset of the epidemic. Particularly relevant cases are the experiences recorded by David and Sageman (1987) at Bellevue Hospital in New York; the first art therapy groups coordinated by Bartholomew (1998) at the London Lighthouse—a residential and support center for AIDS patients—in 1989; a 2-year project run by Beaver (1998) that ended in 1993 with prisoners with HIV and AIDS at the Scottish Prison Service; and a single art therapy session registered by Michele Wood (1998) in 1990, with a man dying of AIDS.

With the closing of the 20th century a project started in Germany by Merz, the "HIV Art Project," addressed many of the issues that affect the quality of life of PLWHA. Art therapist Merz (2006) carried this project into the new century and wondered, as part of her 2006 doctoral studies, if HIV specific parameters are actually visible in HIV-positive/AIDS patients' paintings. In 2000, a community hospital in Champaign, Illinois, the Carle Hospital, launched a pilot expressive arts program for HIV-positive/AIDS patients coordinated by Kellman (Mitchell, 2005). Since 2001, the charity run by volunteers under the coordination of Brown and Gurney, MADaboutART, which combines art therapy for children living with HIV in South Africa with arts-based workshops in U.K. schools, has been challenging the stigma associated with HIV (Elliot, 2006). Since 2003, the United Nations Children's Fund (UNICEF) has sponsored an art therapy camp for children in Thailand, run by the NGO We Understand Group, which stresses the need to rebuild the kids' self-esteem and confidence (Few, 2007).

In 2006, art and photo therapist Weiser revisited her 1996 article on HIV-positive/AIDS in view of the changes and challenges posed by the new drug therapies. Weiser (2006) has been a long-term researcher in this field. In 2009, a randomized clinical trial on symptom management for PLWHA was conducted by Rao, Nainis, Williams, Langner, Eisin, and Paice (2009), who concluded by stating how beneficial one session of art therapy was for those who participated in it. In 2009, art therapist Saunders launched an art therapy project at the Haven Youth Center in Philadelphia, raising HIV/AIDS awareness among young people by working on the self-evaluation that facilitates self-acceptance (Rollins, 2009). In 2010, Dr. Alex Leão Flores Xavier, who has been working with AIDS clients in Rio de Janeiro, recorded his findings and experience in a monograph (personal communication, November 2010).

EVIDENCE-BASED PRACTICE AND ART THERAPY

In my particular case, on the one hand, I chose to follow the Art Therapy Level of Evidence (Brooker et al., 2005, cited by Gilroy, 2006), which centers on case studies, art-based and collaborative studies, among other sources. On the other hand, my choice of qualitative research was based on the fact that it allows for a holistic view that takes the following parameters into account:

1. Questionnaires (provided to each client at the end of every project).
2. Discourse analysis and client observation (recorded in my transcripts of the art therapy session, which I print and bind every year for permanent consultation).
3. Content analysis (reviewing the images produced by each client and contextualizing them within the whole set of images of each client's production) that considers changes in symbolic representations and in the formal elements within them.

I favored case studies due to the fact that they are conducted within the same population and their members share the same pathology, which allows for cumulative evidence based on the efficacy of the art therapy interventions (Gilroy, 2006). This approach will inevitably result in cohort studies, since at this stage of the project I am able to document the appearance and frequency of particular patterns in the images produced.

GENERAL CHARACTERISTICS OF THE PROJECT

In a large part of Argentine society, the social representation of HIV-positive/AIDS is a basically conservative (Kornblit et al., 2000), commonly held belief. PLWHA are seen as being responsible for having contracted the virus, and this amply justifies the need for those individuals to avoid openly disclosing their serological status. The infection took hold in what originally was considered to be a risk groups (i.e., homosexual males). However, according to the Joint United Nations Program on HIV/AIDS (UNAIDS), recent statistics show that by 2009, of 110,000 PLWHA in Argentina, 36,000 were women over age 15.

Due to these prejudices, the only places where the issue can be freely addressed are the departments of infectology in hospitals, peer groups, meetings organized by support networks, and psychology consulting rooms. In most other places, the person who declares that he or she is living with the virus risks discrimination, mainly based on ignorance. Thirty years on, little appears to have changed.

For the purposes of my project, the results of a recent research study, sponsored by UNAIDS and presented at the National AIDS Conference in the province of San Juan, Argentina, during the last week of August 2011, were of particular significance (Lipcovich, 2011). The study measured both the external and internal "stigma index." I found the latter to be especially relevant since the study revealed that 43.8% of interviewees said that they blamed themselves for having contracted the virus, while 39.4% reported "low self-esteem." Of the total, 35.9% said that they felt guilty, and 27.8% claimed to have feelings of shame.

THE ART THERAPY WORKSHOP IN ACTION: INTERVENTIONS AND THEMES

The art therapy workshop is a mixed, open group of an average of 14 clients per week, both heterosexual and homosexual, ages 18–60 years. The first session of the workshop was held July 3, 2004, and although clients tend to come and go, some have been attending the workshop since the first meeting. They represent the "memory" of the activity and have helped to build the "myth" that tells the history of the workshop from day one, with anecdotes, their impressions of the first artwork they produced, and the ongoing remembrance of the three regular clients who have since died, although only one of these died from AIDS-related causes.

Those who came to the activity on that very first day were clearly unsure as to why they were coming or what they were going to find, although I had previously held a preliminary meeting with a small group at an HIV prevention center. However, the general atmosphere was one of curiosity mixed with a certain excitement. Some of them recognized each other from visits to health centers or hospitals, which lent to the event the feeling of a reunion between old friends but in a totally different setting, an art therapy room. I knew that my role as art therapist would be to provide suitable stimuli to allow them to connect with their inner worlds and their relationships (Fernandez Cao & Martinez Diez, 2006). However, there was something else that had to do with the particular characteristics of the group: A bond of trust had to be built with these clients. It would have to be articulated within specific parameters, such as understanding that after a positive test result, a PLWHA might feel that his or her life would never be the same again, and that for such a client establishing new relationships might involve feelings ranging from plain rejection to conditional acceptance by a new partner. As a member of a helping profession, the art therapist needs to promote self-care and, through the production of artwork by PLWHA, make it easier for them to face fears, doubts, uncertainties, and prejudices.

From the outset, the idea was to meet for eight to 10 meetings, each of which would include clearly defined themes with objectives in keeping with the spirit of the workshop. This would facilitate group dynamics and lend a sense of purpose to the overall work. Themes and/or projects emerged as follows.

Initial Sessions

The first project, titled "Toward New Horizons," gave the group an opportunity to explore the idea of projection and continuity. In fact, the first three meetings were not theme-based, in order to give the group members enough time to become acquainted with the different art materials available and help them to relax and enjoy the activity.

I believe that an ideal starting point for any art therapy workshop is to suggest that clients produce a scribble. There is not only a sense of play to this, but it also allows participants to create with no predefined ideas. It provides clues as to how individuals organize themselves spatially; how they accommodate perceptions to find hidden unconscious images within the chaos of lines; and how, by observing the images brought to the foreground, they make sense of those findings.

However, regardless of the sense of play, a scribble may reveal unexpectedly powerful images. A particularly poignant example of this occurred at the beginning of 2009, when a client discovered in her scribble the silhouette of a baby and promptly started crying, saying, "Not again, not again." I suggested that she step outside the art therapy room and we sat in a small, empty consulting room. She then explained to me that when she became pregnant with her baby, she sensed that something was not right. Neither she nor her husband had ever been tested for HIV, because they did not deem it necessary. When the baby was born, she did not want to breastfeed him, and she felt that something was still wrong. Three months later, the baby died. The autopsy revealed that he had had AIDS, which is how my client learned that she had been infected by her husband before she became pregnant. Although she was under the impression that she had been able to overcome her baby's death during the time she had been in psychotherapy, art therapy provided her with the emotional understanding that she had not actually completed the mourning process. Months later, she shared this story with the group, saying that only now did she feel that she had been able to process the situation completely.

"How I See the World"/"How I See My Own World"

Other themes I worked on with the group were "How I See the World" and "How I See My Own World," articulating aspects of what is public and what is private, and how PLWHA relate to both areas. Many PLWHA tend to shy away from public exposure and to become more introspective, which implies restricting social interaction in a variety of fields.

After producing a complex piece of work that comprised three panels, one young man wrote: "Those of us who have any kind of infection in our bodies, and choose to make use of our creative resources, have one more tool with which to say that life is not paralyzed by the infection. . . . With creativity we have the best possible weapon, the best possible antidote. We will not be that easy to defeat." This kind of statement proved to be very uplifting for the whole group, since it sums up what many of them had indeed reported after doing art therapy over a long period of time.

"My Imprints"

"My imprints" proposed that clients make a journey through their own history to seek out a memorable yet positive event that forged a change in their lives (e.g., their wedding day). Such a mark or imprint could contribute to reinforcing the self, especially in the case of a PLWHA. As an example of this, one of my clients arrived one day with the bad news that his medication was having no effect on him. He painted a landscape with a cross and wrote: "My imprints can be found on the mountain where the cross of life stands, the cross which gives me the strength to carry on walking while projecting light on my footsteps, which are also illuminated by the sun of life." As he read, he started to cry silently. I stood behind him with my hands on his shoulders, while another client held his hand.

I have frequently seen reactions of this kind over the years. Clients coming to the group at different stages of the infection has allowed me to identify three key moments in the life of any PLWHA, on which to work through different art therapy themes: (1) receiving a positive result confirming that one is infected and will henceforth need to prepare for a new, different pattern of life; (2) starting to take the cocktail of drugs, and perhaps suffering unpleasant side effects; and (3) poor adherence to the medication regimen (e.g., the treatment may not be working because one is not taking the pills as advised, or is participating in risky behaviors that render the drugs ineffective). The art therapist must be aware of these situations in order to find creative ways to help clients best cope with them, and reduce the level of anxiety and fear that these produce.

"My Book of Dreams and Desires"

Another project, "My Book of Dreams and Desires," involved putting together a personal diary with text and images, as a form of projecting the self. A 35-year-old male client drew his body as if reflected in a mirror, alternating positive and negative signs, thus expressing the wish "to get rid of the virus by reducing its presence in blood." This image was discussed by the group at large, since it not only refers to good adherence to the treatment but it also modifies the impression that many PLWHA have of themselves: that of being a sort of time bomb. His work promoted self-care. On the back of his work he wrote: "Future tasks: to search for a future and secure one."

An 18-year-old client wrote: "As I go over the dates in the calendar, many mark the beginning of a new kind of fight, maybe the most difficult one. An October 18th reminds me that I am mortal. On that day I felt that my dreams faded away, darkness came back into my life, night took over my days, and an unwanted tenant took over my 'body.' Living side by side, day with night, darkness with light, and my body, with this intruder in it, my fight for life began once again."

This poses another issue to consider: The infection does not have the same effect on somebody who has had an active life and is over age 40 or 50, as it does on a young boy or girl who faces harder challenges for the future. Art therapy allows the PLWHA to explore their fantasies and fears in a safe environment, where the sense of projection in life is still more urgent and necessary.

SUMMARIZING THE FIRST PROJECT

The last of the first series of meetings included a group theme called "The Tree of Life," in which clients were invited to paint real and imaginary tree leaves that, combined with true ones, became part of a huge tree that hung for months and months in the art therapy room, constantly reminding the group that life regenerates itself throughout the seasons, the same way our bodies do.

Future projects addressed other relevant issues through themes such as "How I See Myself Today." A 32-year-old male client wrote:

> It is confusing to understand what is happening inside me, but I would like to bring together all the images that appear right now. But although I've always believed that shapes and color best represented me, I feel more comfortable writing about my present. And my present is

peculiar, shared, sustained and, what is more important, valued. I am like a whirlwind of sensations, and for the first time I see a different life. I have found the real value of wanting to do the things I like most. This change is due to the search for those images that I have always had in my mind, and today, here, I can try to make them come to life, and they make me happy, put life into my life. The projects we work on (at art therapy) are the engine, and you (the group), the chassis that helps me to move and reach some of the goals I set for myself.

This reveals that some of the clients not only express their feelings through painting but that sometimes they also attempt to write about their emotions.

To explore the importance of medical checkups, with regular tests of their CD4 cell count (i.e., the type of immune cell attacked by HIV) and the viral load (the amount of HIV circulating in the blood), I suggested a theme called "Routes," designed to visualize the spaces or places that form part of the PLWHA daily routine and how they reach them (i.e., either in a straight line, or by taking alternative routes, or perhaps in a confused roundabout way). They used different colored wool to identify the various routes, and eight out of 10 participants identified the hospital where they were being treated as a relevant part of their routes.

Finally, through "My Stamp Collection," each participant created a series of stamps based on a theme of interest during the eight meetings. One client chose to tell his life, beginning with images of his violent childhood home, his aimless adolescence, his time in jail, the infection, the suffering, and the cocktail of drugs. This proved to be a powerful statement that helped him to heal a damaged inner child born out of serious family conflict in his early years. However, it also allowed me to construct a certain profile of those who become infected, which strengthened the connection I had made between low self-esteem originating in the early years and exposure to risky situations as a means of finding a limit.

GROUP ACTIVITIES

Group activities have always been greatly appreciated by participants. They usually take place at the end of the year. One of the most popular group themes is an activity I designed, "Leaving Our Rucksacks Behind." It consists of the group painting on a large sheet of thick brown paper some 3 yards long, a sea with two opposite shores, and an island in the middle. Individually, each person prepares a small plasticine rucksack and thinks about what to put inside, mostly things (emotions, memories, situations, etc.) that he or she feels a need to cast off. Then, the person makes and paints a paper ship, puts the rucksack inside it, and places them both on the departure shore. One by one, the clients then move their ship over the sea to deposit the rucksack on the island, returning with an empty ship to the arrival shore, where the coordinator and the clients who have already made the journey are waiting. Each new arrival is greeted with a hug and applause. It is a very moving experience, which for a group of 15 involves some 2½ hours of work.

Another successful group activity was "The Circus," for which a text based on Picasso's painting of circus characters was the stimulus. Once read, participants divide into two groups, and members of each group paint their circus memories on a sheet of brown paper some 4 yards in length. Both sheets of paper are then used as a background for a circus performance. Each group has to prepare its own show, featuring circus music with, for example, clowns, trapeze artists, conjurers, and lion tamers. This theme promotes the recovery of early childhood memories and puts clients' resources to work. It has proven to be a good exercise in expressive arts, since it combines painting, dance, psychodrama, and music. Hats, wigs, and noses, along with all sorts of objects with which music and noises can be made, must be provided by the coordinator.

"A New Skin," based on the myth of Iansã, Afro-Brazilian goddess of the winds, was another stimulating activity for group participants. Patients are given a sponge with which to caress their bodies, brushing it over their clothes as if cleaning themselves. This must be done in silence, and with full concentration. However, on one occasion I discovered that after a while the group members were sitting in a circle, and each was rubbing the back of his or her companion with the sponge. After this ritual of symbolically getting rid of the old skin, each client is given a square sheet of thick brown paper (I recommend 1 square yard). First, the client cuts a circle in the center, so that it can later be worn as a sort of poncho. Then the client paints it with the colors and textures that he or she will wear over the following year, thus creating a new skin to serve as protection.

This activity demands great attention on the part of the art therapist. For instance, in one session, a client fell into a sort of trance and he rubbed the sponge on his right arm so strongly that it began to bleed. I assumed that he felt the need to clean off the stigma of living with HIV. In such cases it is advisable to call the client aside and explain the purely symbolic meaning of the theme, and the importance of not acting it out and putting oneself, or others, at risk.

"The Bridge" proved to be another moving experience. Each client received a small cylinder of cardboard. Participants had to paint the cylinders and place them on a large platform along with those painted by group members. These became the columns that held the main structure of the bridge. As with any bridge, it was understood that it would connect two areas, in this case, two concepts chosen by the group, such as illness–health, sadness–happiness, darkness–light, and so on. Each client painted the image that best represented him- or herself on a small sheet of paper and placed it at one of the ends, or on the bridge itself, which symbolized the transition from one state to the other. This activity allowed each client actually to see what is perceived as an internal state. The session closed with suggestions and ideas for those who placed themselves on the negative side of the work/bridge.

"Rewriting Fairy Tales" was another favorite theme. The objective was to deconstruct certain archetypes by placing them in different settings and situations. Participants were divided into three small groups and each group chose a popular fairytale to rewrite, after which they had to paint the story on a large sheet of thick brown paper. One by one, each group presented its own version to the other groups, which became the audience. This theme also combined painting with writing.

I close this section with a statement written by one of the clients we lost last year. It was on the occasion of his remembering the first theme he had explored on his first day with the art therapy group. The theme was "My Inner Treasure," and I had read a story called "The Rabbi's Treasure." He remembered the reception he had had from the group and also the idea of something homey (e.g., the hearth at the center of the story). He wrote: "The workshop, that much loved space on Saturday afternoons whose sweet taste lasts throughout the week. Here I have found affection, warmth, joy and a connection with my ancestors; my friends, my childhood and myself. That is what the workshop means, all summed up in the warmth emanating from that 'home' that we all built together on one of those Saturdays" (November 26, 2006).

CASE EXAMPLE

David came to the first session and his scribble, made with shy, restrained movements, took up a small section of the page. He entitled it "The One Who Suffers" (Figure 13.1). When the clients shared their comments on their work during the last part of the session, David explained that he had many ideas in his head but found it difficult to put them into words. However, he did say that his work represented a kind of confusion and, picking up on a suggestion by one of his companions, he became aware of a little black figure with flames coming out of its head, which he had not previously noticed. David could not say anything else.

The theme of the following session was "Do a Painting in the Style of. . . . " The group was given a selection of reproductions of paintings by well-known early 20th-century artists. David chose *I and the Village*, by Marc Chagall. He focused his attention

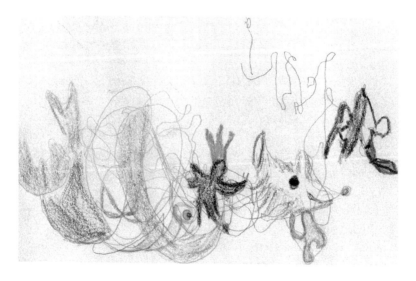

FIGURE 13.1. "The One Who Suffers."

on the top right-hand section of the original, in which several houses in a row are upside down. He called it "Crisis," although he had originally given it another title, "Viewpoints," which he had then erased. When presenting it to the group he said, "I chose that part because it shows how when things are running smoothly they can suddenly change dramatically."

He was absent from the next session but sent a message saying he was depressed. However, the following week, his change of mood was evident in the theme "How I See the World" (Figure 13.2). He began by painting a sort of semicircle on the left side of the page in black and grey, followed by a middle section in brown in the upper and lower parts of the page.[1] He then went on to paint another sort of semicircle on the right side of the page using a generous variety of other colors. Finally, he spent some time thinking about how to connect both surfaces before deciding that blue glue was the solution, and he said: "This is a moment of transition, I am slowly coming out of the well." Once again he erased the first title, of which I could only read the word "truth," before deciding on the final title, which was "Future."

For "How I See My Inner World" David resorted to the use of another small dark figure, which he placed at the bottom of the page. Behind the figure he painted a sun with rays of different bright colors. The title he chose was "Illuminated by Life," and he wrote a small paragraph pointing out that "light radiates from each one of us, as well as a whole spectrum of colors. We must try to obtain the color we wish for our own lives." With the theme "The windows of my soul," my intention was to encourage group members to reveal what they might see if they could look into their souls. David used the

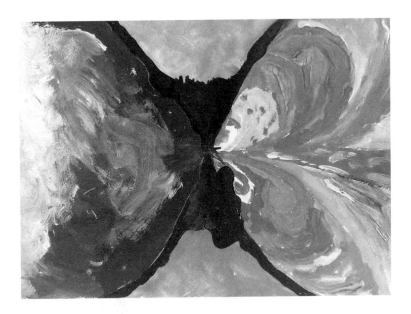

FIGURE 13.2. "How I See the World."

---

[1] Original artwork in this chapter was in color. It is reproduced here in black and white.

technique of frottage to obtain different textures on a long sheet of paper. Next, he laid a sheet of corrugated paper over his work and made little windows that opened to show the paper textured with frottage beneath. However, he then used the technique on the sole of his shoe on a separate sheet of paper, which he joined to the left-hand side of the panel, producing a work that finally measured 54″ × 11″. When explaining it, he said, "I am walking in a certain direction. It is as if my soul had opened up and all these new possibilities were emerging."

For "Painting Love" the idea was for group members to reflect on how they perceived love. David made a colorful piece entitled "Light of the Universe," which consisted of a series of hearts superimposed on each other, with a small red heart at the center. He said nothing about this painting. His "Book of Dreams and Desires" is a powerful statement on his wish to remain healthy. On one of the pages he painted two fiery shapes in red, one of them holding a heart (Figure 13.3), while on another page a crying eye faces a page on which, under a sun, the words "Love," "Family," "Health," and "Security" are written on top of a pyramid, a spiritual symbol. On the back page he wrote: "I wish to learn something new every day, to think more about what I say and say what I feel, to be able to say I need you, I love you, thank you." Once again, he had erased something which I believed to be very significant: "Asking for help."

Successive works show three mandalas: the first one a black star with an eye in the center, called "Watching"; the second one showing a green center surrounded by a blue circle and a red circle, entitled "Universe"; and the third one, a landscape of green pastures and the sun appearing over the horizon against a blue sky, called "Enjoying" (Figure 13.4).

One of David's last works, on the theme "A Place to Call My Own," shows a landscape, a river with small islands and an orange sun on the horizon. But then, in a second

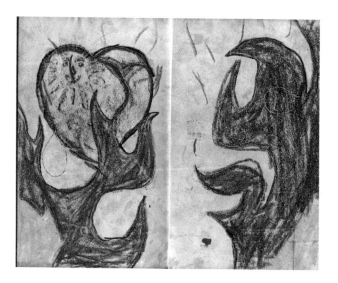

FIGURE 13.3. Image from "Book of Dreams and Desires."

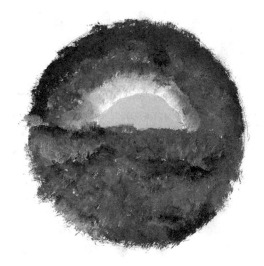

FIGURE 13.4. Mandala image.

work, he zooms into a detail of the first one, portraying two leafy trees against a clear blue sky, as if he had finally been able to focus on what really counts: nature, with its cycles, as an example of the continuity of life. This artwork showed a change in his point of view, and reminded me of that previous work, in which it was no coincidence that he had erased the title "Viewpoints," as if at that moment he had been unprepared to consider alternative views.

This abridged case traces the change from a reduced portrayal of the self to the opening up to new perspectives and possibilities. The use of art therapy made David's journey more significant because it transcended words and helped him to connect with inner aspects in which his desires lay dormant. He arrived at the workshop somewhat confused and depressed, and through the themes proposed, managed to compose a new vision of the world and find a place to inhabit: himself. During the months he attended the workshop David changed from being the one who suffers into somebody who watches and enjoys.

I saw David again on the occasion of my writing this chapter, some 6 years on from that very first day at the workshop. I was pleased to hear that he had made substantial changes in his life. For example, he had decided to move out of his mother's house, where he had always felt secure, to gain independence. After having lived alone for a certain period, he then went to live with a new partner, a young woman with children of her own, to whom he had become a sort of father figure. He was looking healthy and happy, and referred back to his time with the art therapy group as a period of personal growth.

CONCLUSION

The main perceived benefit of the workshop has been the establishment of a network of peers who, besides sharing their memories and experiences through the use of art, have managed to take significant steps in their own lives. For instance, two of the clients recently published a book of stories and poems, illustrated with some of the images produced in the art therapy workshop.

In my case, as coordinator, I have learned important lessons of survival, experiencing firsthand the sometimes devastating effect the virus has in the lives of so many people, and the numerous anonymous stories that have come to life in the art therapy room, and that have found a voice, a name and, most importantly, dignity.

REFERENCES

Bartholomew, A. (1998). A narrow ledge: Art therapy at the London Lighthouse. In M. Pratt, & M. Wood (Eds.), *Art therapy in palliative care: The creative response*. London: Routledge.

Beaver, V. (1998). The butterfly garden: Art therapy with HIV-positive/AIDS prisoners. In M. Pratt & M. Wood (Eds.), *Art therapy in palliative care: The creative response*. London: Routledge.

Branden, N. (1995). *The six pillars of self-esteem*. New York: Bantam.

David, I., & Sageman, S. (1987). Psychological aspects of AIDS as seen in art therapy. *American Journal of Art Therapy, 26*, 3–6.

Elliot, A. (2006). Mad about art, crazy about fighting HIV. Retrieved August 2011, from *www.positivenation.co.uk/issue124/features*.

Fernandez, L., Castro, R., & Pérez, D. (2002). Evolución de la percepción de riesgo de la transmisión sexual del VIH en universitarios españoles/as [Evolution of HIV risk perception in heterosexual relationships in a sample of Spanish university students]. *Psicothema, 14*(2), 255–261. Retrieved September 2011, from *www.psicothema.com*.

Fernandez Cao, M., & Martínez Diez, N. (2006). *Arteterapia, conociminto interior a través de la expresión artística* [Art therapy: Inner knowledge through artistic expression]. Madrid: Ed Tutor.

Few, R. (2007). Art therapy camps build confidence and hope for Thai children living with HIV. Retrieved August 2011, from *www.unicef.org/infobycountry/Thailand*.

Flores Xavier, A. (2010). *A arteterapia diante da AIDS: Um coquetel criativo e holístico* [Art therapy and AIDS: A creative and holistic cocktail]. Unpublished monography, Rio de Janeiro.

Gilroy, A. (2006). *Art therapy: Research and evidence-based practice*. London: Sage.

Kornblit, A., Mendes Diz, A., Petracci, M., Pecheny, M., Vujosevich, J., Gimenez, L., et al. (2000). *SIDA, Entre el cuidado y el riesgo. Estudios en población general y en personas afectadas* [AIDS: Between care and risk: Studies in general population and in people affected]. Buenos Aires: Ed Alianza.

Liebmann, M. (2004). *Art therapy for groups: A handbook of themes and exercises* (2nd ed.). East Sussex, UK: Brunner/Routledge.

Lipcovich, P. (2011). El estigma de los murmullos [The stigma of murmurs]. Retrieved September 2011, from *www.pagina12.com.ar*.

Malchiodi, C. A. (1998). *The art therapy sourcebook*. Los Angeles: Lowell House.

Merz, R. (2006). "Painting is good for your soul!" *Music Therapy Today, 7*(4) 932–938.

Mitchell, M. (2005). Arts program provides services, guidance to HIV-positive/AIDS patients. Retrieved August 2011, from *www.eurekalert.org/pub_releases/2005-07*.

Petrak, J., & Miller, D. (2002). Psychological management in HIV infection. In D. Miller & J. Green (Eds.), *The psychology of sexual health* (pp. 141–161). Oxford, UK: Blackwell Science.

Rao, D., Nainis, N., Williams, L., Langner, D., Eisin, A., & Paice, J. (2009). Art therapy for relief of symptoms associated with HIV-positive/AIDS. *AIDS Care: Psychological and Sociomedical Aspects of AIDS/HIV, 21*(1), 64–69.

Rollins, S. (2009, February 3). Art therapy spreads HIV-positive/AIDS awareness. *The Temple News*. Retrieved August 2011, from *temple-news.com/2009/02/03/art-therapy-spreads-hivaids-awareness*.

Weiser, J. (2006). HIV/AIDS-related therapy—what my clients have taught me along the way. *BC Psychologist*. Retrieved August 2011, from *www.phototherapy-centre.com/articles/2006_hiv_counseling_issues_bcpa_newsltr*.

Winnicott, D. (2005). *Playing and reality*. London: Routledge.

Wood, M. (1998). The body as art: Individual session with a man with AIDS. In M. Pratt & M. Wood (Eds.), *Art therapy in palliative care: The creative response* (pp. 140–152). London: Routledge.

CHAPTER 14

Art Therapy and Hemodialysis
Coping Creatively with Kidney Failure

Rachel C. Schreibman

When the kidneys reach organ failure, called end-stage renal disease (ESRD), dialysis or transplantation is required to live. Hemodialysis (HD) is a medical treatment that keeps the body in balance by removing harmful waste, balancing chemicals, and restoring a healthy blood pressure (National Kidney Foundation [NKF], n.d.). The first primitive dialysis machine, called the Kolff machine, was used in 1948 at Mount Sinai Hospital by Drs. Alfred Fishman and Irving Kroop on a young female patient with acute kidney failure. The machine was a contraption of cellophane surrounding a "large wooden drum set in a bath of fluid designed to attract from the blood those solutes in need of removal" (Peitzman, 2007, p. 86). Following this momentous event in medicine, HD was provided as a routine form of care in the 1940s and 1950s, and the HD machine was updated to become a stainless steel product manufactured and distributed across the Unites States.

In the 1960s, in Seattle, Dr. Belding Scribner invented a Teflon shunt that revolutionized HD care, and he successfully kept a patient alive for more than a decade on HD. The nature of HD shifted into long-term replacement for renal function rather than acute treatment. In 1965, the U.S. Public Health Service created the Kidney Disease Control Program, and 14 outpatient HD units were established, while additional units sprang up around the country without federal backing. The need for dialysis outnumbered the slots available, and so physicians in Seattle came up with the idea of having a panel of persons in the community, termed a "God committee" and headed by clergyman, to determine who would receive the scarce treatment. HD was allocated on the basis of factors such as "working heads of households and those who contributed to community and went to church" (Peitzman, 2007, p. 113).

A public and political sentiment toward lack of dialysis availability evolved after a series of events including the publication of an article in *Life Magazine* titled "They Decide Who Lives, Who Dies: Medical Miracle Puts Moral Burden on Small Committee" by

Shane Alexander (Alexander, 1962), and a plea for funding for dialysis by Shep Glazer, then Vice President of the American Association of Kidney Patients (AAKP), who testified before Congress while undergoing dialysis on the floor of Congress.

In 1972, President Nixon signed Public Law 92-603, a set of Social Security amendments that included a commitment for the federal Medicare program to pay for dialysis due to the "needless" deaths of thousands of Americans suffering from the kidney failure epidemic (Peitzman, 2007). The initiative, called the End-Stage Renal Disease Program, had no precedent; it established reimbursement for dialysis services nationwide for persons with ESRD. Since the 1970s, the number of individuals in the United States needing dialysis has grown exponentially. The NKF (n.d.) reported that in 2009, the number of individuals in the United States on dialysis was more than 367,000 and growing. Diabetes and high blood pressure are the leading causes of ESRD, and African Americans are afflicted at a rate three to four times higher than that of European Americans. Factors such as socioeconomic variables, genetic explanations, and access to care have been cited as reasons for this disparity. Dialysis patients have a 16–37% shorter life expectancy than the general population (Cohen et al., 2007).

MENTAL HEALTH AND EMOTIONAL CONSEQUENCES OF END-STAGE RENAL DISEASE

Research suggests that people enduring HD treatments often face depression, high levels of debilitation, physical deformities, sleep disorders, role impairment, and other serious physical, mental, and emotional problems (Curtin, Sitter, Schatell, & Chewning, 2004; Kimmel & Peterson, 2005). Major stressors such as fatigue, fluid restriction, and interference with social and recreational activities have been named as common problems for this population (Logan, Pelletier-Hibbert, & Hodgins, 2006). Cohen et al. (2007), psychiatrists who study dialysis discontinuation, say that "dialysis patients suffer significant discomfort, inconvenience, and progressive functional disability, in return for which they may sometimes expect a limited prolongation of life on the saw-toothed edge of uremia" (p. 1263). Studies show that 5–22% of HD patients suffer from major depression, and an additional 25%, with subsyndromal depression (Cohen et al., 2007); depression is the most common psychiatric abnormality that patients on HD experience (Kimmel & Peterson, 2005).

Gencoz and Astan (2006) studied psychological well-being, locus of control, and social support of individuals on HD and found that "tailoring treatment to the characteristics and demands of the patients should always be kept in mind, considering the uniqueness of each individual patient" (p. 207). Kimmel (2001) pointed out that relationships among patients, physicians, and dialysis staff have an impact on medical outcomes of dialysis patients. People on HD spend an average of 12 hours per week at their treatment unit. Thus, the staff and unit setting may be seen as a particularly influential social network in which the patient spends time. Kimmel has described a distinct "culture" that arises in each unit, despite the high staff turnover. Furthermore, research shows patients' "satisfaction with staff and their perception that staff cared about them correlated with higher serum albumin levels" (Kimmel, 2001, p. 1608), which is a positive health indication in people with ESRD.

THE BIOMEDICAL MODEL OF TREATMENT

From the time of the ancient Greeks to the 20th century, the belief that the mind can affect the course of an illness has been widely accepted. However, when antibiotics were introduced, a new thinking arose that treatment of infectious or inflammatory disease required only the elimination of the organism that caused the onset, and 20th century medicine began to reject the idea that the mind influences physical illness (Sternberg & Gold, 2002).

The current Western biomedical approach to treating illness usually does not address all of the experience of illness, including psychosocial, emotional, and spiritual parts. Western medicine is "allopathic"; based on a "mechanical, disease-and-drug focused clinical model, it is an approach that largely ignores key healing pathways to body, mind and spirit" (Brown, 2001, p. 34).

Nettleton (2006) outlines five assumptions of the biomedical approach to illness:

1. Mind–body dualism: The mind and body are treated separately.
2. Mechanical metaphor: The body works like a machine and can be fixed or treated as such.
3. Technological imperative: Technological interventions are emphasized (because of assumption 2).
4. Reductionism: Health/illness is explained in biological, not sociological or psychological terms.
5. Doctrine of specific etiology: A disease entity is solely responsible for disease (this emerged out of germ theory in the 19th century).

Nettleton (2006) writes, "Patterns of mortality and morbidity, or a person's 'life chances,' are related to social structures, and vary according to gender, social class, 'race,' and age. Thus the biomedical model fails to account for the social inequalities in health" (p. 5). Also, by promoting evidence-based medicine and highlighting progress, self-care is devalued and a dependency on medical professionals plays out (Nettleton, 2006).

Bringing treatments such as art therapy into dialysis units acknowledges that illness is more than a physiological experience, and approaches treatment of medical disease with consideration for a holistic interplay of wellness aspects (psychological, emotional, spiritual, physical, social). Studies underscore the healing effects of this kind of mind–body approach to illness: "To date, there is strong evidence showing that mind–body interventions are effective in managing many of the chronic medical conditions including post-myocardial infarction, cancer symptoms, incontinence disorders, surgical outcomes, insomnia, headache, and chronic low-back pain" (Samuelson et al., 2010, p. 187).

The biopsychosocial model is one that addresses this complex connection and works from a paradigm rooted in a belief that "the interaction of stressors, coping efficacy, and neuroendocrine function affect disease status (Zautra et al.)" (Sperry, Powers, & Griffith, 2008, p. 371). Sperry et al. point out three constructs of the biopsychosocial model: organ dialect (biological), lifestyle convictions (psychological), and family constellation (social). Psychoeducation and psychotherapy are emerging "as first-line treatments" for chronic medical conditions as care becomes more aligned with a biopsychosocial model (Sperry et al., 2008, p. 373). Art therapy for individuals on HD taps into coping, stress reduction, self-expression, social support, compliance, and other factors of kidney failure, rather than purely approaching ESRD as a biomedical disease.

ART THERAPY AND END-STAGE RENAL DISEASE

Few studies have been published on art therapy with patients on HD, and a scarcity of art therapy programs exist for individuals on HD, despite evidence of the enormous physical and emotional challenges that this population faces. Those studies and programs that do address HD patients show positive outcomes of art therapy. Weldt (2003) presented eight case studies of art therapy with patients on HD and found that with each client, "making art inspired positive attitudes, feelings of power, control, and freedom, and the drawings gave them [the clients] a sense of achievement" (p. 98). Participants in the study were asked to create three pieces of art to elicit reactions and expressions on varying topics: a free drawing (to elicit self-expression without a directive), a self-portrait (to elicit body image or self-concept), and a drawing of "what you most like, what you wish for, or desire" (to elicit goals and aspirations). Art therapist researchers then conducted two interviews with each participant to discuss his or her artworks and process. Participants consistently expressed that the intervention helped them to reflect on their lives and illness. One client said that the experience "changed me a little because I keep things locked up inside, and when I put them on paper, I get a different perspective" (Weldt, 2003, p. 95).

Nishida and Strobino (2005) found that eight art therapy sessions with a client on HD created an opportunity for self-expression and communication through art, and resulted in self-reported increased feelings of control, accomplishment, and self-confidence. In this study, each art therapy session was structured with specific materials, and themes and goals for each session were identified. After the eight sessions were complete, the art therapist researcher conducted an interview with the client. The client reported that the intervention offered an opportunity for engaging in a new activity (art), which "helped the time pass more quickly" while dialyzing (p. 224). During the art therapy sessions, the client spoke about personal topics such as relationship issues, hobbies/skills, memories, and overcoming challenges.

In an arts-in-medicine (AIM) program implemented for 6 months in an outpatient dialysis unit, Ross, Hollen, and Fitzgerald (2006) found improved scores for pain, social function, and laboratory parameters; better quality of life (QOL); and a trend toward less depression among patients who participated. Over the course of the study, dozens of HD patients worked with two resident artists and ad hoc volunteers to engage in a variety of creative activities including drawing and watercolor, crafts, crochet, music, creative writing, and shared written journals. Carts with art materials were available to patients when resident artists were not present, and often dialysis patients became active in handing out materials when HD shifts began. The results of the study included positive objective and subjective findings. Compelling comments by participants and the staff reflect an enthusiasm and excitement for the AIM program; while treatment in HD is usually perceived as a burden to the patient, with the AIM program, patients "seemed happier" and "looked forward to coming here [to dialysis] for some of the activities" (Ross et al., 2006, p. 465).

Social support has been associated with longer survival and improved patient outcomes for HD patients in many studies (Gencoz & Astan, 2006; Spinale et al., 2008). Since art therapy may serve as a type of social support for an HD patient, further research is needed to examine how art therapy might impact health outcomes for HD patients.

Goals of art therapy with patients on HD include the following:

- Stress reduction
- Self-expression
- Positive recreation
- Social support
- Increased coping skills
- Increased compliance and disease management

ART AS A NARRATIVE IN AN OUTPATIENT DIALYSIS UNIT

I spent approximately 1 year providing art therapy at a suburban outpatient HD unit. (Figure 14.1 is a photograph of a client working in art therapy with me.) The unit had not previously had counseling or art therapy services available to patients. Patients at the unit were local residents with kidney failure, mostly middle-aged to older adult African Americans.

Upon introducing the idea of art therapy sessions to patients in the unit, many reported feeling excited about art therapy for the simple reason that it introduced something new and stimulating to do during treatments. Many HD patients report feelings of boredom during treatment, and often choose to sleep or watch television to pass the long treatment time. Patients who participate in art therapy often have commented to me that they enjoyed the novelty of working with art media that included watercolor, clay, and drawing. Art therapy provided a positive recreational experience during time that was usually spent idle.

When working with patients, I use an eclectic approach to art therapy that blends humanistic and existential approaches. A humanistic approach emphasizes art therapy as a shared journey, and underscores the need for the therapist to create a nonjudgmental

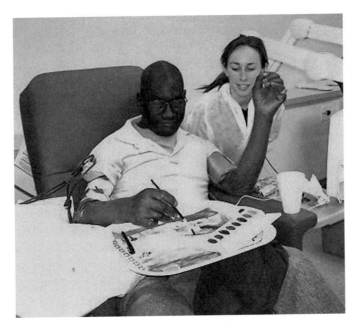

FIGURE 14.1. Author Rachel Schreibman works with a client in art therapy who is receiving dialysis. For more information about the Art Therapy Dialysis Project, visit the Renal Support Network's website: *www.rsnhope.org.*

setting (Garai, 2001). An existential approach to art therapy considers and honors four ultimate concerns common to living: death, freedom, isolation, and meaninglessness (Moon, 1995). It also values art as a medium that leads to mindfulness.

Patients who participate in art therapy often express that they are facing serious physical, emotional, and spiritual challenges tied to illness and loss. Whether art therapy was provided over one session or over many months, I witnessed the power of art making as a medium through which a patient may express reaction to trauma through images.

IMAGES THAT TELL A STORY

The benefits of creating an avenue for self-expression of emotional experience of illness spans diagnoses and disabilities. Collie, Bottorff, and Long (2006) suggest that art therapy empowers the patient to get a clearer view of the emotional experience and clear the way emotionally with regard to processing difficult emotions. Malchiodi (1999) points out the importance of accessing emotions both nonverbally and verbally in medical art therapy, and highlights the ability of art media to tap into emotional material that is often unspoken.

Pennebaker, author of nine books and more than 250 articles, has contributed a large body of clinical research on the healing power of expressing emotions. Pennebaker's studies report on the effects of both inhibiting and expressing thoughts and emotions.

His work shows that inhibition creates immediate biological changes (e.g., perspiration), and over time serves as a stressor that contributes to increased illness and stress-related conditions (Pennebaker, 1997). Pennebaker's research on "opening up" supports the phenomenon that expressing emotions leads to improved physical and mental health. In a similar fashion, art therapy gives kidney dialysis patients an opportunity to benefit from emotional expression.

The images here (Figures 14.2, 14.3, and 14.4) represent artwork by patients who worked with me in art therapy at a suburban outpatient dialysis unit. Figure 14.2 is a watercolor painting by an elderly patient, Norma. Norma used the art materials to depict her painful experience of having both legs amputated due to complications of diabetes. She was, like many dialysis patients, dealing with comorbid conditions, including heart disease, glaucoma, and kidney failure. After our many months of working together, she talked about her memory of undergoing amputations three separate times. She asked that I draw an outline of a foot for her to paint in (bottom right, Figure 14.2), and as she painted, she described her experience with gangrene ("It looked like black pearls," she said). Her story seemed to be filled with sadness, regret/shame (due to noncompliance with diet and medication), and a sense of impending doom (She often said to me, "I ain't gonna make it one of these days [sic]"). While telling her story, she lifted her pant leg and asked me to touch the end of her amputated limb. I felt as if she were asking me to recognize her loss, and to affirm to her through touch and a nonjudgmental relationship that her physical disabilities should not be barriers to connection and acceptance.

Norma also explored her strengths and positive coping skills in art therapy. In Figure 14.3, she depicts flowers. When asked about the significance of the image, she spoke about taking care of plants as a hobby that brought joy to her life. Also, to her, flowers represented hope for getting better with fluid restriction and insight into how lifestyle

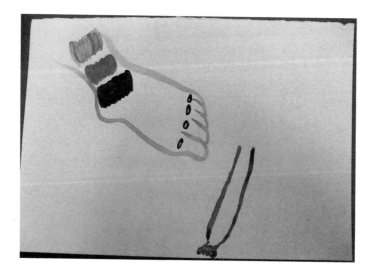

FIGURE 14.2. A painting made by a patient and art therapist in art therapy to explore the patient's story about having her legs amputated.

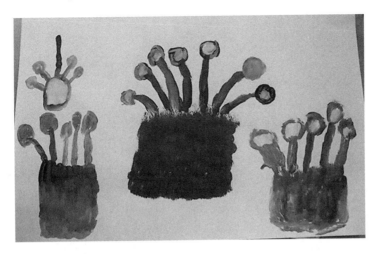

FIGURE 14.3. A painting of flowers made in art therapy by a patient on HD.

habits impacted her illness ("It's just like if you water your flowers too much or too little," she remarked).

The image of flowers also brought to her mind the relationships in her life she valued, and that served as social supports for her. Norma enjoyed talking about her son and other family members on whom she could rely during difficult times. She made several pieces in art therapy that she wanted to give to her son, including a "life book," with poetry about their relationship.

Adam, a middle-aged patient, participated in brief art therapy with me. Adam shared with me his involvement in Narcotics Anonymous (NA), a support program for individuals recovering from narcotic addictions. He had been highly involved in NA for 18 years. Adam began using cocaine, crack, and heroin when he was 16 years old, and said he "grew up in the 'hood' [sic]." Adam spoke about using his experience of recovery to motivate other men with addiction to make changes and get help. The day that I met with him for our first art therapy session, he was scheduled that night to give an inspirational speech about his story to an NA group in a prison. He served as a sponsor for others working toward recovery, and said he had been completely drug- and alcohol-free since joining NA.

Adam also spoke about the challenges he faced in life and used art therapy to express anguish (Figure 14.4). He had recently lost his job as a construction worker. A year earlier, Adam's body rejected the kidney his sister donated to him, and he had to go back on HD after the transplant failed. Adam told me this figure was him, "in the dark, away from the things outside the doors," which includes "God, faith, belief, courage, and hope." Shelter, food, and transportation were things that Adam said he still had. I was concerned to see Adam's depiction of himself lacking emotional and psychological supports such as faith, courage, and hope. I inquired about suicidal ideation, which he denied.

Adam's image brings to mind a feeling of being overwhelmed. His rather quick disclosure of painful emotions and circumstances also signaled that he might be dealing

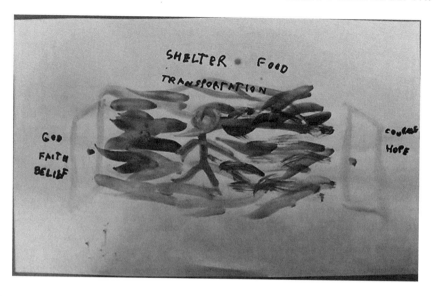

FIGURE 14.4. A painting made in art therapy by a patient on HD who explored such themes as job loss, failure of transplant, recovery from addiction, and faith.

with intense feelings of depressiveness or hopelessness. I asked Adam what thoughts or people helped to buffer his suffering and contribute to positive coping and resilience. He again spoke about his deeply personal connection to the NA support program and shared inspiring stories about his participation.

Although I only shared a brief time with Adam, we were able to work together to confront some of his difficult emotions. He gave me permission to ask the social worker at the unit to check in with him about his financial hardship and job loss. Before I left that day, Adam told me he felt that the doors in his painting (Figure 14.4) were open, and that although he was in darkness, there was "light at the end of the tunnel."

ADDITIONAL ART THERAPY APPLICATIONS ON HEMODIALYSIS UNITS

Art therapists have worked with the staff in a variety of medical settings to address the emotional impact of caring for chronically ill patients and experiencing loss as a part of the occupational environment. Art therapy programs and services have been implemented with oncology staff (Italia, Favara-Scacco, DiCataldo, & Russo, 2008; Nainis, 2005), medical residents (Julliard, Intilli, Ryan, Vollman, & Seshadri, 2002), hospice and palliative care workers (Murrant, Rykov, Amonite, & Loynd, 2002), and others. Staff in HD units are at risk for burnout and emotional distress: In a large study conducted in the United States, Flynn, Thomas-Hawkins, and Clarke (2009) found that burnout among American HD nurses is "unacceptably high," (p. 578) with one nurse in three reporting symptoms of burnout.

I facilitated two single-session art therapy groups with the dialysis staff at the HD unit, which included dialysis nurses, the unit manager, a technician, the dietician, and the social worker. The purpose of the groups was to use art to process loss and to remember patients who had passed away. I started by explaining the concept of vicarious trauma and burnout, then asked the group members to create art reflecting their thoughts and emotions regarding working with chronically ill patients. Staff members then took turns sharing their images and words with the group.

Most participants included images related to a particular patient who had passed away (a memory), or to thoughts about death and dying. A central theme that emerged was spirituality as a way of coping. Figures 14.5 and 14.6 are images by the dietician and a technician (respectively). In Figure 14.5, the words at the bottom of the page read "free like a butterfly," with the name of a patient who died at the top of the page (covered for confidentiality). During the session, the artist of Figure 14.5 became emotional and cried. Others in the group appeared supportive and expressed sadness, as well as hope, and positive memories they had of patients. The art therapy group gave staff members a unique opportunity to connect with each other about common experiences and emotions related to working with very ill or dying individuals. It also provided a space for using imagery to process loss and honor the lives of patients who had passed away. At the end of the sessions, participants expressed that the group was helpful and they enjoyed taking part in it. The art was placed into a scrapbook (a "memory book") and kept at the HD unit for staff members to look at and/or add to by creating additional artworks or writings for as desired.

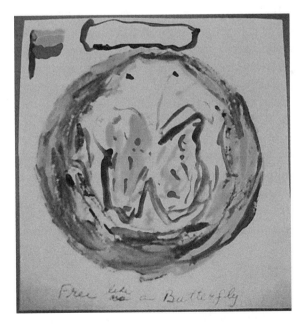

FIGURE 14.5. A painting by a dietician made in art therapy to honor a patient on HD who passed away.

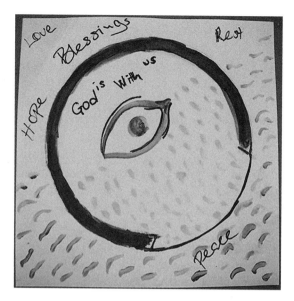

FIGURE 14.6. A painting made in art therapy by a dialysis technician who spoke about his faith.

Creating group artwork is another way to incorporate art therapy on an HD unit; often this type of collaborative art is displayed in a lobby or other venue. One particular group project I facilitated began with one client, who painted an image of "a doorway to heaven." The piece was circulated to two other clients who took turns adding to the image. The clients were all receiving HD during the same shift and sat within earshot of each other. They appeared enthusiastic about sharing their art with each other, and although they each had separate narratives about their portions of the painting, the piece had a high level of coherence in style and content.

By incorporating art therapy approaches beyond individual treatment (i.e., with staff members and in a group project), art therapy also tapped into HD as a collective experience. Cukor, Cohen, Peterson, and Kimmel (2007) describe a unique culture that exists in each dialysis unit despite high staff turnover. They propose that research be conducted on "the impact of social work groups on the unit or organized social activities," because "it is clear that the culture of the dialysis unit and the connectedness the patient feels to the dialysis staff are important factors and may mediate differential outcomes in dialysis programs with similar patient populations" (p. 3049). The additional applications of art therapy that I implemented drew on the strength of group cohesion within the HD unit. Staff members and patients were able to reframe themselves as a positive, healthy social network and were open-minded, and willing to try something new.

CONCLUSION

Art therapy offers patients on HD a medium for both nonverbal and verbal self-expression; a positive recreational activity to engage in during often idle time while receiving treatments; and a supportive, nonjudgmental experience of social support. The program I created at the dialysis unit succeeded in many ways by providing connection, novel activity, and encouragement for patients to explore their journeys introspectively. Many patients on HD were coping with very challenging and debilitating physical and emotional circumstances; I was told throughout my time working on the unit that having the opportunity to express themselves in confidence about these stressors was highly valued.

Miller (1997) states that "the process of illness and suffering awakens something inside of us which not only longs to be heard, but must be heard" (p. 42). She goes on:

> The steps toward healing and self-care appear to be subtle; yet, like germinal seeds of awareness, it is our task to listen, to study them and to allow them to speak to us. Not only is the listening subtle, but the hearing must allow for uncertainty. (p. 42)

All of the patients in the unit who participated in art therapy had the opportunity to be heard, to be witnessed, and to speak their truths. Their artwork and stories are testimony to their courage and resilience. It is my hope that art therapy services and programs increase in HD units in order to provide individuals with kidney failure an opportunity to self-reflect and to find hope while coping with a debilitating chronic disease.

REFERENCES

Alexander, S. (1962, November 9). They decide who lives who dies: Medical miracle puts moral burden on small committee. *Life Magazine*, pp. 102–125.

Brown, L. (2001). East meets West and Western medicine takes a back seat: Why Ayurvedic and traditional Chinese medicines are at the core of all that's right with holistic healing today. *Better Nutrition, 63*(12), 34–40.

Cohen, M., Bostwick, M., Mirot, A., Garb, J., Braden, G., & Germain, M. (2007). A psychiatric perspective of dialysis discontinuation. *Journal of Palliative Medicine, 10*(6), 1262–1265.

Collie, K., Bottorff, J. L., & Long, B. C. (2006). A narrative view of art therapy and art making by women with breast cancer. *Journal of Health Psychology, 11*(5), 761–775.

Cukor, D., Cohen, S., Peterson, R., & Kimmel, P. (2007). Psychosocial aspects of chronic disease: ESRD as a paradigmatic illness. *Journal of American Society of Nephrology, 18,* 3042–3055.

Curtin, R. B., Sitter, D. C., Schatell, D., & Chewning, B. A. (2004). Self-management, knowledge, and functioning and well-being of patients on hemodialysis. *Nephrology Nursing Journal, 31*(4), 378–396.

Flynn, L., Thomas-Hawkins, C., & Clarke, S. (2009). Organizational traits, care processes, and burnout among chronic hemodialysis nurses. *Western Journal of Nursing Research, 31*(5), 569–582.

Garai, J. E. (2001). Humanistic art therapy. In J. A. Rubin (Ed.), *Approaches to art therapy theory and technique* (pp. 149–162). New York: Brunner/Routledge.

Gencoz, T., & Astan, G. (2006). Social support, locus of control, and depressive symptoms in hemodialysis patients. *Scandinavian Journal of Psychology, 47,* 203–208.

Italia, S., Favara-Scacco, C., DiCataldo, A., & Russo, G. (2008). Evaluation and art therapy treatment of the burnout syndrome in oncology units. *Psycho-Oncology, 17,* 676–680.

Julliard, K., Intilli, N., Ryan, J., Vollmam, S., & Seshadri, M. (2002). Stress in family practice residents: An exploratory study using art. *Art Therapy: Journal of the American Art Therapy Association, 19*(1), 4–11.

Kimmel, P.L. (2001). Psychosocial factors in dialysis patients. *Kidney International, 54*(4), 1599–1613.

Kimmel, P. L., & Peterson, R. A. (2005). Depression in end-stage renal disease patients treated with hemodialysis: Tools, correlates, outcomes, and needs. *Seminars on Dialysis, 18*(2), 91–97.

Logan, S. M., Pelletier-Hibbert, M., & Hodgins, M. (2006). Stressors and coping of in-hospital haemodialysis patients aged 65 years and over. *Journal of Advanced Nursing, 56*(4), 382–391.

Malchiodi, C. A. (1999). *Medical art therapy with adults.* Philadelphia: Jessica Kingsley.

Miller, W. (1997). Imagery, art and health: Excerpts from a series of presentations on art as complementary medicine. *Journal of the Creative and Expressive Arts Therapies Exchange, 6,* 41–46.

Moon, B. L. (1995). *Existential art therapy: The canvas mirror* (2nd ed.). Springfield, IL: Thomas.

Murrant, G., Rykov, M., Amonite, D., & Loynd, M. (2002). Creativity and self-care for caregivers. *Journal of Palliative Care, 16*(2), 44–49.

Nainis, N. (2005). Art therapy with an oncology care team. *Journal of the American Art Therapy Association, 22*(3), 150–154.

National Kidney Foundation (NKF). (n.d.). Website. Retrieved September 5, 2011, from *www. kidney.org.*

Nettleton, S. (2006). *Sociology of health and illness* (2nd ed.). Cambridge, UK: Polity Press.

Nishida, M., & Strobino, J. (2005). Art therapy with a hemodialysis patient: A case analysis. *Art Therapy: Journal of the American Art Therapy Association, 22*(4), 221–226.

Peitzman, S. J. (2007). *Dropsy, dialysis, transplant: A short history of failing kidneys.* Baltimore: Johns Hopkins University Press.

Pennebaker, J. W. (1997). *Opening up: The healing power of expressing emotions.* New York: Guilford Press.

Ross, A., Hollen, T., & Fitzgerald, B. (2006). Observational study of an arts-in-medicine program in an outpatient hemodialysis unit. *American Journal of Kidney Disease, 47*(3), 462–468.

Samuelson, M., Foret, M., Baim, M., Lerner, J., Fricchione, G., Benson, H., et al. (2010). Exploring the effectiveness of a comprehensive mind–body intervention for medical symptom relief. *Journal of Alternative and Complementary Medicine, 16*(2), 187–192.

Sperry, L., Powers, R., & Griffith, J. (2008). The biopsychosocial model and chronic illness: Psychotherapeutic implications. *Journal of Individual Psychology, 64*(3), 369–376.

Spinale, J., Cohen, S., Khetpal, P., Peterson, R. A., Clougherty, B., Puchalski, C., et al. (2008). Spirituality, social support, and survival in hemodialysis patients. *Clinical Journal of the American Society of Nephrology, 3*(6), 1620–1627.

Sternberg, E. M., & Gold, P. W. (2002). The mind–body interaction in disease. *Scientific American Special Edition, 12,* 82–89.

Weldt, C. (2003). Patients' responses to a drawing experience in a hemodialysis unit: A step towards healing. *Art Therapy: Journal of the American Art TherapyAssociation, 20*(2), 92–99.

CHAPTER 15

Focusing-Oriented Art Therapy with People Who Have Chronic Illnesses

Laury Rappaport

Focusing-oriented art therapy (FOAT; Rappaport, 2009) integrates mindful awareness, compassionate listening, and access to the body's innate knowing with art therapy. It is based on renowned philosopher and psychologist Eugene Gendlin's (1981a, 1996) mind–body Focusing method that he developed out of research with Carl Rogers on what leads to successful psychotherapy. FOAT is especially applicable to people with chronic illnesses because it helps clients learn to befriend their illness, reduce stress, work through unresolved emotional issues, and access well-being.

This chapter provides an overview of chronic illness and the significant literature that supports a FOAT approach with this population. A brief history of FOAT is presented along with the main concepts of Focusing that are essential to know in order to understand FOAT. The primary FOAT approaches for working with people with chronic illnesses are presented—the Focusing Attitude, Clearing a Space with Art; Theme-Directed FOAT, and Focusing-Oriented Art Psychotherapy—along with case examples to illustrate each method.

OVERVIEW

There are numerous types of chronic illnesses, such as cancer, heart, disease, diabetes, AIDS, chronic pain, fibromyalgia, chronic fatigue syndrome, and so forth. "Chronic illness" is defined as "a lifelong process of adapting to significant physical, psychological, social, and environmental changes" as a result of illness (Bishop, 2005, p. 219). Chronic illnesses are often accompanied by feelings of loss, grief, depression, and anxiety, and typically impact self-esteem and identity (Livneh & Antonak, 2005; Livneh, Lott, & Anonak, 2004). In a first-person account, Freeza (2008) shares, "The flow of my life had stopped. I was no longer myself. I became my PAIN . . . " (p. 328). In another first-person narrative, Keane (2008) stated, "I did not know how to reassess my life that included the illness that I wanted to so badly to reject and be rid of" (p. 345).

Livneh and Antonak (2005) identified the following commonalities among people experiencing chronic illness: interference with daily activities and roles; uncertain prognosis; functional limitation; prolonged treatment and/or rehabilitation; psychosocial stress; impact in relation to family and friends; and financial losses due to a diminished ability to work, as well as an increase in medical expenses.

Both Focusing and art therapy have made positive contributions to people living with chronic illnesses. In the most researched Focusing method, "Clearing a Space," clients are invited to sense inside the body to what is in the way of feeling at ease, or at peace. As each issue or situation is kinesthetically sensed from within the body's experiencing, the client imagines placing it at a distance outside of the body. The issues are not the client's entire life issues or stressors, but rather those that the person is carrying in the present. After metaphorically "placing" the issues outside of the body, the client senses the place within that is at ease or "all fine." Clearing a Space has been found to decrease depression in women with cancer (Grindler Katonah & Flaxman, 1999; Klagsbrun, Lennox, & Summers, 2010); reduce anxiety, depression, and pain in chronic pain patients (Ferraro, 2010); and improve body attitudes (Antrobos, 2008; Ferraro, 2010; Grindler-Katonah & Flaxman, 1999; Klagsbrun et al., 2005), as well as overall quality of life (Klagsbrun et al., 2010). Focusing has also helped people with chronic illness to form a more caring relationship with their bodies and illness, to access meaning, and to make choices for treatment (Frezza, 2010).

In art therapy, several studies on people with cancer have demonstrated beneficial results, including decreased depression and fatigue (Bar-Sela, Atid, Damos, Gabay, & Epelbaum, 2007), reduced anxiety and tiredness (Nainis, 2008); and improvement in a broad range of symptoms, including overall anxiety (Nainis et al., 2006). Art therapy has also fostered increased states of relaxation and calmness (Curry & Kasser, 2005; Nainis, 2008), improved quality of life in people with cancer (Monti et al., 2006; Svensk et al., 2009), and has helped to resolve existential and spiritual issues that arise from living with a chronic illness (Gabriel et al., 2001). Although FOAT is relatively new, Clearing a Space with Art has shown promising results to reduce stress in sign language interpreters (Castalia, 2010) and graduate students (Weiland, 2011).

FOCUSING-ORIENTED ART THERAPY

FOAT is based on 30 years of integrating Focusing with art therapy with a wide variety of clinical populations (Rappaport, 2008, 2009). To understand FOAT's clinical application to chronic illness, it is necessary first to understand the history and main concepts of Focusing and the foundational principles of FOAT.

Focusing

Gendlin and Rogers's research on what leads to effective psychotherapy concluded that the theoretical approach is not the crucial factor. They found that successful clients naturally accessed a bodily sense, or what Gendlin (1981a) termed "felt sense," described as follows:

> A bodily experience of a situation, person, or event. An internal aura that encompasses everything you feel and know about a given subject at a given time—encompasses it and communicates it to you all at once rather than detail by detail. (p.32)

As I learned Focusing, it was clear to me that access to a felt sense occurred through art making. The felt sense informs one about which color or media to use, guides the unfolding of the artistic process, and signals when the art making is finished. Gendlin (1981b) seemed to know this connection, too. He stated, "Creative people have probably always used this method. What is really new in it is the specificity with which we can describe the steps and teach them" (p. 16).

The steps to which the previous quote refers are Gendlin's original Focusing method that he developed to teach how to access and listen to the innate wisdom of a felt sense. It comprises the following six steps:

1. Clearing a space (previously described).
2. Choosing an issue and getting a felt sense.
3. Finding symbol/handle: a word, phrase, image, gesture, or sound that describes or matches the felt sense.
4. Resonating: checking the symbol/handle against the felt sense for a sense of rightness.
5. Asking: The therapist may invite the client to ask the felt sense (or art) a question inwardly. This elicits an inner dialogue to access meaning and inner knowing (e.g., What does it need? or what's a good step in the right direction?).
6. Receiving: the client receives the body's answer.

It is helpful to understand Gendlin's steps as they are integrated with art therapy to create the basic FOAT method (expressing a felt sense in art), and the three main approaches—clearing a Space with Art; Theme-Directed FOAT, and Focusing-Oriented Art Psychotherapy—described after the foundational FOAT principles.

Foundational Principles of FOAT

The most important principle of FOAT is based on Gendlin's approach—the safety of the client comes first, before any intervention. Gendlin (1996, p. 287) reminds us that "there is always a person in there." The concept of "the person in there" is especially important when working with people who have chronic illness and have lost a sense of their identity, or have lost themselves to an illness identity.

To support the safety of the client, therapeutic presence, clinical sensitivity, grounding, empathic reflection, and the Focusing Attitude are paramount. Therapeutic presence begins with the therapist's ability to become aware of his or her own state, to set his or her issues aside in a healthy way, and to transmit an openness to connect with "the person in there."

It is essential to be mindful of the unique needs of each client and clinical population, and to adapt FOAT accordingly. Since FOAT includes a somatic component in which looking within the body can bring up surprising or buried issues, it is important for clients know how to "ground" themselves, especially prior to inner guided Focusing. Grounding exercises include being aware of the breath coming in and out of the body, and body awareness, such as noticing the feet touching the floor, where the hands are resting, and so forth.

Focusing can include closing the eyes in order to notice the body's felt experience, similar to meditation or guided imagery. However, it is advisable always to offer a choice to clients to keep their eyes open or closed, whichever is most comfortable to them. If the eyes are closed, it is important for clients to know that they can open their eyes at any time, without needing to wait for the therapist's instruction. In the beginning of treatment with clients who have trauma and severe mental illness, it is important that they focus with the eyes open and only be invited to close their eyes after the therapist knows they ground themselves and self-regulate (Rappaport, 2010).

Empathic reflection is interwoven throughout FOAT sessions. Reflection can be verbal (experiential listening), artistic mirroring (e.g., drawing a shape, using a color, or creating an image that matches the client's experience), and movement whereby the therapist conveys understanding through nonverbal body movement or gesture.

The Focusing Attitude begins with mindful awareness toward the bodily *felt sense* experience and being "friendly" to whatever is there—stresses and difficult feelings, as well as peaceful or uplifting qualities. The Focusing Attitude also is directed toward the creative process and art product.

Basic FOAT Method

A basic FOAT method is to express a felt sense in art. Clients are invited to bring mindful awareness and a "friendly" attitude toward the bodily felt sense of an issue,

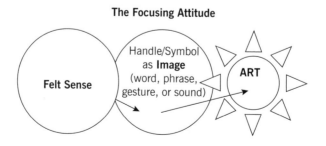

FIGURE 15.1. Expressing the handle/symbol in art.

experience, or situation. They are then guided to see if there is a symbol or handle—an image (or word, phrase, gesture, or sound)—that matches the felt sense. Clients resonate with or check the image for a feeling of rightness. They then express the felt sense image through art (Figure 15.1).

CLINICAL APPLICATION TO CHRONIC ILLNESS

Befriending Illness though the Focusing Attitude

The Focusing Attitude of being "friendly" or welcoming to one's experience is especially beneficial for people with chronic illness, since many feel angry at their illness and betrayed by the body. Bringing the Focusing Attitude toward the bodily felt sense helps to pave a pathway for increasing kindness and compassion toward the body and self.

In the following example, the Focusing Attitude is integrated with the basic FOAT step for accessing a felt sense and expressing it in art.

Heather was in her late 20s when she unexpectedly was diagnosed with a rare chronic illness that caused chronic pain and affected her autoimmune system. FOAT has helped Heather to transform her relationship to her body and to access its wisdom for healing and health-related decisions. She shared:

> "Before I began Focusing with art, I thought of my pain with anger and hatred. FOAT has helped me to pay attention to the parts of myself that I would typically prefer to ignore—my body and pain."

Focusing Attitude and Check-In Exercise

> "Take few deep breaths down into your body, being friendly and accepting to whatever you notice inside. It may be warm, or jumpy, or calm. When you're ready, ask inside, so how am I on the inside right now? [pause] See if there's an image that matches the inner felt sense. Check it for a sense of rightness. If it's not right, let it go and invite a new image to come. When you have it, use the art materials to create your felt sense image."

Heather began to draw an image of a red outline of a body with a small, black clawing figure within it.[1] Short red strokes emanate from the head, hands, and feet of the small figure (Figure 15.2). Heather describes her art and felt sense:

> "I drew a red outline of a human figure with a creature with sharp black claws inside of it. The creature was clawing and scratching inside the body, leaving bloody, red scratch marks. As I brought an attitude of 'being friendly' to it, I began to understand, that the creature was clawing and scratching inside the body because it was

---

[1] Original artwork in this chapter was in color. It is reproduced here in black and white.

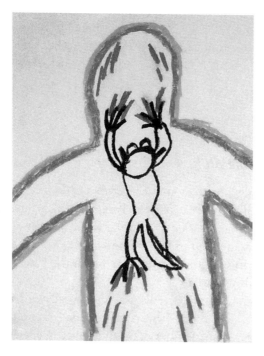

FIGURE 15.2. Focusing attitude and felt sense 1.

trapped and scared and confused. It wasn't evil and it meant no harm. It was innocent and as terrorized as I . . . and it was simply trying to get free."

As can be seen, Heather began to see the "creature" inside as scared, confused, innocent, and terrorized instead of evil and intending harm. This begins a more compatible and compassionate relationship with her body, rather than feeling victimized by a foreign creature.

Heather continued to work with the Focusing Attitude and bringing greater friendliness to the illness. During another FOAT exercise, Heather received the felt sense image of a blue figure holding a small figure; the larger figure is surrounded with bright, yellow light (Figure 15.3).

Heather described her experience: "Now the figure is blue and is cradling that same creature, now curled and sleeping softly in its arms. The claw marks from the previous drawing are still visible inside the figure but now they are black instead of red, symbolizing healing scars rather than fresh wounds. Seeing my pain as innocent and frightened led me to have more compassion for myself as I came to understand the pain as an aspect of myself. In cradling the creature, I was actually cradling the vulnerable part of myself that was frightened and hurting."

The healing power of the Focusing Attitude is palpable and clearly seen in the art and in Heather's descriptive words. The creature is no longer a creature but a vulnerable part of self that was frightened and hurting. Instead of being angry at the illness and in

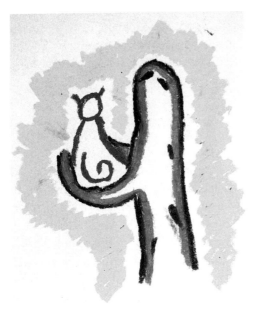

FIGURE 15.3. Focusing attitude and felt sense 2.

conflict with her body, Heather is able to access a part of self that can feel compassion toward it. Similar to meditation and relaxation methods that bring greater results with practice, the Focusing Attitude cultivates greater self-acceptance and compassion over time. In addition to integrating the Focusing Attitude with a guided art exercise, the therapist can offer suggestions during a client's sharing, such as "I hear the difficulty. Can you take a moment and be friendly to that." The therapist also needs to transmit that quality of "friendliness" and acceptance. The Focusing Attitude is more than a technique—it is a way of being for the therapist while teaching clients to cultivate a gentle, accepting attitude within themselves. The Focusing Attitude is an intrinsic part of FOAT and is also seen in the remaining case examples and FOAT approaches.

Clearing a Space with Art

In Clearing a Space with Art, an effective stress reduction method that helps the client to access a state of wholeness, the client identifies the issues that are in the way of feeling "all fine" and imagines placing them at a distance outside of the body. Imagery is incorporated in helping to set the issues at a distance that feels right in order to "clear the space." For example, the client might imagine wrapping each issue in a package and placing it at a comfortable distance, or putting a concern or problem on a boat and letting it float out on a lake. Art is incorporated in order to concretize and symbolize the felt sense of the issues being set aside. After clearing the issues, the client gets a felt sense of the "all fine place" and symbolizes it in art.

Depending on client needs, Clearing a Space with Art can be done with either a guided Focusing process (similar in feel to guided imagery) or without the guided process, using art materials only (Rappaport, 2009, 2010).

The following example is from a 4-week support group for people with cancer. In the first week, I led the group in a guided Clearing a Space with Art exercise. Each woman was given a blank journal in which to draw and write about her experience.

Guided Clearing a Space with Art Exercise

"Take a few deep breaths inside to your body . . . being friendly and accepting to whatever is happening within right now [Focusing Attitude]. Imagine yourself in a peaceful place. When you're ready, ask, "What's between me and feeling "all fine" right now?' As each concern comes, up, just notice it, without going into it. Imagine a way to set the issues at a distance from you outside of your body—such as wrapping up each concern and setting it at a distance from you. As you put each thing aside, sense how it feels inside. Check again . . . except for all of that, I'm 'all fine'? Once you set aside the concerns or stressors, notice how you are inside. See if there is an image that matches your inner felt sense of the 'all fine place.' When you're ready, express your experience in art. Some people prefer to only create the 'all fine place,' while others like to include the stressors they are setting aside and the 'all fine place.' Trust what is right for you."

Sheila, a 53-year-old woman diagnosed with breast cancer, drew a figure with bright blue eyes surrounded by greenery and a yellow light in the sky. In front of her are blocks of blue, representing a ledge (Figure 15.4). Sheila describes the art and Focusing:

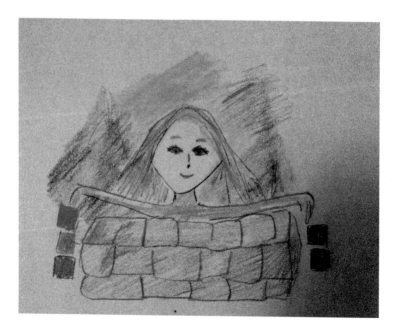

FIGURE 15.4. Clearing a Space with Art: Sheila.

"I imagined being at a serene villa in Tuscany that had a swimming pool. As each issue came up, I imagined wrapping it up in a package and dropping it over the ledge. It felt wonderful to get space from them. In my 'all fine place' I felt safe and protected. I received an image of myself basking in the light and green rolling hills. A word came—'blessed.'"

With clients who may be overwhelmed with feelings or are not able to self-regulate, it is best to use Clearing a Space without the inner guided Focusing process. Clients can decorate a box to hold their stressors or anything that's in the way of feeling "All Fine." They can draw or write their stressors on cards and place them in the box (Figure 15.5). They can close the box, then move it to a place in the room that gives them some space from it. After, they can create something to represent their "all fine place" (Figure 15.6).

Clearing a Space with Art can be done as a regular self-care practice. A student of mine who has suffered migraines for approximately 25 years, began to use a CD recording of Clearing a Space (Rappaport, 2011). She described the benefits as follows:

"Clearing a Space helps me to be friendly to the pain. I used to fight it, which made my body more tense, which created more pain. The relaxation helps to soften the pain. The art helps to me to feel each stressor in my body and to separate it out. When I look at the 'all fine place' [Figure 15.6] of feeling relaxed and light, it brings me back to that felt sense quality in my body–mind. Overall, I don't suffer the same amount of time and the pain is less."

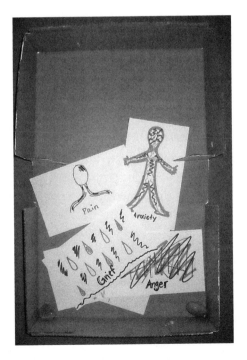

FIGURE 15.5. Setting stressors and issues aside.

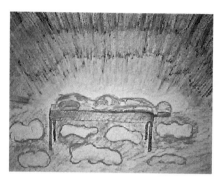

FIGURE 15.6. "All fine place."

Theme-Directed FOAT

Theme-Directed FOAT is frequently used in groups and provides common topics for social support. Examples of themes to be explored when working with chronic illness might include topics that harness resilience and positive energies, such as sources of strength, resources and supports, illness as teacher, and self-care. Clients are guided to take a moment to become aware of a particular theme, to sense the whole feel of it (felt sense), then to see if there is an image that matches the felt sense (symbol/handle) that is then expressed in art.

The second week of the previously described cancer support group addressed the theme "source of strength." The goal was to help members identify a source of strength that would help in coping with their illness. Ideas of sources of strength included an actual memory, something from nature, a pet, spiritual resources, people, an inspirational author, or something imagined.

Source of Strength Exercise

"Take a few deep breaths down into your body . . . breathing in . . . breathing out. Become aware of your body where it meets the chair, of your feet touching the floor. Feel how your body is supported. . . . I'd like to invite you to become aware of something in your life that has been a source of strength. It may be a specific memory, a natural landscape, a beloved pet, a spiritual teacher or teaching, a person known or unknown to you . . . anything that you experience as a source of strength. [pause] Describe this source of strength to yourself . . . seeing its image and feeling its strength. Turn your attention inside to your body and notice how it feels inside as you focus on this source of strength. [pause] See if there's an image that matches the inner felt sense. [pause] Check it against your body for a sense of rightness. If it's not right, let it go and invite a new image [or word, phrase, gesture, or sound] to come. [pause] When you're ready, bring your attention to being in this room, stretch, and gently open your eyes. Use the art materials to express your felt sense of your source of strength." (Rappaport, 2009, p. 174)

After the guided Focusing, 63-year-old Cindy drew a small circular shape with rays reflecting a larger green shape, colored with a thin marker. The words "creativity, happiness, and energy radiate from the smaller circle to the larger shape" (Figure 15.7). At the bottom of the drawing she wrote, "A wonderful French film about the magical effects of a green moon." Cindy shared:

> "I remembered a French film about the magical effects of a green moon. I don't remember the details of the film, but there was a magical quality of the green moon and it had an incredible beauty. I felt the strength and magic of the green moon, taking in its energy of creativity, happiness, and energy. The experience was extraordinary as I could feel the magical energy from the green moon pouring into my body." (Rappaport, 2009, p. 178)

As illustrated in this example, the art externalizes the energies from Cindy's source of strength—the green moon radiating into the larger shape—through which Cindy feels the "extraordinary" magical effects throughout her body.

Focusing-Oriented Art Psychotherapy

In Focusing-Oriented Art Psychotherapy with chronic illness, FOAT is helpful to work through unresolved issues such as fear, grief and loss, as well to explore ways to take steps toward self-care and healing. The following example illustrates a moment-by-moment unfolding of a FOAT psychotherapy session with a client who wanted to work on her fear of a recurrence of cancer. In addition to the basic FOAT step of expressing the felt sense in art, questions are posed to the felt sense as the client listens inwardly to the body's answers (Steps 5 and 6 in Gendlin's Focusing method). Experiential listening is interspersed with Focusing and art making. It is also possible to integrate dialogue with the art.

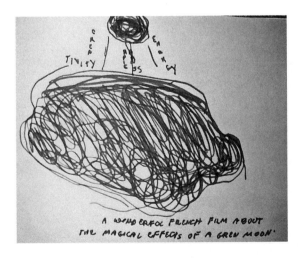

FIGURE 15.7. Source of strength: Cindy.

Sarah, a 48-year-old cancer survivor, came to see me for expressive arts therapy. Her goals were to learn tools for stress reduction and reexamine her life in order to prioritize what has meaning. To demonstrate the facilitation and unfolding of an individual FOAT session, excerpts of the session transcript are presented, along with how Focusing steps and listening responses are interspersed.

Choosing an Issue

THERAPIST: Would you like to take a moment to check inside and ask, "What's needing my attention today?"

SARAH: The fear of recurrence of cancer.

Felt Sense

THERAPIST: Let your attention come down inside your body to the place of fear of the cancer recurrence. See if you can be friendly to it [Focusing Attitude]. Imagine sitting down next it . . . sense the whole feel of it [felt sense].

Symbol/Handle

THERAPIST: See if there's an image (or word, phrase, gesture, or sound) that matches the inner felt sense.

SARAH: Sarah opens her eyes, creates a rolled thin shape using model magic with a balloon shape at the end [Figure 15.8]. It feels tight in my throat. That's where the fear is.

Resonate

THERAPIST: Check to see if the image and art materials match the felt sense.

Asking the Felt Sense

THERAPIST: Go back inside to the felt sense, keeping it company. Can you ask it, "What makes it so afraid?"

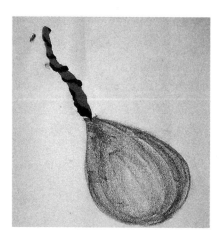

FIGURE 15.8. Felt sense of fear: Sarah.

Receive

SARAH: It says it gets afraid that when any stress comes, it will cause the cancer to come back.

THERAPIST: There's a fear inside that when you have any stress, it will cause the cancer to come back [listening reflection].

SARAH: Yes.

THERAPIST: Can you ask it what it needs?

SARAH: (*Takes a moment to sense inside.*) It says singing helps.

THERAPIST: Singing helps. Would you like to sing now or imagine singing? [Sara was a singer in a band.]

SARAH: I'd rather imagine singing.

THERAPIST: Imagine a time when you have sung. Bring that experience into the present moment and feel what it feels like in your body to sing [felt sense]. See if there's an image that matches the inner felt sense of singing [symbol/handle].

SARAH: (*Picks up a green oil pastel and draws from the bottom of the page upward and outward, with flowing open movements. She adds other colors—yellow, red, purple, and blue [Figure 15.9].*) When I imagine singing, the energy just kind of went up—there was a release.

THERAPIST: (*Sets the two drawings next to each other. We are both amazed with the change—from the tight restricted fear to the open, light-filled radiance [artistic reflection].*)

SARAH: Just the difference in feeling. It's such a healing feeling. I need to give this to myself. During those times when I am afraid, or worrying . . . this is something I can do—just imagining myself singing can change the feeling. It just keeps telling me, you can't forget this. This is going to save your life.

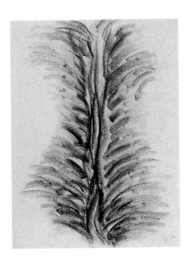

FIGURE 15.9. Felt sense from singing: Sarah.

THERAPIST: Yes—this is something that you have all the time. You can always imagine . . . it takes just a moment. Doing this releases the stress so it says, don't forget this, because this is going to save your life!

In Focusing-Oriented Art Psychotherapy, there is often an alternation among Focusing, listening, and art making. Focusing helps the client to access the answers from within, while the art serves to externalize the felt sense and carry it forward toward healing. As Gendlin (1981a) states, "Our body knows the direction of healing and life. If you take time to listen to it through Focusing, it will give you the steps in the right direction" (p. 78).

CONCLUSION

FOAT provides a way for a client with a chronic illness to form a more positive relationship with his or her body and access its inner wisdom and creative intelligence. Both the Focusing Attitude and Clearing a Space help clients to access a part of themselves that is inherently whole, that can be in a relationship with the illness or pain rather than being consumed by it. FOAT attends to the relational and attachment dimensions of the therapeutic relationship by establishing the safety for the "person in there" as paramount and integrating reflective listening. A Theme-Directed FOAT approach helps to build psychosocial support, while Focusing-Oriented Art Psychotherapy addresses more in-depth needs for clients oriented toward insight.

REFERENCES

Antrobos, J. (2008). *Focusing and you: Effects on body weight*. Unpublished dissertation, The American School of Professional Psychology, Chicago.

Bar-Sela, G., Atid, L., Danos, S., Gabay, N., & Epelbaum, R. (2007). Art therapy improved depression and influenced fatigue levels with cancer patients on chemotherapy. *Psycho-Oncology, 16*, 980–984.

Bishop, M. (2005). Quality of life and psychosocial adaptation to chronic illness and disability: Preliminary analysis of a conceptual and theoretical synthesis. *Rehabilitation Counseling Bulletin, 48*, 219–231.

Castalia, A. (2010). *The effect and experience of clearing a space with art on stress reduction in sign language interpreters*. Unpublished master's thesis, Notre Dame de Namur University, Belmont, CA.

Curry, N., & Kasser, T. (2005). Can coloring mandalas reduce anxiety? *Art Therapy: Journal of the American Art Therapy Association, 22*(2), 81–85.

Ferraro, M. (2010). *Focusing used as an intervention for chronic pain*. Unpublished dissertation, American School of Professional Psychology, Argosy University, Chicago.

Freeza, E. (2008). Focusing and chronic pain. *The Folio: A Journal for Focusing and Experiential Therapy, 21*(1), 328–337.

Gabriel, B., Bromberg, E., Vandenbovenkamp, J., Walka, P., Kornblith, A. B., & Luzatto, P. (2001). Art therapy with adult bone marrow transplant patients in isolation: A pilot study. *Psycho-Oncology, 10*, 114–123.

Gendlin, E. T. (1981a). *Focusing.* New York: Bantam Books.

Gendlin, E. T. (1981b). Focusing and the development of creativity. *The Folio: A Journal for Focusing and Experiential Therapy, 1*, 13–16.

Gendlin, E. T. (1996). *Focusing-oriented psychotherapy: A manual of the experiential method.* New York: Guilford Press.

Grindler Katonah, D., & Flaxman, J. (1999). Focusing: An adjunct treatment for adaptive recovery from cancer. Retrieved October 30, 2011, from *www.focusing.org/adjunct_treatment.html.*

Keane, J. (2008). Narrative focusing: Discovering the person in chronic illness. *The Folio: A Journal for Focusing and Experiential Therapy, 21*(1), 345–359.

Klagsbrun, J., Lennox, S., & Summers, L. (2010). Effects of "clearing a space" on quality of life in women with breast cancer. *United States Association for Body Psychotherapy Journal, 9*(10), 48–53.

Klagsbrun, J., Rappaport, L., Marcow-Speiser, V., Post, P., Stepakoff, S., & Karmin, S. (2005). Focusing and expressive arts therapy as a complementary treatment for women with breast cancer. *Journal of Creativity and Mental Health, 1*(1), 101–137.

Krycka, K. (1999). The recovery of will on persons with AIDS. *The Folio: A Journal for Focusing and Experiential Therapy, 18*(1), 80–92.

Livneh, H., & Antonak, R. (2005). Psychosocial adaptation to chronic illness and disability: A primer for counselors. *Journal of Counseling and Development, 83*, 12–20.

Livneh, H., Lott, S., & Antonak, R. (2004). Patterns of psychosocial adaptation to chronic illness and disability: A cluster analytic approach. *Psychology, Health, and Medicine, 9*(4), 411–430.

Monti, D., Peterson, C., Shakin Kunkel, E. J., Hauck, W. W., Pequignot, E., Rhodes, L., et al. (2006). A randomized controlled trial of mindfulness-based art therapy (MBAT) for women with cancer. *Psycho-Oncology, 15*, 363–373.

Nainis, N. (2008). Approaches to art therapy for cancer inpatients: research and practice considerations. *Art Therapy: Journal of the American Art Therapy Association, 25*(3), 115–121.

Nainis, N., Paice, J., Ratner, J. Wirth, J., Lai., J. & Shott, S. (2006). Relieving symptoms in cancer: Innovative use of art therapy. *Journal of Symptom Management, 31*(2), 162–169.

Rappaport, L. (2008). Focusing-oriented art therapy. *The folio: A Journal for Focusing and Experiential Therapy, 21*(1), 139–155.

Rappaport, L. (2009). *Focusing-oriented art therapy: Accessing the body's wisdom and creative intelligence.* London: Jessica Kingsley.

Rappaport, L. (2010). Focusing-oriented art therapy with trauma. *Journal of Person-Centered and Experiential Psychotherapy, 9*(2), 128–142.

Rappaport, L. (2011). *Focusing for wellbeing: Guided exercises* [CD]. Santa Rosa, CA: Focusing and Expressive Arts Institute.

Svensk, A. C., Oster, I., Thyme, K. E., Magnusson, E., Sjodin, M., Astrom, S., et al. (2009). Art therapy improves experienced quality of life among women undergoing treatment for breast cancer: A randomized controlled study. *European Journal of Cancer Care, 18*, 69–77.

Weiland, L. (2011). *The use of clearing a space with art to reduce stress in graduate students.* Unpublished master's thesis, Notre Dame de Namur University, Belmont, CA.

CHAPTER 16

Art Therapy and Medical Rehabilitation with Adults

Marcia Weisbrot

Acute medical rehabilitation is a unique setting for the practice of art therapy and is different from the traditional mental health, social service, and education settings in which many art therapists work. This chapter describes the most common situations that bring patients to medical rehabilitation, then illustrates how art therapy can play an important part of their treatment, facilitating healing and understanding. Art therapy has much to offer in this setting.

There are some specific challenges and profound opportunities to provide art therapy in medical rehabilitation. The greatest challenge is in working with patients who have lost body function and helping them in the process of adjustment to disability (Liebmann, 2008). In the beginning, patients are focused solely on their bodily losses, usually mobility and cognitive function, and it takes time for emotional and/or spiritual concerns to emerge. These most pressing core issues are common to almost all patients in medical rehabilitation (Alyami, 2009; Michaels, 2005; Michaels & Weston, 2007). Patients may have limited hand and upper extremity mobility, an aspect that must be addressed with each patient prior to beginning art therapy. These challenges and patients' progress are explored in this chapter.

WHAT IS MEDICAL REHABILITATION?

"Medical rehabilitation" (medical rehab) is the process of helping people achieve their most functional levels of ability after a disabling illness or accident. While there may be physically disabling issues, mental health issues are also present. The medical specialty of physiatry is also part of medical rehab and is defined as a branch of medicine that specializes in diagnosis, treatment, and management of disease primarily using "physical" means, such as physical therapy and medications. Essentially, physiatrists specialize in a wide variety of treatments for the musculoskeletal system—the muscles, bones and associated nerves, ligaments, tendons, and other structures—and the musculoskeletal disorders that cause pain and/or difficulty with functioning. Additionally, nursing, physical therapy, occupational therapy, speech therapy, case management, recreation therapy, peer counseling and, in the cases presented in this chapter, art therapy make up the medical rehab treatment team.

Many situations bring people to a medical rehab unit. During the time I worked in rehab, I worked with patients who had strokes; closed head injuries from extreme accidents (motorcycle, bicycle, automobile accidents, falls); brain injuries from tumors; drug overdoses and/or chronic drug use that affected the brain; disabling rheumatoid arthritis, complex multiple medical problems that resulted in mobility changes; severe burns; and spinal cord illness and/or injury that left them paralyzed. Some of the patients had been victims of violence, and their rehabilitation was a bit more complex. The learning curve about this type of medical practice is huge and fascinating. Some of the major conditions found in medical rehab settings include the following:

- *Stroke.* Briefly, a person in medical rehab who has had a stroke experiences some kind of difficulty with blood supply, blood clot, and bleeding in the brain. The affected part of the brain is usually on the side of the body opposite where the disabling symptoms occur (Edmans, 2011). In other words, a person who had a stroke on the left side of the brain, depending on the severity, might have mobility problems on the right side of his or her body. Strokes vary from person to person depending on many medical factors, age, previous medical history, and how quickly the stroke is treated (Edmans, 2011).

- *Head injuries.* Like strokes, head injuries also affect the brain, but the results are not as uniform. They may take more diverse shapes and forms. Whether from brain tumors, accidents of all kinds, violent injury to the head, or chronic drug use, these injuries manifest differently than a stroke, but the recovery issues are very similar: loss of previous function and adjustment to a new way of life.

- *Spinal cord injuries.* Spinal cord injuries are most often caused by accidents, with motor vehicle accidents accounting for the highest percentage (Holtz & Levi, 2004). The late actor Christopher Reeves, a most famous and dramatic example, sustained his spinal cord injury while riding a horse and unsuccessfully jumping over a bar. While spinal cord injury follows a specific and predictable structure, depending upon where on the spinal cord the injury took place, each patient has different medical, social, and emotional needs. One important factor is whether the cord is severed partially or completely. In physiatry terms, a spinal cord that is severed completely is known as a "complete injury," resulting in a greater level of paralysis. One that is partially severed is called an "incomplete injury," and the range of mobility is more unpredictable (Holtz & Levi, 2004). Briefly, an injury to a cervical (C_1–C_7) area at the top of the spine results in the most paralysis if it involves a complete break of the spinal cord. The other parts of the spine are the thoracic, T_1–T_{12} area; the lumbar, L^1–L_5 area; and finally, at the very bottom, the sacral area, followed by the coccyx (Selzer & Dobkin, 2008). Again, to use Mr. Reeves as an example, his injury was complete and was very high up on the cervical spine at C_2. Thus, he sustained a very high level of paralysis, including difficulty breathing, because the muscular supports to his lungs were affected. It is important to understand spinal injuries in order to realize what mobility function patients will have and how they will be able to accomplish activities, including those in art therapy. It is also central to helping with a patient's emotional and psychosocial issues.

MAJOR TREATMENT GOALS AND OBJECTIVES

Treatment issues for art therapy include but are not limited to functional improvement and addressing emotional and traumatic issues associated with physical injuries. Functional improvement is the primary goal of all staff members working with medical rehab patients. The physical therapist has goals for regaining function of limbs as much as possible. The occupational therapist hopes to get the patient to be as independent as possible with his or her daily activities and needs. The speech therapist hopes to get patients to speak as much as they did before, or to improve their poststroke/head injury speech. In most cases, time is of the essence here, as the return of function takes place for most people in the first 6 months, although many people continue to improve in specific areas over a longer period of recovery (Gillen, 2010).

Dealing with a trauma of any kind is overwhelming and frightening, but especially so if the trauma is within or to one's own body and if it means one's body has been permanently changed. Confusion, anger, and fear are only a few of the emotional responses to trauma to the body; the question "Why me?" is constant during early stages of physical injury. If the trauma was sustained by violent means, there is added fear and anger, apprehension about repercussions or repeat violence, and a sense of powerlessness. Gradually, patients realize that changes are permanent: They experience loss, and realize that their lives may be ruined or irrevocably altered, and never be the same again. Very often, depression, anger, and anxiety take hold (Gillen, 2010; Liebmann, 2008).

In brief, art therapy goals with medical rehab patients are designed to augment functional goals wherever possible; to provide the structure and means for expressing experiences of trauma and loss; and to help patients understand, resolve, and adjust to their experiences and body changes. As with any complex traumatic event and recovery, these goals are not always reached before the patient returns home, but are instead accomplished outside of hospitalization.

IMPLEMENTING ART THERAPY ON A MEDICAL REHAB UNIT

There are many ways that art therapy can help patients in medical rehab. First and foremost, the art therapist can help with functional mobility, as determined by the treatment team. For example, art therapy can be designed to encourage patients to reach for and use materials in ways that augment the goals of physical and/or occupational therapy. Painting and drawing with wide movements use the hand and upper body movements that complement physical and occupational therapy goals. Assisting a patient in organizing colors and materials before and after painting can help improve visual and spatial abilities; encouraging verbal communication about artwork individually or within a group supports speech therapy goals and builds confidence (Horovitz, 2005).

Adapting art materials and methods and creating assistive tools for art making are central to successful art therapy in medical rehab settings. Assistive devices may be very simple—for example, using tape to hold a paper for painting when the patient has only one mobile arm. Some patients may be able to use only sponges for painting; I often cut sponges into all sizes, so patients can experiment with what feels most comfortable for them to use.

With the assistance of occupational therapists who enjoy this challenge of creating assistive devices, we created a cuff that holds a paintbrush. It has an adjustable band that uses Velcro. The brush itself is inserted into the cuff and held in place with a Velcro strap. This is especially helpful for quadriplegic patients who have no hand mobility but have some limited wrist or shoulder movement. It is also useful for other patients with varying hand and arm mobility, who may start out using the cuff, then gradually put it away if or when their mobility increases, providing a measurement of success as well.

Plastic polymerized vinyl chloride (PVC) pipe (found in hardware and plumbing stores) can be adapted for art therapy use and is popular with patients who have brain injury and limited hand mobility. The pipe has a small hole drilled on one side so that a Cray-Pas or chalk can be inserted and held in place with a screw. Someone who is able to grip the pipe but does not have the fine motor coordination can use this to draw (see information at the end of this chapter; also see Chapter 1 for more information on adaptive art therapy techniques and Very Special Arts Washington/Creative Activities—Adaptive Equipment [*www.creativeactivities.org/resources/adaptive-equipment*]).

Finally, sometimes the most effective adaptive art mechanism is a method I call "art director." The patient becomes the art director as I, another staff member, and/or a volunteer executes the art for them. This is an especially good adaptive device for collage. Collage is a relatively nonthreatening medium to work with, as well as one that offers a great deal of control—control being an important aspect for a patient who is newly disabled. In addition, collage allows examination, sorting, and choosing, all of which contribute to emotional and cognitive integration (Hass-Cohen & Carr, 2008). Patients choose magazine or photo images and instruct the art therapist as to where to place and to adhere them to paper or poster board. In addition, almost all patients are working on learning to give directions to others, to help them with their daily needs and care. "Art directing" helps to fulfill some of that goal.

Some patients are ready to work on psychosocial issues immediately, while others are not; some are resistant to the idea that they need help with mental health and emotional issues. Even though it seems obvious that anyone who has experienced such profound body changes would need support and therapy, patients are generally focused on physical rehabilitation in the beginning of their treatment. In other words, if patients' abilities to walk, talk, and think are compromised, then these take precedence; depression or anxiety may not always be apparent to patients.

CASE EXAMPLES

The following case studies include one long-term patient and two shorter-term patients, and illustrate different aspects of treatment depending on length of stay and type of illness. (Names have been changed to protect privacy, and identifying information has been altered.)

Darin

Darin, a 27-year-old man, was in a serious auto accident that resulted in an incomplete injury to his spine at the cervical level (C_4–C_5) and left him paralyzed. He also had a history of drug and alcohol abuse, behavioral issues, and family conflict. I first introduced myself to him about a week after his admission. I visited with him briefly over the next few weeks, taking time to do this slowly because I knew that he would be at the facility for a long time, and because he seemed suspicious of me.

My goals at this time were simply to build rapport and trust with him. The first session with Darin included collage with images of his choice (he "art directed" and I did the work) and some general conversation about his experiences in the hospital. He was open about his hospital experiences but guarded when I asked about his life prior to the accident. His collage was very scattered and primarily dark imagery, but the experience seemed to give him a sense of control, something that is crucial to a person with his kind of injury (Malchiodi, 2007). The second time we met he created a collage that was quite playful. Darin remarked that each collage portrayed a different side—his dark side and his light side. He also attempted to use a marker but was quite frustrated by his inability to do so.

Next, Darin participated in a group session where he tried to paint. Painting seemed to make him regress, as evidenced by his cursing and trying to provoke the therapists. It took myself, the peer counselor, and a volunteer to contain him. It seemed that painting did not offer the same amount of control as collage. This lack of control was what made his behavior change in a negative way. It might not have been an appropriate medium for him at this stage of treatment.

By this time I had formulated treatment goals for Darin. These included using collage to build rapport, to provide structure and a sense of control; encouraging choice of images related to disability issues; encouraging appropriate social interactions in group settings, with attention to group dynamics and improved interpersonal relations; working on adjustment to disability (e.g., denial, anger, acceptance of loss); and understanding functional abilities through the use of art. During the next individual session Darin created a large collage across two sheets of paper. It included an image of a man reflected in the water. It also included several heads that were severed from their bodies (in my experience, a common image for quadriplegics to choose). In a group collage session the following week, he also chose more severed heads but was unable to talk about the meaning of his collage images when group members asked about them.

Figure 16.1 is a commonly seen image painted by numerous patients adjusting to quadriplegia while in medical rehabilitation. While the color version shows more connection of the head to the body (yellow just below the neck, not white), the overall visual impression is that of a head floating above the body.[1] This may express a feeling of separation of the head, which is still mobile, sensitive, and "working," from the immobile body that has little movement and even less sensation.

In group session 2 weeks later, Darin chose the words "the anxiety of being incomplete" from a disability magazine. I conjectured that at this point he was able to relate this to his own injury, and that this was an important breakthrough in his self-understanding of his disability. At this time, Darin and I went for an outing to the park across the street; all therapists were encouraged to do this, as it helped patients learn to be more independent of the hospital, as well as practice outdoor mobility. Several children were throwing a volleyball nearby, and one yelled out, "Hey, look out for the dude in the wheelchair!" Darin recognized this with surprise but also realized that this is how he would be seen in the outside in the world.

A few weeks later, he created a very large collage with black and white images from a black and white publication that included the words "a beginner" and a picture of an infant. We talked about how he was a beginner, feeling infantilized and needing to be cared for by others. There was a brightness and lightness about this collage that was significantly different than the others. Also, his mother and grandmother were present in the activity room during part of the session when he worked on this image.

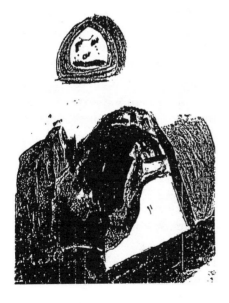

FIGURE 16.1. Image by a patient with quadriplegia.

---

[1]Original artwork in this chapter was in color. It is reproduced here in black and white.

In the subsequent weeks, prior to his discharge from the hospital, Darin attended the group regularly and got angry when we did not want him to paint. I considered that it might have been a mistake to ask him not to paint. Although it had some value for him, it also stimulated regressive behavior. I was also concerned about the needs of other group members who might be impacted by his behavior. He tried to paint anyway and became quite regressed, painting a curse word, and putting his fingers in paint and into his mouth.

Darin's final art piece while at the facility was a large collage of relief objects that he collected over a period of several weeks. He worked on it for several sessions very patiently and since it was a hanging piece, asked if I could draw a picture of him on the other side. I've often drawn simple portraits of patients over the years and have found that it is a positive connecting experience for both of us and can also be an excellent termination/goodbye exercise. This was true in his case, as Darin was delighted with the portrait I drew and felt it added so much to his work. I felt privileged to make that contribution at the end of his hospital stay. During the months that I worked with Darin in art therapy, he was able to increase his ability to express himself visually, to give excellent directions to me about his artistic preferences and ideas, and to use collage to gain some self-awareness. He was also able to use collage to express and integrate feelings about his life, and to communicate some acceptance of his disability. I recommended that he continue art therapy at home using collage and markers (he was resistant to this, though he did have enough hand mobility to do so). In addition to disability issues Darin had many issues of self-esteem and family conflicts to work on.

Elisa

Elisa, a 77-year-old stroke patient, was seen by the art therapy intern for two sessions, a week apart, during her stay on the rehab unit. She said she had never painted before and chose to paint with sponges rather than brushes, as do many patients whose mobility in their dominant hand has been affected by their stroke. Elisa chose bright colors and painted with diligence and great concentration. She painted four small images (see Figure 16.2, the first in the series) and said that these paintings expressed how she felt. She titled her images "Frustration," "Confusion," "Rest," and "Laughter." Her stroke had left her speech quite impaired and it was obvious that she was deriving pleasure from this experience of painting. Perhaps she was even finding a new voice.

During the following week, in another session, Elisa was eager to paint and created more boldly, taking up more space on the paper. One of her goals was to try and write her name with a marker. She did this three times on each of three paintings she produced; her letters were legible and fully formed. The art therapy intern made a meaningful connection with Elisa in just two sessions and encouraged her to keep painting when she arrived home, suggesting various supplies and directives to help her continue. The intern also worked with the occupational therapist to devise ways to set up a painting workstation at home. Elisa's case is a good example of short-term treatment, in which a patient achieved a difference in functional improvement, affect, and, self-esteem in two carefully structured sessions.

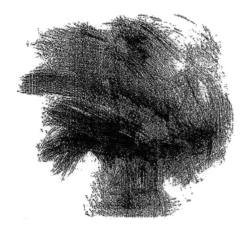

FIGURE 16.2. Image by a stroke patient.

Bob

Bob, a 35-year-old man, was assaulted with a knife by his lover of 2 years. His injuries to his lower spine, various muscles, and back were extreme. As a result, he experienced anger, trauma, and feelings of victimization and betrayal of trust; the injuries and distress greatly impacted his preexisting mood disorder and personality issues. Bob's assailant was a health care professional, making the work with all therapists on the unit even more challenging, as he was most distrustful of us all. In addition, Bob's case drew unwanted local media attention.

Because of his intense emotion surrounding his situation, it took a while to engage Bob in art therapy. But he drew easily with a marker and was quick to speak (Figure 16.3). He pointed out that he was the depressed patient in the wheelchair, alone in the

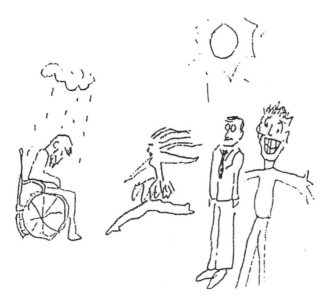

FIGURE 16.3. Bob's drawing of himself in wheelchair, physical therapy, and doctors.

corner and under a rain cloud. His physical therapist was constantly trying to get Bob to do the difficult things he didn't want to do. He portrayed the doctors with sunny, phony dispositions, looking the other way, grinning, and not understanding him at all. Bob appeared quite pleased with this drawing and stated that it made him feel vindicated in his feelings about being in the hospital. It gave him a sense of control to put all the players in the hospital drama together.

Bob was discharged to another facility because of insurance regulations before we were able to provide any further interventions. His case is an example of the complexity of rehabilitation from a disabling attack that involves responses to violence, as well as preexisting health conditions.

GROUP ART THERAPY

A weekly art therapy group is recommended as an option for patients in medical rehabilitation. A group setting offers the following patient benefits: a sense of self-esteem and social skills through group participation (Smith, 2007), and a place to share emotions with others (Liebmann, 2004, 2008), knowing that they are not alone in their feelings. Group work can also assist the process of finding meaning in the accident or illness itself. Finding meaning in a horrific life event can alter the way one feels about it, and help with adjustment and subsequent life wellness; it can also facilitate acceptance and understanding of one's medical situation (Coetzer, 2006).

The peer counselor, a man in his 40s who had sustained a C_5–C_6 complete spinal cord injury at the age of 31, was a tremendous resource for both staff and patients on this unit. He lived independently with the assistance of in-home support aides, drove an adaptive van, and was a great role model for the patients.

We worked together to plan the structure of each group and set goals for each patient. We were quite flexible about all of this due to the loosely structured format, and because it took place in a room with others moving in and out and about. We encouraged staff members to participate, and sometimes they did. Most often it was nurses, who took time out from working behind the nearby nursing station. Their pleasure in doing art with us was helpful for patients to observe, and their interactions with all of us in the group provided additional perspectives on using art in the group.

We (including the peer counselor) usually painted for about 30–40 minutes. We used large sheets of paper, approximately 18″ × 24″; water-based paints; and the adaptive devices mentioned earlier. The peer counselor was a very important role model, because all of the patients knew that he had less upper body mobility than they, and if he could paint, so could they.

We then taped paintings up on the wall to look at and discuss. Why? One reason is that work looks different from a distance and provides another perspective. Another, more important reason is that opportunities to connect with others are greater—patients see similarities between their own work and others (Gonen & Soroker, 2000). They also can see growth and change. For patients who were working on speech improvement, this was a good opportunity to practice talking with others, and to talk about their work and their feelings in a safe place.

Patients help one another sometimes more than staff, because we are not in their shoes. We would send work home with patients as inspiration to keep painting and as a transitional object from hospital to home. Mostly we focused on painting in the group, because it was the easiest and most immediate medium to use, but for those who were able some drawing and collage also took place, and occasionally printmaking and work in three dimensions. When it was possible we also did collaborative mural painting and even a three-dimensional (3D) collage that covered a broken pinball machine in the activity room.

The peer counselor and I would suggest various topics to paint related to the treatment issues discussed earlier. Sometimes patients would take to that; other times they did not. How much insight-oriented work was taking place varied, and the group membership changed constantly. The average length of stay for stroke patients was 3 to 4 weeks. Patients with more complex rehab, such as head or spinal cord injuries, were there much longer, sometimes 6 months to a year. Older group members would instruct the new ones. And we always paid extra attention to those who were being discharged to go home, focusing on review and termination issues.

At times, drop-in studio groups with patients, family, and staff took place informally before or after dinner, depending on who was on the unit, and included both staff members' and patients' families. There were no directives or assignments, but "suggestions" evoked a lot of conversation between family members of various patients. This was my goal—to help them connect with each other, and to provide each other support and understanding about their particular family member's situation and the commonalities they shared, using the group to build rapport, support, and understanding. Staff members would come by and participate in the activities, which most often focused on collage, art journals, and some painting. Again, this group met during the weeks when active family members were present on the unit.

ART THERAPY AND MEDICAL REHAB INSERVICE TRAINING FOR STAFF

Because art therapy is not always entirely understood in medical rehabilitation and other hospital settings, providing staff training can be important. Once I had a better understanding of patient needs and the treatment team, I offered many inservice programs about art therapy, underscoring how it could be an active part of the treatment team. Typically, I would start out with a brief overview of art therapy, discussing the role of art therapists in different settings, in order to explain what I was contributing to patients' health care. As a result, staff members would often respond with new ideas for art therapy that I could apply to work with patients. This also made a noticeable difference in how the staff responded to me and how art therapy was understood. Because I was the first art therapist to work at the medical rehab unit, this was very important. All of the inservice programs were experiential (yes, there was some resistance to this) and focused on functional, as well as emotional, needs of patients that could be addressed through art therapy. I included patients' art products in the discussions to demonstrate methods and outcomes.

When art therapy is provided as part of a team approach to medical rehab, the staff should be aware of the following goals of art therapy: (1) Art therapy supports the functional goals of other therapists who are working with patients; (2) it can improve visual perception and cognition, and increase motor activity (Kim, Kim, Lee, & Chun, 2008); (3) it can improve sensory integration, access memory, and engage parts of the brain early in the rehabilitation process (Pratt, 2004; Van Lith, Fenner, & Schofield, 2010); and (4) it can provide one of few opportunities in rehab to process feelings about physical injuries and associated trauma, and to help patients learn how to understand their emotions while they adjust to their new lives (Mackenzie & Rakel, 2006).

CONCLUSION

The art therapist's work in a medical rehabilitation unit begins with building relationships with patients by providing verbal support and getting to know them soon after admission. It develops when the art therapist invites patients to use art materials (adapted where appropriate) to continue working on their functional goals. The use of adaptive devices and methods to create art and provide functional gains, and adaptation to a higher degree of flexibility are critical in this setting. This begins the process of expression of loss, strengths, and adjustment to disabilities, both through individual and group art therapy experiences.

This chapter ends with the words of a spinal cord patient who was at first resistant to art therapy, but then came to embrace it: "This art therapy has helped make my hand stronger and it's been a good place to understand what's happened to me. It's fun. And knowing that other people are going through it, helped me." The art therapist has much to offer in this setting.

REFERENCES

Alyami, A. (2009). The integration of art therapy into physical rehabilitation in a Saudi hospital. *The Arts in Psychotherapy, 36*(2), 1–7.

Coetzer, R. (2006). *Traumatic brain injury: A psychotherapeutic approach to loss and grief.* New York: Nova Science.

Edmans, J. (2011). *Occupational therapy and stroke.* Oxford, UK: Blackwell.

Gillen, G. (2010). *Stroke rehabilitation: A function-based approach.* St. Louis, MO: Mosby.

Gonen, J., & Soroker, N. (2000). Art therapy in stroke rehabilitation: A model of short-term group treatment. *The Arts in Psychotherapy, 27*(1), 41–50.

Hass-Cohen, N., & Carr, R. (2008). *Art therapy and clinical neuroscience.* London: Jessica Kingsley.

Holtz, A., & Levi, R. (2004). *Spinal cord injury*. New York: Oxford University Press.

Horovitz, E. (2005). *Art therapy as witness: A sacred guide*. Springfield, IL: Thomas.

Kim, S., Kim, M., Lee, J., & Chun, S. (2008). Art therapy outcomes in the rehabilitation treatment of a stroke patient: A case report. *Art Therapy: Journal of the American Art Therapy Association, 25*(3), 129–133.

Liebmann, M. (2004). *Art therapy and groups*. East Sussex, UK: Routledge.

Liebmann, M. (2008). *Art therapy and anger*. London: Jessica Kingsley.

Mackenzie, E., & Rakel, B. (2006). *Complementary and alternative medicine for older adults: A guide to holistic approaches to healthy aging*. New York: Springer.

Malchiodi, C. A. (2007). *The art therapy sourcebook*. New York: McGraw-Hill.

Michaels, D. (2007, February). *Case study: The role of art therapy as a potential space for the processing of psychological and physical experience following a stroke*. Paper presented at the National Health Service, Sheffield, UK.

Michaels, D., & Weston, S. (2005, April). *Art therapies in the stroke pathway*. Paper presented at the Brain Injury Stakeholders meeting, National Health Service, Sheffield, UK.

Pratt, R. R. (2004). Art, dance, and music therapy. *Physical Medicine and Rehabilitation Clinics of North America, 15*(1), 829–830.

Selzer, M. E., & Dobkin, B. H. (2008). *Spinal cord injury: A guide for patients and families*. New York: Demos.

Smith, C. (2007). Innovative rehabilitation after head injury: Examining the use of a creative intervention. *Journal of Social Work Practice, 21*(3), 297–309.

Van Lith, T., Fenner, P., & Schofield, M. (2010). *Art therapy in rehabilitation*. Center for International Rehabilitation Research Information and Exchange, University of Buffalo, State University of New York. Retrieved August 30, 2011, from *http://cirrie.buffalo.edu*.

CHAPTER 17

Art Therapy, Creative Apperception, and Rehabilitation from Traumatic Brain Injury

Margaret M. McGuinness
Kathy J. Schnur

Art therapy is most often used to improve the emotional well-being of the client. Measurable goals and objectives are scientific approaches often underutilized when working with emotions. Therefore, professionals often find that measurable outcomes are difficult to conceptualize. But goals, objectives, and outcomes are paramount when working with neuropsychiatric impairments from a traumatic brain injury (TBI) event.

As art therapists working within the confines of insurance company reimbursement, we designed a multimodal program to measure executive functioning (cognitive skills) and self-regulation (affective skills) with adult clients who have sustained a TBI. Included in this design was assessment of each client's needs, implementation of individual patient data collection charts, and maintenance of monthly progress levels as prescribed by the therapeutic treatment plan. Key to this program was establishing a therapeutic relationship with the client using a model based on combining the theory of creative apperception and mirror neurons system theory.

TRAUMATIC BRAIN INJURY

In the United States, approximately 1 to 2 million people sustain a TBI yearly (Silver, McAllister, & Arcinegas, 2009). Silver et al. define TBI as a physiologically significant disruption of brain function resulting from the application of . . . external physical force. . . . Evidence of disrupted brain functions at the time force is applied may include loss of consciousness; loss of memory for events immediately before . . . or after . . . collectively called posttraumatic amnesia; an alteration in mental state; a focal neurological deficit. (p. 653)

Being a unique organ the brain responds to injury in a complex manner. Unlike injuries experienced elsewhere in the body, which heal and regain previous functioning, injuries to the brain affect physical abilities, mental abilities, as well as personality (Sohlberg & Mateer 2001). These changes in personality and cognitive functioning impact the client's daily living skills and relationship to family, social groups, and community.

Therefore, recovery from brain injuries can be overwhelming in nature and require complex short-term and long-term treatment. The emotional and social support from TBI clients' treatment team professionals provide a key in understanding these changes and allow for development of new identities and personalities. Unfortunately, some clients and their families may not be aware of the extent of clients' deficits in cognitive, social, and emotional functioning until the client attempts to return to normal activities at home or at a job (Weiss, 2011). As art therapists working with this population, we notice that clients' sense of identity (McGraw, 1999) suffers as a result of this uncertainty, due to both physical and psychological trauma (Malchiodi, 2003).

NEUROBIOLOGY

It is important for art therapists and anyone working with adult clients diagnosed with TBI to understand the neurobiology of the brain. Due to the scope of this chapter, it is impossible to review all the neurological and biological anatomical systems of the brain. By reviewing basic brain anatomy and functions, explaining the theory of brain plasticity (Sohlberg & Mateer, 1989, 2001; Nudo, 2003) and interpreting expected resulting behavior deficits as not uncommon results of injury, we found that our clients felt reassured that their deficits could be retrained or repaired. The prevailing belief about the ability of the brain to form new pathways, or "neuroplasticity," helped us explain to our clients about the possibility of making new neural pathways during art activities.

The neurobiology of the adult brain involves a large prefrontal cortex (PFC). In evolutionary terms, the PFC is the most recently developed part of the brain, the last to evolve from childhood to adult. It is linked to decision making and other executive functioning skills (Sohlberg & Mateer, 1989). According to therapists Galbraith, Subrin, and Ross (2008), our more primitive brain includes the hippocampus, the entorhinal cortex located near the temporal lobes and the amygdala. These primitive areas are responsible for attaching emotions to memory and work together with the PFC when utilizing executive functioning skills. Our multimodal approach of art therapy was designed to help clients to attach the relearning of executive functioning skills to their long-term memories, which may have not been impacted by the trauma of the TBI event.

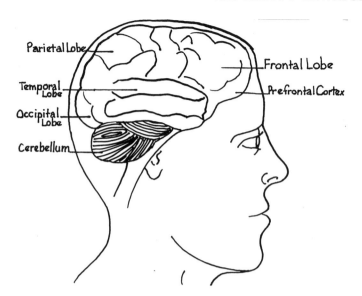

FIGURE 17.1. Brain diagram to help patients understand brain changes during or after a TBI.

Figure 17.1 was designed to help our clients understand what changes in their brain may have occurred during and after their TBI event, thereby normalizing the deficits. Explaining the anatomy of the brain and its functions to clients was accompanied by descriptions of what we thought were important duties of particular areas as related to selected art activities (Lehr, 2011).

1. *Frontal lobes.* Divided into right and left sides, the two frontal lobes are responsible for the regulation of emotion and personality. It is thought that the left frontal lobe controls language, and the right frontal lobe controls nonverbal behavior, such as emotions. Functions affected by damage to the front of the head include problem solving, memory, initiation, judgment, and impulse control. In art therapy sessions, we have frequently noted long-term problems with attention and focus affecting short-term memory recall.

2. *Temporal lobes.* Hearing, memory acquisition, and visual perception are major responsibilities of the two temporal lobes. Impairments of interest to art therapy may include difficulty categorizing objects in the visual field, especially facial recognition; difficulty with the selective attention to what is seen and heard; short-term memory loss; and if the right temporal lobe is damaged, inappropriate, persistent talking.

3. *Parietal lobes.* Two functions of the parietal lobes are cognition (integrating what we sense and what we perceive) and perception of the world around us. Language disorders and denial of problems must often be addressed by the entire treatment team. However, damage to the parietal lobes resulting in an abnormal body image can be addressed in art therapy sessions. During the initial assessment, the client's deficits of perception combined with the inability or resistance to draw or to make things are observed by the

art therapist and communicated to the treatment team, because clients often overcompensate for sensory and perception deficits in traditional treatments.

4. *Occipital lobe.* The occipital lobe, located at the back of the skull, is where vision resides. Even when the impact of the external force is initially applied to the frontal lobes, the acceleration and deceleration effect known as contracoup (whiplash) may result in bruising in this area. Sometimes the initial whiplash damage, along with the lack of oxygenation from the swelling and bruising, may cause additional damage not only to the initial affected area but also other areas (Weiss, 2011). Some of the visual injury deficits displayed include visual field neglect (right or left), inability to recognize colors, reading and writing impairments due to word blindness, and visual hallucinations. We noticed that clients with an injury to the vision area were often unaware of visual deficits, and our long-term goals included teaching clients to be aware of deficits and to request assistance as needed.

5. *Cerebellum.* Located at the base of the skull, the cerebellum is responsible for the coordination of voluntary movement and memory for reflex motor actions. People with injuries to this area may be seen to sway or stagger as they walk. Adaptive tools and activities may be needed in art therapy sessions.

6. *Brain stem.* The brain stem attaches the brain to the spinal cord. It affects the client's level of alertness, ability to sleep, and sense of balance. The brain stem also controls blood pressure, breathing rate, swallowing, sweating, digestion, body temperature, and startle response. Special arrangements in sessions for deficits seen here would include limiting or adjusting stimuli such as noise, lighting, and environment temperature. We adjust art therapy session length if clients demonstrate low levels of alertness.

TESTING

Diagnostic imaging studies can be performed many times during the recovery process of a TBI. Magnetic resonance imaging (MRI), computed tomography (CT) scans, and positron emission tomography (PET) scans assist in acute and nonacute physical phases of brain healing. Neuropsychological testing is performed after the client stabilizes. The neuropsychological testing is an arduous and lengthy psychological examination that usually takes two days for the client to complete. Rehabilitation is a long-term process after an acute event and can take many paths. In day treatment for adults diagnosed with TBI, our focus of testing is on cognitive remediation skills.

COGNITIVE REMEDIATION SKILLS

Due to the complex nature of TBI, executive functioning, creative apperception, and mirror neuron system theories are important in order to provide cognitive remediation. "Executive functioning," necessary for everyday living skills, is a set of cognitive and affective processes that help connect past experiences with present actions. These include planning, organizing, strategizing, paying attention, remembering details, self-regulation of emotions and behaviors, and the management of time and space (Sohlberg & Mateer, 1989). Executive system disorders are new to neuropsychological theory (Bell & Halligan, 2009). If executive functioning of a client is significantly impaired, the very things that make us human, such as the ability conceptually to process abstract thoughts and ideas, regulate emotions, and govern social interactions, may also be impaired (Zillmer, Spiers, & Culbertson, 2008). Introspection, the ability to be able to look at and have a feeling "of knowing," is a newer posit of repair theory necessary for executive functioning (Bell & Halligan, 2009; Sohlberg & Mateer, 2001).

Wunt (see Hergenhahn, 2009), known as the father of experimental psychology, identifies the ability to examine one's own thoughts and feelings as apperception. This complex philosophical idea has roots in early childhood development and education. "Apperception" is defined as the unconscious ability to become aware of something through the senses, in terms of a person's emotional outlook, prior knowledge, and past experiences (Abram & Hjulmand, 2007). "Apperception quickly scans large networks of associations. There it detects a clue which links past with present" (Austin, 1999, p. 523). Although this ability for scanning large networks appeared to have been compromised for some of our clients, linking past to present often remained possible.

"Creative apperception," a term used by Winnicott (Abram & Hjulmand, 2007) describes the infant–mother relationship in apperceptive terms as the perceived anticipation that allows an infant to know they are seen by the mother, then affirms the infants' perception that they exist (Amendt-Lyon, 2001; Kuspit, 2009; Simon, 2005) . "When I look/I am seen, so I exist. I can now afford to look and see" (Abrams & Hjulmand, 2007, p. 8). In a therapeutic space, this visual gaze and perceptive affirmation of existence between individuals appears to mirror the mother–child dyad as explained in object relations theory (Schaverien, 1999) and allows apperception by the client through anticipation. Another theory posited by Wundt, is that attention and apperception go hand in hand, that "what is attended to is apperceived" (Hergenhahn, 2009, p. 245). As a mother attends to her infant, her gaze provides the space of safe holding that allows the infant to grow.

Therefore, it seemed natural to associate the changes seen in our clients' sense of self and need for re-creation of identity with creative apperception. When the client knows he or she is being seen in a safe, structured, art therapy holding environment, a client–art therapist trusting relationship is attended to, the client can apperceive that he or she exists and begins to anticipate an acceptance of deficits and/or reconstruction of missing aspects of personality (McGraw, 1999). As art therapists, we attended to our clients' need to reconstruct identity.

Additionally, this ability to create or reconstruct appears to be related to newer theories about *mirror neurons* and the development of empathy. As mother and child interact, the growing brain develops multiple mirror neuron systems that specialize in understanding and carrying out not just the actions of others, but their intentions, the social meaning of their behavior, and emotions involved (Buccino, Binkofski, & Riggio, 2004).

Mirror neurons enable us to recognize someone else's actions as something we can learn and do (Hass-Cohen & Carr, 2008). Mirroring is only part of a larger social interaction system called "empathy" (Gerdes, Lietz, & Segal, 2011). Iacobini and Dapretto (2006), the founder of mirror neuron systems theory, notes that "the more a person imitates others, the more empathic he or she is likely to become" (p. 949). Therefore the actions of each individual in a relationship can shape or mirror a response to their own previous action as well as the anticipation of the others' reaction. We feel that this anticipation is the same anticipation that is vital to understanding creative apperception. We found by improving executive functioning skills while using creative apperception and empathy, identity can be reconstructed with clients.

ART THERAPY PROGRAM FOR ADULT CLIENTS DIAGNOSED WITH TRAUMATIC BRAIN INJURY

There are few recent publications on art therapy and TBI describing measurable goals and objectives (Sell & Murrey, 2006; Pratt, 2004). In the conceptualization of our design, we decided to utilize the Executive Functioning Scales model presented by Sohlberg and Mateer (1989), because this seminal work divides up the necessary skills in such a manner that art therapy objectives and outcomes can be easily tracked in a measurable way for each client. The design of the art therapy program includes individual client sessions of 50 minutes up to three times weekly for approximately 1 year. Individual assessment and team treatment planning with other therapies is also included.

Because private insurance reimbursement mandated no duplication of services at the facility, art therapy was designated for remediation of executive functioning disorders. Other ancillary therapies were categorized accordingly: music therapy for memory and dysarthria (word finding) and yoga for physical conditioning, self-regulation of emotion and behaviors, and stress reduction. Each client had a primary psychotherapist for individual sessions focusing on emotional behavior and beginning social skills management. Group psychotherapy focused on knowledge of diagnoses, cognitive restructuring, co-occurring disorders, and practicing social skills. The treatment team determined a need for physical and occupational therapies to be added to the choices of services offered. The clinical director, a psychologist, administered pre- and posttesting according to standards of care, focusing on measurable outcomes for efficacy of treatment in each client's treatment plan. According to clients' diagnostic needs, not all clients received all therapies. Treatment was individualized and determined by the treatment team. Prior to admission, neuropsychological testing was performed by an outside agency, and diagnosis of TBI and a prescription for day treatment services were provided from either the client's psychiatrist or physiatrist.

As soon as possible upon admission to the program, the art therapists administered the Diagnostic Drawing Series (DDS; Cohen, Mills, & Johnson, 2010) to each client. The ability to abstract, conceptualize, follow directions, tell a story, and express emotions and thoughts was measured by the DDS. While administering the DDS, we evaluated executive functioning skills; gross and fine motor abilities, including dexterity skills; visual–spatial relationships, including field neglect; and speaking skills, including expressive and receptive abilities, noting clients' strengths and deficits. Using the Executive Functioning Scales (Sohlberg & Mateer, 1989) we could easily track art therapy objectives and outcomes in a measurable way with a simple chart for each client. For example, attention could be recorded as a breakdown of time into measurable units using a Likert-type scale. As a result of art therapy data collection, changes were discernible in a broad perspective in either a desirable or undesirable direction. For example, with several clients who had seizure disorders (not uncommon in our clients with TBI) the data collection on attention skills suggested undesirable attention changes in data tracked pre-event and desirable attention changes postevent.

Subsequently, multimodal, client-chosen and strength-based art therapy sessions were designed for each individual, carefully constructed to safely explore issues relevant to the individual treatment plan. For example, we might recommend that one client focus on 3D media, while another might require figure /ground remediation utilizing simple black-on-white calligraphy; still another client might benefit from "homework," later to return with the artwork in hand for discussion. Although a desirable goal of executive functioning skills is to have clients self-initiate as much as possible, very often it was necessary for us to guide the sessions in content and media. Flexibility in the variety of approaches was also necessary. At times, a cognitive approach worked for some; for others, a more expressive approach was utilized. While for other individuals a more education-based approach was necessary.

In rehabilitation of clients who have sustained a TBI, goals and objectives are established, and education of the clients is stressed. While executive functioning goals were designed around rehabilitation models, the theoretical and practical applications of studio art therapy also provided education models, using a teacher-based individual educational plan (IEP). The IEP objective requires measurable behavior changes designed by staff for each person. For example, a goal might read, "The client will work at his or her maximum attention ability." Objectives were planned using the Bush (1997) IEP-educational model. Our objective may read "using the art based intervention of figure/ground black and white calligraphy, client will demonstrate concentration. Possible outcomes were defined as predetermined measurable increments (e.g., client will show attention sustained in measured time units: 0–5 minutes, 5–10 minutes, 10–15 minutes, 15–30 minutes, or entire session).

We found that what appeared to be immeasurable goals simply required reframing of objectives into smaller sequential steps of skills needed to perform each task. Our second goal of increasing organization and planning demonstrates this finding. One objective of this goal is to self-initiate art making. The skill set for self-initiating art making that we used includes skills such as showing up on time for the session, finding or asking for needed art supplies, and follow through to completion of art. Keeping in mind that the outcomes are always observable states, measurable outcomes were recorded in this manner:

1. Not possible at this session.
2. Possible with hand-over-hand assistance and guidance from the art therapist.
3. Client only requires verbal prompts from art therapist for completion of task.
4. Client is completely an independent initiator of task.

Our third executive functioning goal was improving self-regulation of emotions and behavior. One objective of a self-regulation goal that we used was having the client tolerate increasing frustration inherent in the process of art making. The measurable outcomes of frustration tolerance were similar to the above cited for organization and planning, ranging from "not possible" to "can tolerate more frustrating art processes." This moved the client from least complex to more complex projects.

In summary, we looked at the skill sets necessary to measure executive functioning. Our three main goals were:

1. Improving client attention and focus.
2. Organization and planning.
3. Self-regulation of emotions and behavior.

We found that if clients could not attend and focus, the outcomes of the other goals were recorded as Level 1, "not possible at this session." In addition, the goal of organization and planning needed positive outcome measurements to continue working on frustration tolerance. We followed the method of recording these changes as utilized in client medical records, regarding outcomes in percentages. For example, the first objective for the goal of self-initiating would be written as "client showed up for sessions 100% and is a complete initiator of task." The second objective for the above goal, asking for or finding art supplies, would be written as "client demonstrated 75% ability" as indicated by requiring verbal prompts. Combining a multimodal approach in an open studio model, careful assessment of each session was observed and behavioral changes recorded over a long time-frame meeting individual client needs.

THE ART THERAPY OPEN STUDIO

The physical environment for art therapy was an old fire station garage converted into an activity area with two pool tables, a modern kitchen, and an eating area with snack and pop machines; the space was attached to a smaller area divided into individual therapy offices and a reception area. Two commercial overhead heaters, located at the front and back of the activity space, provided heat in winter but caused significant hearing problems due to the noise emanating from them. There was a large overhead garage door that could be opened in warm weather to allow airflow; however, the space overlooked a large asphalt parking area, barren of trees, so the summer heat was intolerable. The art therapists provided fans to keep the air moving, and allowed clients to decide whether they wanted to work in art therapy that day or not, depending on the heat. We did try to use the small, air-conditioned therapy offices, but oftentimes they were in use.

Despite the inconveniences, we designed a safe, structured oasis by arranging large wooden bookshelves and metal shelving as outside boundaries to limit intrusions. A large cement block wall provided excellent exhibition space for completed artwork, and large commercial easels provided not only an appropriate place for a large work in progress (paintings, mixed media, drawings), but a special place for viewing work. It was here that establishment of the safe holding space for working through treatment goals and creating the therapeutic relationship was generated. Here, the therapists and clients could practice the seeing and being seen necessary for creative apperception.

CASE EXAMPLE

Will, a 57-year-old male, at the first meeting wore sunglasses, appeared disheveled, and was talking into the Bluetooth device in his left ear. Initial status assessment revealed he was withdrawn, apathetic, and distractible. His language appeared pressured, his communication was fragmented, and his attention was preoccupied. His constricted affect, anxious mood, and minimal awareness indicated that he was not reality-based. His records noted multiple motor vehicle accidents and two diagnosed TBIs over a period of 8 years.

The art therapist presented the simple drawing directives included in the DDS, emphasizing the request to not talk during the art making. It was clearly explained that after his art assessment he would be able to speak about himself and the artwork. Unable to comply with this, Will talked continuously throughout the session. Will's disorganized artwork and behavior demonstrated significant indicators for depression, anxiety, trauma, and poor self-regulation of emotions, evidenced by erratic use of color, poor problem-solving skills, and a lack of boundaries. Upon request by the therapist to limit distractions, he complied when asked to remove both the Bluetooth device and the glasses. During the process of the assessment the therapist noted that his trance-like approach to the drawings diminished his attention and focus, requiring repeated verbal cues from the therapist regarding time. Poor use of time caused processing of artwork and talking to be postponed until the next scheduled session.

At the next scheduled session, the therapist consistently reinforced that the emotions and behaviors Will presented were normal and to be expected. He was eventually able to decide that art would be a new skill he wanted to master to improve focus and reduce his anxiety. At this time, he showed both minimal awareness of deficits and a limited attempt at acceptance of acknowledged deficits. In many future sessions, Will shared his problems with reality, reinforcing his apparent denial of deficits. He was proud of the fact that he could recall everything the art therapist stated, possibly due to his ability to mimic and/or imitate what was said during sessions, while the art therapist provided a nonjudgmental witness. Will especially enjoyed the beginning relationship, referring to the art therapist as his "mentor," as he perceived mentorship as part of an overall "inspired design of a larger world order." Will was comfortable enough to reveal a pre-TBI substance abuse history, and a history of trying nonconformist religious rituals, especially out-of-body experiences. He continued to come to every session despite overwhelming physical pain, lack of sleep, and loss of appetite due to digestive problems.

Will helped to establish goals and objectives for art therapy based on building on his perceived strengths. His initial treatment plan included the following:

- *Goal 1.* Demonstrate improved attention.
- *Objective 1.* Using two-dimensional materials, client will create a series of drawings of maps of "Where You Are Right Now," from start to finish (Figure 17.2). Outcome will be measured in time by requiring less direction to complete tasks in each session.

The first goals and objectives were met very quickly as Will completed tasks during the session and asked for homework to keep working on his art at home. New goals and objectives were added, following the treatment plan, as Will maintained his levels of improved attention over 30 days. Through initial simple tasks that could be built upon, and repetition of basic skills, Will was able to meet simple goals and objectives, and gradually moved toward planning and organizing, and the more difficult goals of self-regulation of emotions and behaviors, and mental flexibility to solve problems and understand social cues.

The data collected during every session were helpful, showing the client his progress levels and how possible external events might influence his progress. For example, Will's increasing anxiety over multiple doctor appointments, lawyers and insurance adjusters

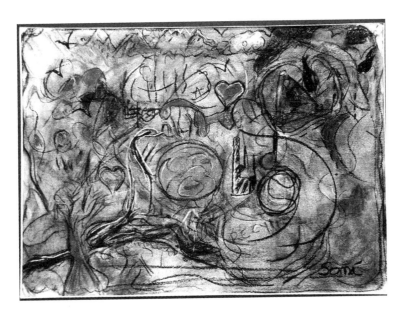

FIGURE 17.2. Map drawing of "Where You Are Right Now."

interrupting scheduled services, and growing responsibilities at home with being a single parent seemed to thwart his progress; these could be shown in his data charts as an erratic up–down progression. Care conferences were established to address these concerns with the case management staff, the outside primary therapist, and other treatment team members, including a speech and language pathologist. The consequent establishment of a therapeutic relationship was maintained through the consistent reassuring tone and demeanor of the art therapist and the supportive atmosphere within the art studio. This allowed further exploration and problem solving through expanding the role of Will's art and self-expression toward decreasing anxiety and increasing acquisition of skills and compensatory strategies, as well as beginning to accept loss of function and reconstructing his new perceived sense of self.

Multiple art therapy approaches seemed appropriate to assist with Will's treatment plan. An art educational approach was used to teach skills development and helped to increase his self-esteem on small success steps. New learning was attached to old memories and previous experiences. Educational techniques included a drawing of the brain (Figure 17.1) and focusing on appropriate areas each session. It was noted that by reviewing brain functions, Will reduced his anxiety as he met his goals and set new ones. Color theory was introduced after Will managed maximum attention goal setting. Will began to identify with being an artist as he learned to control his color choices and application. His immersion into understanding figure/ground, structure, and composition through an intense and long-term study of Diego Rivera's Detroit Industry Murals began during art therapy field trips to the local museum. This enabled him to begin self-initiating improved compositions at home. Discussions of imagery and therapeutic feedback in the studio thereby increased Will's feelings of safety.

During the subsequent sessions, Will began to discuss his imagery in depth, and nascent insight into some of his past traumas emerged. An art psychotherapy approach allowed Will to begin self-exploration into past, pre-TBI events, so collaboration with the music therapist and yoga instructor was initiated to support and safely structure this journey for Will, as was constant communication with other members of his expanding treatment team. What brought this to fruition was Will's voluntary revelation of collaborative complex traumas from early childhood into adolescence, beginning with early loss of primary caregivers. In a structured art psychotherapy session, after 1 year of intense work, Will was able to reveal that he had an alter identity. He stated that this other identity, which at times was violent and fought back, had not been around since his initial treatment at this current facility.

With the help of the music therapist, an intensive 8-week program was begun to address Will's early childhood traumas and give closure to losses. Music therapy focused on writing new lyrics to a familiar song depicting the strengths and accomplishments of the client's involvement in all three therapies. Moreover, increasingly challenging themes were soon requested in art thereby solidifying Will's artist identity. This became evident when Will initiated a large figure/ground painting using a variety of media that explored coming to terms with his loss. Transforming himself through the use of art, he metaphorically depicted the creation and the birth of this new identity. At the same time, yoga was used to help with creating meditations and intensifying *asanas* (poses) to deepen his meditations on acceptance of loss and transformation of self. The culmination of this effort was acceptance of this particular artwork in a public art exhibition on the healing power of art. At the artist reception, Will demonstrated appropriate new skills when he interacted with strangers appropriately, and beamed with pride as he recognized his new self as artist.

As Will's new artist identity took hold and he became increasingly comfortable and secure in his identification with "being an artist," a Gestalt art therapy approach was utilized to keep him in the present moment. Discussing the imagery in his art and recognizing it as self-imagery enhanced his ability to imagine more realistic, day-to-day themes. In one session, Will described the willow trees around his residence and revealed how much he identified with abilities of trees to bend and flex, withstand overwhelming storms, and continue to grow. When Will continued to request homework, it was suggested that he create a drawing of himself as a willow tree. He began what for him turned into a major artwork in terms of identity, healing, and acceptance of the present moment. The completed portrait now hangs in his therapist's office and is continually well received by new clients.

As Will became less reactive to perceived threats, he announced a desire "to be an advocate to others with TBI." He agreed to attend more often, so he was now seen three times weekly for the three therapies, and he joined the biweekly 1½-hour cognitive-behavioral psychotherapy group. Will developed a more assured sense of who he was (an artist) and felt safe allowing his defenses slowly to take a lesser role (his incessant talking abated). At the same time, Will was increasing his nonverbal communication, as well as participating in songwriting and creating his own meditations. Will's next mixed-media composition included three figures based on an earlier work. In the first work there was one figure; now the three figures were falling toward earth (Figure 17.3). Looking at this artwork he indicated that the figures were himself and his daughters. The art piece itself showed understanding of perspective, complex intentional composition, and narrative in nature. His acceptance of complex traumas and losses became a benchmark toward greater independence. Will's treatment began to focus on slowly decreasing his 24/7 attendant care, with an ultimate goal of semi-independent living within 1 year.

CONCLUSION

From initial assessment of impaired reality to acceptance of the possibility of falling toward earth, along with a transformed sense of self as "Artist . . . and advocate," over the course of treatment, Will visibly changed in his demeanor and his artwork. Accompanied by nonjudgmental, compassionate therapists who provided for safe containment of his feelings, and adequate time and space with which to practice new concepts, Will's journey began to provide self-acceptance of a new identity. By using creative apperception, mirror imaging, and empathy, we worked on the rehabilitation of executive functioning skills in Will's sessions. We found that the art therapy process resulted in

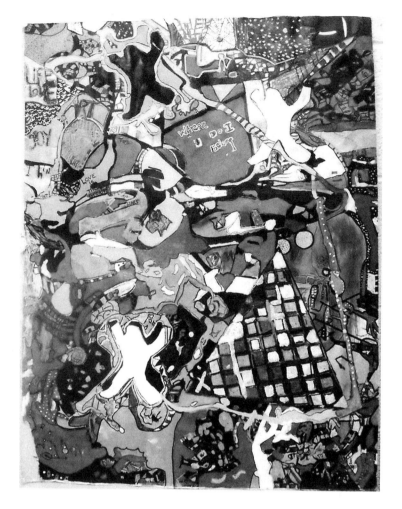

FIGURE 17.3. Will's mixed media composition with three figures falling toward earth.

measurable outcomes, while providing psychological insight. Our hope is that additional art therapy, research-based studies using measurable outcomes will allow clients diagnosed with TBI to accept deficits, focus on strengths, and reestablish identity.

REFERENCES

Abram, J., & Hjulmand, K. (2007). *The language of Winnicott: A dictionary of Winnicott's use of words* (rev. ed.). London: Karnac Books.

Amendt-Lyon, N. (2001). Art and creativity in gestalt therapy. *Gestalt Review, 5*(4), 225–248.

Austin, J. H. (1999). *Zen and the brain: Towards an understanding of meditation and consciousness* (rev. ed.). Cambridge, MA: MIT Press.

Bell, V., & Halligan, P. W. (2009). Cognitive neurology. In G. Bernston & J. J. Cacioppo (Eds.), *Handbook of neuroscience for the behavioral sciences* (Vol. 2). Hoboken, NJ: Wiley.

Buccino, G., Binkofski, F., & Riggio, L. (2004). The mirror neuron system and action recognition. *Brain and Language, 89,* 370–376.

Bush, J. (1997). *The handbook of school art therapy: Introducing art therapy into a school system.* Springfield, IL: Thomas.

Cohen, B., Mills, A., & Johnson, K. (2010, April). The Diagnostic Drawing Series: Two-day workshop. Wayne State University, Detroit, MI.

Galbraith, A., Subrin, R., & Ross, D. (2008). Alzheimer's disease: Art, creativity and the brain. In N. Hass-Cohen & R. Carr (Eds.), *Art therapy and clinical neuroscience* (pp. 256–257). London: Jessica Kingsley.

Gerdes, K. E., Lietz, C. A., & Segal, E. A. (2011). Measuring empathy in the 21st century: Development of an empathy index rooted in social cognitive neuroscience and social justice. *Social Work Research, 35*(2), 1–23.

Hass-Cohen, N., & Carr, R. (Eds.). (2008). *Art therapy and clinical neuroscience.* London: Jessica Kingsley.

Hergenhahn, B. R. (2009). *An introduction to the history of psychology.* Belmont, CA: Wadsworth.

Iacoboni, M., & Dapretto, M. (2006). The mirror neuron system and the consequences of its dysfunction. *Nature Reviews Neuroscience, 7,* 942–951.

Kuspit, D. (2009). Falling apart and holding together: Kandinsky's development. *Artnet Magazine.* Retrieved March 21, 2011, from *www.artnet.com/magazineus/features/kuspit/vasily-kandinsky9-22-09.asp.*

Lehr, R. (2011). Brain function and map. Retrieved June 30, 2011, from *www.neuroskills.com.*

Malchiodi, C. A. (2003). Art therapy and the brain. In C. A. Malchiodi (Ed.), *Handbook of art therapy* (pp. 16–24). New York: Guilford Press.

McGraw, M. K. (1999). Studio-based art therapy for medically ill and physically disabled persons. In C. A. Malchiodi (Ed.), *Medical art therapy with adults* (pp. 243–262). London: Jessica Kingsley.

Nudo, R. (2003). Adaptive plasticity in motor cortex: Implications for rehabilitation after brain injury. *Journal of Rehabilitation Medicine, 35*(41), 7–10.

Pratt, R. R. (2004). Art, dance, and music therapy. *Physical Medicine and Rehabilitation Clinics of North America, 15,* 827–841.

Schaverien, J. (1999). *The revealing image: Analytical art psychotherapy in theory and practice.* London: Jessica Kingsley.

Sell, M., & Murrey, G. (2006). Art therapy within a TBI rehabilitation program. In G. Murrey (Ed.), *Alternative therapies in the treatment of brain injury and neurobehavioral disorders: A practical guide* (pp. 29–40). Binghampton, NY: Haworth Press.

Silver, J., McAllister, T., & Arcinegas, D. (2009). Depression and cognitive complaints following mild traumatic brain injury. *American Journal of Psychiatry, 166,* 653–661.

Simon, R. M. (2005). *Self-healing through visual and verbal art therapy.* London: Jessica Kingsley.

Sohlberg, M. M., & Mateer, C. A. (1989). *Introduction to cognitive rehabilitation: Theory and practice.* New York: Guilford Press.

Sohlberg, M. M., & Mateer, C. A. (2001). *Cognitive rehabilitation: An integrative neuropsychological approach.* New York: Guilford Press.

Weiss, R. (2011, May). *Understanding traumatic brain injury.* Paper presented at monthly meeting of professionals in TBI Rehabilitation, Southfield, MI.

Zillmer, E. A., Spiers, M. V., & Culbertson, W. C. (2008). *Principles of neuropsychology* (2nd ed.). Belmont, CA: Wadsworth.

CHAPTER 18

Art Therapy with Patients Who Have Early-Stage Alzheimer's Disease and Mild Cognitive Impairment

Angel C. Duncan

Mild cognitive impairment (MCI) and early-stage Alzheimer's disease have become a national health care crisis. Approximately once every 69 seconds a person is diagnosed with Alzheimer's disease. That's nearly a new patient per minute. At this rate of growth, today's pool of 5.4 million affected Americans will triple by 2050 (Alzheimer's Association, 2011a). This number does not reflect the millions of families that are also affected.

With no cure in sight, caregivers and medical practitioners shouldering the burden of care need all the help they can get. Art therapy can and should be a key tool in their arsenal. Using it well, however, requires first understanding the implication of the disease and the needs of patients and their families. With that understanding, art therapy can then be valuable as a diagnostic aid and as an intervention therapy for patients alone or together with their families.

ALZHEIMER'S DISEASE AND MILD COGNITIVE IMPAIRMENT

What exactly are Alzheimer's disease and MCI, and how do they differ? The answer depends somewhat on where one looks for information. They are debilitating brain diseases outside of the normal aging process. More specifically, Alzheimer's disease (U.S. National Institutes of Health, 2010a, 2010b) is an irreversible, progressive brain disease that slowly destroys memory and thinking skills, eventually undermining a person's ability to carry out the simplest tasks. MCI, in contrast, is defined by the Mayo Foundation for Education and Research (2010) as an intermediate stage between the expected cognitive decline of normal aging and the more pronounced decline of dementia. It involves problems with memory, language, thinking, and judgment that are greater than typical, age-related changes.

With MCI, an individual will be more forgetful than others in his or her age group. More than just "Where did I leave my car keys," an MCI patient can have moments of significant memory loss. Typically, though, and in contrast to Alzheimer's disease, MCI does not significantly interfere with the person's ability to participate in daily activities (Alzheimer's Association, 2011b). It can, however, affect many areas of thought and actions. Attention, reasoning, reading, and writing skills all can be impaired.

Another important difference between the two diseases is progression. Alzheimer's disease is always progressive but MCI is not. Some people with MCI go on to develop Alzheimer's disease. Others are at increased risk for developing Alzheimer's disease or another form of dementia, and still others do not further progress in the diagnosis at all, remaining stable throughout the rest of their lives. Some people with MCI never get worse and a few eventually get better (Mayo Foundation for Education and Research, 2010). A number of studies are underway, testing treatments that might prevent or delay dementia in people with MCI, but currently science lacks the predictive tools to determine when, or in which patients, MCI will or will not progress.

DEFINING THE NEEDS

Alzheimer's disease and MCI are complex diseases affecting a wide range of people, targeting both genders and even different ethnicities and age groups. Dementia is often identified as a senior citizens' disease, yet an alarming number of new patients with MCI and early-stage Alzheimer's disease are adults in their 40s and 50s. Many of these sufferers still parent children, are productive in the workforce or, at the time of diagnosis, are otherwise living full lives. Unfortunately, with no cure and an often rapid advancement of the disease, major adjustments are frequently required. Some may be forced to quit jobs; others may need long-term care or otherwise be forced to divert energy toward planning for decline in the future. As the disease progresses, the problems only compound.

Too young for older adult day programs and poorly suited for assisted living facilities because they are still cognizant and in-tune with surroundings, these patients need other types of support. Common issues can include marital/family discord, financial hardship, isolation, heightened confusion, helplessness, and hopelessness that could lead to major depressive disorder. Challenges also extend to their families, which are relied on heavily for caregiving and financial contributions. The Alzheimer's Association estimated that total time of unpaid provided care added up to 17 billion hours. The value of that time is estimated to be worth over $202 billion (2011a). The financial drain on individuals and society may be one of the most staggering implications of the disease. Financially pressed, socially stigmatized, and medically underserved, those with early-stage Alzheimer's disease and MCI need help.

RESEARCH

There is limited research on art therapy within dementia populations, and even more limited research on MCI and early-stage Alzheimer's disease; however, the studies that have been conducted consistently validate the power of art for treatment interventions. In one notable example, art therapist Toni Morley, MFT, ATR-BC, collaborated with Stanford University School of Medicine for an art therapy research study of patients with Alzheimer's disease. The study found that participants who engaged in art had increased positive interaction and attention to detail, and experienced a heightened sense of awareness, accomplishment, and productivity (Krisztal, Dupart, & Morley, 2003). Physician Gene Cohen (2007) also has contributed to greater understanding of how art therapy can impact older adults. He conducted a 25-year study of creativity and aging, utilizing art as treatment in people with illnesses from depression to dementia. His findings revealed that there were increases in participants' physical health, morale, and activity level, and decreases in the number of doctor visits, depression, and medication usage. Cohen notes, "Creativity increases with the latter years in life and Alzheimer's disease might not affect imagination as harshly as it devours memory."

ART THERAPY AS A DIAGNOSTIC AID

One of the major challenges of MCI and early-stage Alzheimer's care is effective detection and diagnosis. Part of the problem is similar to that in any ailment: A sufferer may write symptoms off as inconsequential, saying, "I'm stressed and tired; not a big deal," or not seek medical attention until much later, if at all. When patients do seek treatment, medical professionals have a reasonably high level of accuracy with diagnosis, but the complexities of the diseases (and similarities to other ailments in how they present), can sometimes lead to misdiagnosis.

Often physicians not specialized in the fields of gerontology or neurology do not have a precise understanding of Alzheimer's disease; brain scans are not completely reliable in picking up brain changes in some patients. Neurological testing is dependent on the person's affect and a number of other factors that interfere with a proper diagnosis. Current diagnostic protocols involve a number of elements that include a detailed medical history, Mini-Mental State Exam, physical exam, chest x-rays, laboratory tests, imaging tests (i.e., brain scans, such as magnetic resonance imaging [MRI]), and neuropsychological tests (WebMD, 2005–2011).

Art therapy offers methods that can help physicians and other health care professionals reach a diagnosis and treatment plan for patient care. In early-stage Alzheimer's disease and MCI, patient artwork can be assessed, processed, and evaluated for clues of brain dysfunction. The clock-drawing test is one method used to compliment other types of cognitive assessments. Participants are given a piece of paper and asked either to draw a clock from memory or to draw in the time in numbers on the clock face, oftentimes 10 minutes past 11 o'clock. The clock-drawing test requires verbal understanding, memory, and spatially coded knowledge, in addition to constructive skills (Agrell & Dehun, 1998). Typically, individuals with dementia struggle to draw the clock correctly compared to those with normal cognitive abilities. The test is considered to be a good predictor of executive functioning, including sequencing, planning, and organizing that directly affect a person's ability to live independently (Malchiodi, 2012; Richardson & Glass, 2002). With few exceptions, it is an effective evaluation to screen for cognitive impairment and dementia. The one shortcoming of the clock-drawing test is that when the Alzheimer's patient is only mildly symptomatic, the results can be normal (Agrell & Dehun, 1998).

The Formal Elements Art Therapy Scale (FEATS; Gantt & Tabone, 1998) is an alternative method for use with earlier stage presentations of Alzheimer's or MCI. The FEATS assessment asks participants to draw a Person Picking an Apple from a Tree (PPAT). In developing the protocol, the scale developers theorized that valuable diagnostic information could be found in seeing how art is created. In their view, drawings could be evaluated to determine psychiatric symptoms, and if the formal elements of the art reflected these psychiatric symptoms, the art elements would change when or if the symptoms did. Stewart (2004) observed that the FEATS is helpful in tracking the disease in dementia progression and regression, zeroing in on graphic indicators, and assessing general cognitive and problem-solving ability.

Other types of drawing directives may help therapists identify brain disorders or injuries. For example, a male patient received a diagnosis of psychosis NOS (not otherwise specified) based primarily on abrupt, erratic behavior that was deemed to put him in danger of hurting himself and others. I asked him to create whatever came to his mind (free association) within the framework of a sand mandala. The mandala form was intended to provide him enough structure to feel safe. Free association was intended to help him dive deeper into his subconscious. When the patient completed his image (Figure 18.1), I asked him to describe his work. Explaining it, he said, "This is my brain.

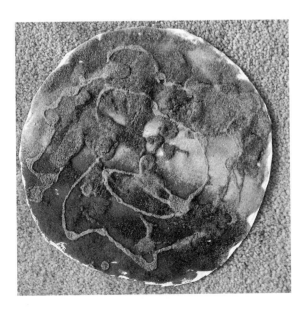

FIGURE 18.1. Sand mandala: "My Brain."

I don't feel right. Something is wrong." Through observation and additional evaluation, it was recommended that he get a brain scan. The scan revealed evidence of a prior head injury that had damaged one side of his brain and was the cause of the erratic behavior and depression. The content of the artwork and his statements contributed to this patient obtaining a proper diagnosis and effective treatment. Wald (1999) and Kim, Kim, Lee and Cyun (2008) report similar experiences using art as a source of supplemental information on organic brain injury, stroke, and psychiatric disorders.

ART INTERVENTIONS FOR PERSONS WITH EARLY-STAGE ALZHEIMER'S AND MILD COGNITIVE IMPAIRMENT

Due to the stigma of memory loss, patients with Alzheimer's disease or MCI tend to feel a sense of helplessness and hopelessness. Oftentimes, those with early-stage Alzheimer's disease are forced to retire from their jobs or asked to step down from positions when the workload becomes unmanageable. This can be demeaning, difficult to accept, and hard to talk about, causing a sense of isolation. Many people with both MCI and early-stage Alzheimer's disease often feel ostracized by their family, friends, and work associates.

A woman with MCI, "Jane," is an example. At the age of 63, Jane was working as an advertising director for a high profile corporation. Due to her lapse in memory, Jane was struggling to keep on top of her fast-paced demands. After 10 years with the company, she was asked to take an early retirement. Participating in my Early Memory Loss Enrichment Group, Jane said, "I feel embarrassed. I don't want anyone in my work to know what happened so I keep a low profile. I don't know what to do with all my free time now; I've never had this much time before to do whatever I wanted, yet I can't do whatever I want because of my memory." With Jane, the process of creating art gave her a hands-on, functional outlet for her angst and emotion. Discussing the inspiration behind the art gave her a safe format to explore her thoughts, gain insight into her condition, and find empowerment. The art ultimately helped her effectively communicate and cope.

Art can create a space in which feelings may be fully encouraged and expressed in a safe environment, and it can help address the stigmas at hand. There are three main objectives in art therapy for people with Alzheimer's disease or MCI:

- *Offer choice.* From the small things to the big things, autonomy is a human right. Try to give the person as many choices as possible to offer a sense of ownership. Let the individual decide which color of paper, pencil, marker, oil pastel, or other art media he or she wants to use.

- *Reduce anxiety.* Patients with early-stage Alzheimer's disease and MCI can become easily frustrated or discouraged. It is best to try to identify situations that might cause anxiety in advance, then preemptively work around them. For example, individuals can sometimes get overwhelmed or distracted if asked to find pictures from a magazine for a collage project; there are simply too many choices. By planning ahead and having precut images and words, participants still have choices without the anxiety of having too many decisions or stimulation.

• *Promote dignity.* People coping with early-stage Alzheimer's disease and MCI often confront societal stigma. They often feel like they are treated like children, having to be watched and told what they can and cannot do. To create a welcoming environment and promote self-esteem, it is extremely important to offer adult art supplies, not child-like arts-and-craft tools to support an atmosphere of dignity.

CASE EXAMPLES OF ART DIRECTIVES

Figures 18.1, 18.2, 18.3, 18.4, and 18.5 illustrate several examples of art directives used with people with early-stage Alzheimer's disease, using a circular format (mandala) as a structure. Whatever directives are used, always keep in mind that the overall goal is for individuals to feel secure and freely express the positive and the negative aspects of their experiences. Be prepared to talk about, or allow the person with MCI or early-stage Alzheimer's disease to verbalize the negatives of the loss (relative to memory, work, relationships, social activities, reading, driving, etc.). It is acceptable to grieve and necessary to release such feelings of loss. But within the negatives, at the closing of any session, emphasize the positives. Reaffirm what participants can still do and celebrate those

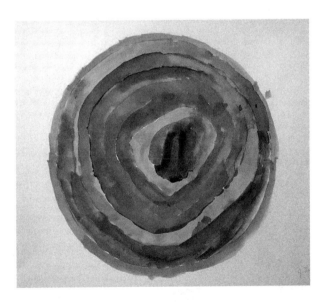

FIGURE 18.2. *Create your supports: Using words, symbols, or color(s), create an image to express who and what supports you.* Jenny has early-stage Alzheimer's disease and used colors to represent specific people, pets, hobbies, and places that are important to her. The goal is for Jenny to think about and appreciate her support systems and understand that she is not alone in this disease, but that she has connections of the love, friendships, and bonds in life.

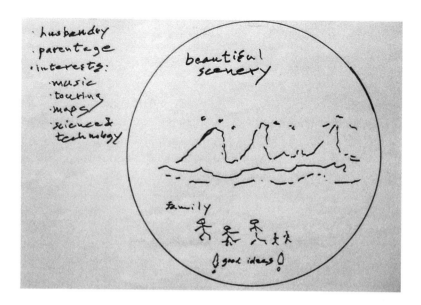

FIGURE 18.3. *Draw or write the things you never want to forget.* Darryl has MCI and wanted to emphasize the importance of nature (beautiful scenery of the mountains) and family (image of wife and children). Outside the circle he listed other elements: husbandry, parentage, and interests (music, touring, maps, science and technology). His mandala communicates what having faith represents while hoping for a cure for MCI. Not losing his "good ideas," represented by two exclamation marks on either side and in the middle at the bottom center, was extremely important to Darryl.

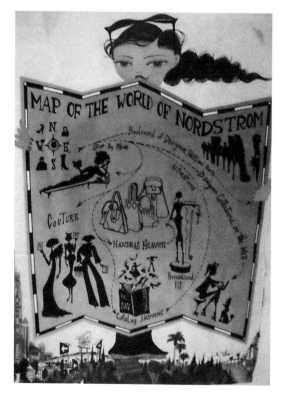

FIGURE 18.4. *Create what gives you personal strength (e.g., mandala, collage, free form).* Susan has early-stage Alzheimer's disease and created a collage of an image of a woman with sunglasses on her head, holding a very large map that is almost bigger than she is. The map is filled with dotted lines mapping out places to go and leading to various places of culture and fashion. Below the map, the woman is standing on top of a park; she is bigger than the skyscrapers, highways, trees, and land mass. The idea was the feelings of being "larger than life," the ability still to do for herself and to remain active, young, and beautiful. She wanted to map out where she desires to go and "go there."

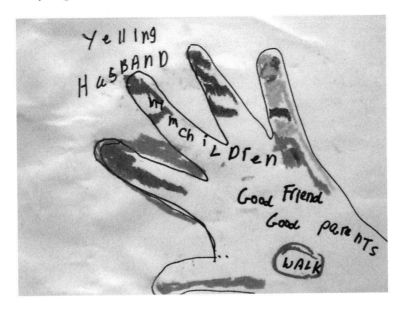

FIGURE 18.5. "My Supports Inside My Hand."

talents, reminding participants that they are not their diagnoses. The experience of Alzheimer's disease and MCI is unique to each person; there is no designated time when the progression will happen. End each session on a positive note.

ART THERAPY GROUPS WITH EARLY-STAGE ALZHEIMER'S AND MILD COGNITIVE IMPAIRMENT

Over several years of practice, I have conducted many art therapy groups for patients with early-stage Alzheimer's disease and MCI. Though often challenging, these groups were some of the most rewarding experiences of my life. Participants were as young as 48 years of age and came from a wide range of careers: football players, engineers, professors, architects, musicians, physicians, social workers, and homemakers. Others were high-profile executives, psychiatrists, therapists, and published authors. All lived fulfilling lives and had vibrant careers, and cared for their families; some had children in high school and college. Once diagnosed with Alzheimer's disease or MCI, their worlds were shattered. All came to art therapy with apprehension but found encouragement and empowerment in the experience. Their hope, support, and faith in themselves, and in one another, reflect the potential of human resiliency.

A variety of materials can be used with these groups: paper, markers, colored pencils, oil pastels, chalk pastels, collage, and textured items (i.e., pieces of fabric, sandpaper, cotton, flat wooden sticks). Providing tactile objects allows for sensory stimulation and may also strengthen the ego (Cheston & Bender, 1999). I emphasize directives to help individuals identify adaptive coping skills and find the positives in life. For example, individuals were asked to "create what your strengths are," "create what inspires you," and "trace your hand; on the outside put the things that don't support you, and on the inside put the things that support you." For example, Monica, who has early-onset Alzheimer's disease, did not like to talk much in my Early Memory Loss Enrichment Group. Instead, she preferred to paint and express her feelings in her art. Sometimes her message was abstract; other times, the message was much more direct: "Yelling Husband," "Good Friends," and "Children" (Figure 18.5). The art communicated how Monica felt, and I was able to offer the necessary support, emphasizing her positives and strengths.

Some recurring strengths-based themes to address with participants include family, nature, beauty, music, maps, reading, photography, gardening, friends, involvement, cooking, art, touching, hope, faith, and love. Diane, a woman with MCI, was given the directive, "create a collage of what gives you personal strength." I had a selection for her of precut images and words from which to choose. Every image she chose was deliberate and demonstrative of the underlying emotion and thought behind them. An image of a geisha girl with a jeweled star and seahorse that Diane cut out and glued on the hair for decoration was intended to illustrate the feelings of being beautiful, feminine, and strong. To represent family, Diane placed an image of a man and a woman looking out from a mountaintop, smiling in satisfaction on the top left-hand side of the paper. The word "Beauty" was specifically placed at the top of this image and on the top right-hand side of the paper, Diane placed the words "yearn to retire near the water" under an image of a beach; it reminded her of Cape Cod, a vacation retreat and hopeful retirement. Every choice in her collage was contemplated, and in its own way, descriptive.

With the same directive, "create what gives you personal strength," Martin, who has early-stage Alzheimer's disease, wished to represent the bond between two people, and the support and faith extended from one being to another. At the time, he was living alone and had lost an active life with friends, who no longer came over or invited him out. His drawing was about how believing in someone's abilities, despite having Alzheimer's disease, could help one keep normality. Specifically, he drew a portrait of me as way of connecting with me. We had worked together for 3 months to find coping strategies and meaning for the challenges of his illness.

In all cases, when I have encouraged these individuals with Alzheimer's disease or MCI, they have repeatedly encouraged me. Participants were always able to find beauty and empowerment despite the disease. Because of them, I am always reminded to stay appreciative and present-centered. I also have learned always to be flexible in my approach. There are good days and bad days; listening to each person and making adjustments, case by case, has made for a better experience all around.

ART THERAPY INTERVENTIONS FOR PATIENTS AND THEIR FAMILIES

Caring for a person with Alzheimer's disease or dementia is often very difficult, and many families and other caregivers experience high levels of emotional stress and depression as a result. Caregiving may also have a negative impact on the health, employment, income, and financial security of caregivers. Often, families of those with early-stage Alzheimer's disease and MCI include high school–age adolescents, college students or graduates, middle-aged spouses, and older adult parents. Educating family members about what Alzheimer's disease or MCI is can be benefited by a clear understanding of the disease, of what is happening to their loved one and in their world, and how to better communicate with their loved on and build up coping skills. Art can be a valuable component, because it can communicate the emotions, thoughts, and ideas of family members to each other. Here are some examples:

1. Create a family collage using magazine images, words, and tangible objects that have meaning for the person (i.e., photographs, jewelry pieces, buttons, keys).
2. Create a memory card (a large index- or postcard-size piece of paper) to fill with all the things that are important to each person or that represent a fond or positive memory.
3. Work on a family mandala (a large circle, cut into pie shapes in which each family member draws images); the pie pieces are put back together to recreate the circle.
4. Draw a family bridge or path on which each person adds where he or she wants to go, what family members can do together, or positive family vacation memories or journeys.

There are many empowering ways that families can work together on art projects to express and discover connections and ways to cope. Variations include art with mother and child, father and children, husband and wife, and sibling and sibling (for more information on family art therapy interventions, see Chapter 21, this volume).

CONCLUSION

Without a cure for Alzheimer's disease and MCI, and with limited treatment options, medical professionals and families are turning to non-drug-related interventions to handle the stresses of the diagnosis and to maintain patient quality of life. Art therapy has proven to be a valuable complement to existing resources. For the medical staff, it can aid in diagnoses. It also offers insight into the individuals' worlds, especially when their words become difficult or impossible. For patients and their families, art therapy encourages better communication and increases patients' sense of dignity and self-esteem. Art therapy should not be overlooked in the treatment of Alzheimer's disease and MCI, and it should a part of noninvasive treatment. Ultimately, art can provide organization to a disorganized mind as it provides a window to the soul of the individual that science will not find on an MRI or PET scan. Science needs art just as much as art needs science.

REFERENCES

Agrell, B., & Dehun, O. (1998). The clock-drawing test. *Age and Ageing, 27*, 399–403.

Alzheimer's Association. (2011a). Alzheimer's disease facts and figures. Retrieved June 2, 2011, from *www.alz.org/downloads/facts_figures_2011.pdf*.

Alzheimer's Association. (2011b). What is mild cognitive impairment? Retrieved July 5, 2011, from *www.alznyc.org/nyc/earlystageservices/mci_ad_other_dementias.asp*.

Cheston, R., & Bender, M. (1999). *Understanding dementia: The man with the worried eyes*. Philadelphia: Jessica Kingsley.

Cohen, G. (2007). The Creativity and Aging Study: The impact of professionally conducted cultural programs on older adults. Retrieved June 2, 2011, from *www.nea.gov/resources/accessibility/cna-rep4-30-06.pdf*.

Gantt, L., & Tabone, C. (1998). *The formal elements art therapy scale: A rating manual*. Morgantown, WV: Gargoyle Press.

Kim, S.-H., Kim, M.-Y., Lee, J.-H., & Chun, S. (2008). Art therapy outcomes in the rehabilitation treatment of a stroke patient: A case report. *Art Therapy: Journal of the American Art Therapy Association, 25*(3), 129–133.

Krisztal, E., Dupart, T., & Morley, T. (2003). *Emotion in dementia patients: Effects of a fine arts group on well-being*. Unpublished manuscript, Stanford University School of Medicine, Palo Alto, CA.

Malchiodi, C. A. (2012). Creativity and aging: An art therapy perspective. In C. A. Malchiodi (Ed.), *Handbook of art therapy* (2nd ed., pp. 275–287). New York: Guilford Press.

Mayo Foundation for Medical Education and Research. (2010). *Mild Cognitive Impairment (MCI)*. Retrieved July 7, 2011, from *www.mayoclinic.com/health/mild-cognitive-impairment/DS00553*.

Richardson, H. E., & Glass, J. N. (2002). A comparison of scoring protocols on the clock drawing test in relation to ease, diagnostic group, and correlations with mini-mental state examination. *Journal of American Geriatric Society, 50*, 169–173.

Stewart, E. (2004). Art therapy and neuroscience blend: Working with patients who have dementia. *Art Therapy: Journal of the American Art Therapy Association, 21*(3), 148–155.

U.S. National Institutes of Health: National Institutes on Aging. (2010a). *Alzheimer's Disease Education and Referral (ADEAR) Center* (NIH Publication No. 08-6423). Retrieved July 5, 2011, from *www.nihseniorhealth.gov/alzheimersdisease/toc.html*.

U.S. National Institutes of Health: National Institute on Aging. (2010b). Early Alzheimer's disease. Retrieved June 2, 2011, from *www.ahrq.gov/clinic/alzcons.htm*.

Wald, J. (1999). The role of art therapy in post-stroke rehabilitation. In C. Malchiodi (Ed.), *Medical art therapy with adults* (pp. 25–42). Philadelphia: Jessica Kingsley.

WebMD. (2005–2011). Alzheimer's Disease Health Center. Retrieved from *www.webmd.com/alzheimer's/default/htm*.

PART III

ART THERAPY WITH GROUPS AND FAMILIES

INTRODUCTION

This part provides a variety of examples illustrating how art therapy is applied to work with groups and families (see Chapters 1, 4, 10, 11, 12, and 13 for additional examples). Art therapy, like other forms of therapy, often takes place in groups. In brief, group work naturally creates opportunities for interaction and interpersonal exchange. In addition, there are inherent "curative factors" (Yalom, 2005), including universality (learning that others have similar problems), altruism (helping others through difficult times), and hope (learning how others have overcome adversity). Art therapy groups are important in work with individuals coping with illness or disability because they encourage mutual support and problem solving, a sense of belonging, and shared perspectives during stressful life events.

In most medical art therapy groups, practitioners take active roles in facilitating art activities, determining directives or themes, and selecting goals and objectives. These structured groups may include medical art therapy support groups (Malchiodi, 2012) for people with cancer, chronic pain, or other conditions and groups whose purpose is to provide a forum for communication of feelings and experiences with related issues such as grief and bereavement (Chapter 20). Many follow a similar format that includes an opening discussion and warm-up activities, an art experiential, and a discussion period to allow participants to reflect about their artworks and exchange observations. In general, art expression within a group therapy context addresses not only the common concerns of individuals, but also facilitates expression of unspoken aspects of illness, trauma, or loss; provides stress reduction; and encourages mutual support among participants. Because these groups take place within a hospital or outpatient environment, special accommodations may be necessary for participants who have physical challenges, including lack of mobility, fatigue, or pain. Despite these limitations, group work, including art therapy, is widely accepted as an important component in the psychosocial care of patients because of positive outcomes inherent to interaction and social support for individuals coping with illness (Kissane et al., 2007).

If the group is nondirective (no particular theme for art making), participants may work on ongoing paintings, drawings, mixed media, constructions, or other art forms. This is often referred to as an "open studio approach" and has a long history in both art therapy and rehabilitation (Chapter 19). As mentioned earlier in this book, Adrian Hill (1945, 1951) was a strong advocate for art studio work as part of rehabilitation and recovery from illness. The growing "arts in health care" movement in the United States, the United Kingdom, and other parts of the world promotes participation in studio settings within hospitals and other medical settings as an important part of health and well-being (Warren, 2008). Art therapist Mickie McGraw developed one of the earliest and most comprehensive models for studio art therapy in hospitals in the United States, providing patients with opportunities for art making in a normalizing environment where developing an "artist" identity is central to the process in addition to psychosocial intervention (Art Therapy Studio, 2012; McGraw, 1999).

Additionally, families are "groups" and are an important focus in medical art therapy (Malchiodi, 1999), particularly when there is a pediatric patient involved. In fact, art therapists and health care professionals naturally encounter family members at patients' bedsides or waiting rooms, opening up possibilities for parent, grandparent, and sibling participation in art therapy. When a patient is critically ill, immobilized, isolated, or in recovery and unable to engage in art therapy, family members are often those in most need of psychosocial intervention and opportunities for self-expression and stress reduction.

Many of the authors throughout this book also note the importance of evaluating and addressing pediatric patients' family dynamics, particularly in terms of the quality of support received from family members and extended family. In fact, asking family members to examine the types and depth of social support they receive from relatives, friends, and others is a common request from most helping professionals who are involved in patients' psychosocial care. Art therapists generally ask family members or patients to express how they perceive their "support net" through art as a means of exploration (Figure III.1).

In addition, because patients' concerns and experience of illness pervade the entire family system, understanding how hospitalization, chronic illness, or disabilities impact a family is important to how art therapists develop goals and objectives for interventions both for patients and caregivers, parents, and siblings. For example, Councill (1999) notes that a parent's anxiety and pessimism about a child's condition may increase a sense of hopelessness in the patient, compromising the child's capacity for resilience. Similarly, Barton (1999) highlights the importance of using drawing as a method for both children and caregivers to describe perceptions of pain in patients with juvenile rheumatoid arthritis (JRA). Through comparing drawings by both patients and caregivers, Barton learned that caregivers were often confused or inaccurate in their understanding of the patient's experience of pain. By identifying misperceptions through their drawings, the art therapist was able help caregivers provide more effective support for young patients

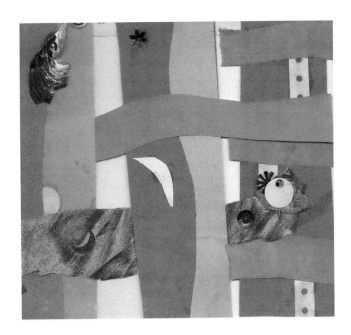

FIGURE III.1. Family's collage depicting their "support network."

with JRA. As explained in Chapter 21, art therapy is a useful form of communication not only for patients, but also for parents/caregivers and siblings to help them clarify perceptions of the patients' illness, strengthen the relationship between the patient and family members, or, in the case of dying patients, assist in the process of grieving.

This section also includes another group of individuals who are also in need of support—health care professionals, including nonmedical personnel such as administrators and executives. It is widely accepted that allied health professionals and support staff who work in emergency rooms or trauma units in particular often experience what is sometimes called "compassion fatigue" (Figley, 1995) or secondary trauma reactions (Wicks, 2005) when working with patients whose physical needs are critical. Chapter 22 highlights some of the benefits of providing artistic self-expression with these individuals, underscoring that providing services to the larger health care system may be just as relevant as the physical and psychosocial care of patients.

In sum, the inclusion of art therapy with groups, whether patients, families, or health care personnel, has a distinct advantage over other psychosocial approaches. By facilitating self-expression through drawing, collage, and other art forms, both therapists and group members can "see" what others are saying (Riley, 2001). It provides a form of communication when words may not adequately describe illness or loss, loss of control and privacy, or the stress of being a patient or the parent, caregiver, or sibling of a patient. As you will read in the chapters that follow, a powerful component of group work is that it helps both those coping with disease or disability and those adjusting to a family member's illness or death of a parent or child by providing empowering experiences of authentic expression.

REFERENCES

Art Therapy Studio. (2012). *About the art therapy studio.* Retrieved May 1, 2012, from *www.art-therapystudio.org/aboutus.html.*

Barton, J. (1999). Comparisons of pain perceptions between children and their caregivers. In C. A. Malchiodi (Ed.), *Medical art therapy with children* (pp. 153–171). London: Jessica Kingsley.

Councill, T. (1999). Art therapy with pediatric cancer patients. In C. A. Malchiodi (Ed.), *Medical art therapy with children* (pp. 75–94). London: Jessica Kingsley.

Figley, C. R. (Ed.). (1995). *Compassion fatigue: Coping with secondary traumatic stress disorder in those who treat the traumatized.* New York: Brunner/Mazel.

Hill, A. (1945). *Art versus illness.* London: Allen & Unwin.

Hill, A. (1951). *Painting out illness.* London: Williams & Norgate.

Kissane, D. W., Grbasch, B., Clarke, D. M., Smith, G. C., Love, A. W., Bloch, S., et al. (2007). Supportive-expressive group therapy for women with metastatic breast cancer: Survival and psychosocial outcome from a randomized controlled trial. *Psychooncology, 16*(4), 277–286.

Malchiodi, C. A. (1999). *Medical art therapy with children.* London: Jessica Kingsley.

Malchiodi, C. A. (2012). Using art therapy with medical support groups. In C. A. Malchiodi (Ed.), *Handbook of art therapy* (2nd ed., pp. 397–408). New York: Guilford Press.

McGraw, M. (1999). Studio-based art therapy for medically ill and physically disabled persons. In C. A. Malchiodi (Ed.), *Medical art therapy with adults* (pp. 243–261). London: Jessica Kingsley.

Riley, S. (2001). *Group process made visible: Group art therapy.* New York: Brunner-Routedge.

Warren, B. (2008). *Using the creative arts in therapy and healthcare.* New York: Routledge.

Wicks, R. (2005). *Overcoming secondary stress in medical and nursing practice: A guide to professional resilience and personal well-being.* New York: Oxford University Press.

Yalom, I. (2005). *The theory and practice of group psychotherapy.* New York: Basic Books.

CHAPTER 19

An Open Art Studio Model

Jill V. McNutt

In this chapter Expressive Arts for Healing, an art in health care and art therapy program bringing visual arts opportunities to the health care system in a large medical center is discussed. Within this program, a community art studio is operated within the medical center meeting the needs of patients, family members, and the staff. This chapter addresses logistics regarding the operation of such a studio within the medical paradigm.

OPEN STUDIO APPROACH TO ART THERAPY

Many different terms are used in reference to an "open studio approach" to art therapy in medical settings, including studio art therapy (Moon, 2002), art as therapy, visual arts in health care, and art-based therapy. The term "open studio" has been used for many decades and can be traced back to early art therapists, including Don Jones (1983), whose work in state mental hospitals, the Menninger Foundation Clinic in Kansas, and Harding Hospital in Ohio, underscores the studio as central to recovery through art expression. Adrian Hill (1945, 1951), considered one of the important figures in art therapy in England, was a strong proponent of art studio work as part of rehabilitation and recovery from illness. The current arts in health care movement in both the United States and England proposes that art making, whether in a studio setting or at bedside, is an important part of health and well-being (Kaye & Blee, 1997; Warren, 2008). More recently, the open studio model has been defined as "sacred" for those who participate and engage in the benefits of art making and art therapy (Allen, 2005; McNiff, 2004).

Art therapist Mickie McGraw's work in medical settings is possibly the most comprehensive model for studio art therapy in hospitals (Malchiodi, 1999). She helped establish the Art Studio–Center for Therapy through the Arts in 1967 to address the

psychosocial and creative needs of individuals with medical illnesses and physical disabilities. It is the oldest hospital-based art therapy program of its kind in the United
States (Art Therapy Studio, 2012; McGraw, 1999). This program has served as a model
for open studios in hospitals, as well as in mental health settings. "Art-centered therapy
works because it actively engages people along a dynamic continuum that provides a
non-verbal contact with the environment" (McGraw, 1999, p. 248; Kahn, McGraw, &
Myers, 1977). In brief, in contrast to art making as a solitary event, a studio approach
adds the element of shared creative experiences, in which the emphasis is on the action
of making art rather than on words (McGraw, 1999).

THE EXPRESSIVE ARTS FOR HEALING PROGRAM

The Expressive Arts for Healing program studio is an adult-centered resource. Children
are welcome to attend alongside a participating parent or guardian but cannot attend
unaccompanied. Some participants benefit from a single time at the open studio. Others
return on a regular basis, and still others come occasionally just to reignite their creativity. The medical system in which the program exists is one that prides itself on the
integration of patient-centered care. Efforts are made to treat the whole person, and care
is taken for family members and health care staff.

People come to hospitals for many reasons and include patients, family members,
friends, outpatients, and the staff. Patients range in diagnosis and acuity; reasons for
hospitalization range from routine interventions and recovery from accidents to life-
threatening or life-changing illness. Patients who attend or benefit from the open studio
format of the Expressive Arts for Healing Program have experienced cancer, stroke,
dementia, heart disease, organ transplant, orthopedic interventions, and more. Family
members and concerned friends have been seen to approach the illness of loved ones in
a variety of ways. Some family members express fear and grief, while others are exploring
new roles as caretakers. Art and art therapy in the format of an open studio approach
are valuable interventions to meet psychosocial needs of all those who pass through the
doors.

Studio attendance generally ranges between 15 and 30 participants. Some artist
participants come regularly and work on a continuing art process; others stop in periodically to "recharge." Some come to pass time, and others take leadership roles within
the setting. Whatever the motivation, or connection, to the health care system, all are
welcome in the studio space. The facilitator/art therapist is adept at creating and maintaining the space and the media. The space itself is inherently healing and comes alive
with the coming and going of artist participants.

Art making in the context of the open studio format provides elements of relaxation and distraction, introspection and self-learning, and healthy catharsis and transformation. The studio facilitation of flow offers artist attendees the opportunity to create
beauty, express hope, relieve pain, soften distress, and spend time in a healing capacity.
It is a place of creativity, potential, and hope; the studio space may be permanent, as

well as temporary, or mobile in nature. Within the Expressive Arts for Healing program, regular studio hours are held open for artist attendees, including hospitalized patients, outpatients or returning patients, family members and friends, the staff, and members of the community. The title of "artist" refers to all who enter the studio, and art experience is not required for attendance or participation. Studio carts are transported to waiting areas and clinics, where patients and family members spend significant amounts of time, and studio materials are made available to patients in their rooms. Through engagement and reflection on the art process and product, artist participants can engage in relaxation and distraction, introspection and self-learning, and transformation or reframing. Whatever the intent or skill of the participants, all are welcome in the open studio format.

DESCRIPTION OF TYPICAL STUDIO

The physical studio requires multiple working spaces, an area to spread out materials for easy access, and adequate lighting and accessibility for patients, family members, and the staff. Cleanliness and order create an atmosphere that is safe and inviting. Background music helps to set the tempo and invitation of the space. It also helps to mask intercom announcements to limit any disturbances to participants' creative expression.

The expressive arts open studio is facilitated by at least one licensed art therapist, a number of graduate art therapy interns, and skilled artist volunteers. It is an opportunity for individual growth, healing, and actualization; for this reason, it is imperative that the lead facilitator hold supervisory status and be educated in a human service with psychological sensitivities. Graduate interns are capable of providing necessary art therapy services within the context of the studio when under the direct supervision of the lead art therapist. Volunteers are able to help with instruction and didactic art processes. When studio attendees reflect and process the work and/or their relationship to the hospital, the volunteer must refer to either an intern or an art therapist.

The studio space is arranged in such a way as to provide a number of separate tables and easy access to material storage and carts. It has regularly scheduled hours, and its location is advertised throughout the hospital. Studio hours are open, meaning that people can come and go at any point during the scheduled time. A variety of media is available to artist participants, including, but not limited to paint, drawing materials, multimedia surfaces, collage, clay, plaster, fabric, beads, and found objects. Participants are free to choose to work in any available media and to bring their own if desired.

Each session is designed around a featured process that involves an art project with enough didactic instruction to ease intimidation and provide enough nondirection to allow personal investment and freedom of the creative energy. The featured processes have easy-to-understand instructions that allow the newcomer to engage quickly and independently. Open studio processes are generally designed to have educational elements, allowing new patients to enter the creative space with a degree of comfort. The process is also open enough to allow the returning patient the opportunity for artistic exploration and metaphoric identification, and to play within the constraints of the featured process. Some examples of featured process include dollmaking, splatter paint-ing, wet-on-wet watercolor, coil building with clay, origami, mask making, and poetry collage, to name a few.

When an artist participant first comes to the open studio, he or she is welcomed by the group facilitators. The new participant is given a brief introduction to the basic tenets of the studio and offered the featured process by means of instruction. The par-ticipant is able to engage in the featured process or pursue work with any other medium available. Once the artist participant has chosen the process he or she would like to practice, the facilitator assesses specific and community needs. Some participants flour-ish at a table by themselves, while others may like to have a facilitator or intern sit and work with them. Some may like to be introduced to other artist participants. It is the role of the facilitator to keep the space safe in both community and materials. In all cases, a personal area should be available for each participating artist.

The perceived success of artists in the studio often facilitates "creative contagion." This contagion can take the form of a new innovation in media application for aesthetic value or illicit psychological connections both between and within artist participants. Through experimentation and play, artist participants have been able to create unique approaches to media. A donation of plastic Petri dishes and experience shrinking plas-tics with applied heat sparked one artist participant's aesthetic eye. The artist, through play with materials, incorporated plastic beads, a permanent marker, and various-size Petri dishes to create ornamental, three-dimensional forms. The success of this partici-pant attracted four other participants, who then engaged in creative problem solving and design of these new forms. The process has been named after the originating artist, and materials for its completion are now available at every open studio event.

Altered books (books that are deconstructed or repurposed with paint, collage and embellishments) are another example of how contagion is manifest within the context of the open studio. A graduate intern was the first to bring an altered book into the stu-dio space. The intern worked on the altered book as a reflection of her experience in the hospital setting. Artist participants became witnesses to the book as it developed over the course of the semester. Two participants requested that altered books become a fea-tured process, so that they could engage in creating their own altered books. Since the initial introduction by the intern, over half of the regular studio attendees have started an altered book to reflect on some aspect of their lives.

Community is also a large part of the working open studio. Connections built through the open studio format take many shapes. Some find long-term friends and build relationships through new commonalities. Other relationships mimic support groups in which personal stories, experiences, and advice are shared. Art therapy groups provide a place where patients can accentuate the positives of art making, as opposed to illness; help others as their own personal needs are being met; and experience a sense of belong-ing (Collie & Kante, 2010). Some participants have used the creative studio space to heal, enhance, or mend existing relationships. Patients who are parents have capitalized on the opportunity to connect with children through the process of co-creation in the open studio. Dyads of parents and adolescent children have made regular visits to the open studio, using art as a common communication tool. Parents diagnosed with cancer have in the open studio a regular opportunity to spend time with children as well. These families benefit from spending creative time together and meeting other families in similar situations. Couples have also used the space to reflect on relationships as they proceed through the illness trajectory.

RELAXATION, INTROSPECTION, AND TRANSFORMATION

The need for relaxation and distraction in the hospital setting is easy to comprehend because of the stressful nature of hospitalization, medical procedures, and illness. Although little evidence-based research is available, engagement in art therapy has been shown to reduce the sensation of pain, reduce anxiety and depression, and increase coping skills (Stuckey & Nobel, 2010). Participation in expressive arts has also been shown to reduce patient's use of call lights and to increase participation in health care decisions (State of the Field Committee, 2009). Many art processes offer patients opportunities to relax and pass time. Care is taken by the art therapist to ensure the successful outcome of art interventions when relaxation and distraction are goals of the process.

Perhaps the most common relaxation-based interventions offered through this open studio model are mandala making and watercolor squares. Mandalas (circular format for imagery) are offered with or without preformed patterns of varying degrees of difficulty. The patient's mobility, vision, and impairments must be considered when offering mandalas for coloring. The creation of watercolor squares is easy and accessible to most patients. Small squares of student-grade watercolor paper (usually four or six inches) are submerged in water. Watercolor paint is applied via brushes in a wet-on-wet technique that allows the paint to run, spread, and blend. The outcome of painting the squares is difficult to predict or control, but the finished work becomes an abstract success. The squares can stand alone as art pieces or can be arranged in family- or community-building watercolor tile art pieces.

Art studio opportunities also offer space for introspection and self-learning through reflection on the art process and product. People are often busy with schedules filled with family, work, and social activity; when illness is thrown into the mix, it makes schedules tighter and more stressful. Time for art and art therapy is often difficult to fit in as well. A specific art therapy directive for introspection is a personal collage. In this directive, clients are asked to select six unrelated images from a variety of magazines. These images should be selected according to the patient's taste and may represent varying aspects of his or her current life and responsibilities. *National Geographic* magazines are preferred because of the artistic photography and relative lack of commercialism. The images are then trimmed and put together as if they were pieces of a puzzle. Using the collage images themselves as a base for this process encourages overlap and unison in the finished artworks. Through this collage process, client artists have been able to find metaphors for personal behaviors, beliefs, and patterns facilitating action and behavioral change.

Introspection and self-learning often becomes the catalyst for personal transformation and reframing in the open studio. Through art making, patients often reframe themselves from being defined as victims of circumstances to being active participants in their own health care and lives. Transformational art interventions are those that start and finish in different forms and become metaphors for change. Crumpled paper becomes sculpture or ash, broken ceramics become mosaics, and medical supplies translate into artwork and symbols of hope, triumph, and memory. The creativity in the studio is able to transcend the bounds of being identified as patients and actualize artist identities (Moon, 2002).

MOBILE OPEN ART STUDIO

The Expressive Arts for Healing open studio was conceived through contemplation of a small art therapy program's expansion to meet the needs of the most people with the least funds. The premise of the studio-based design includes open hours in a dedicated space, where patients, family members, returning patients, and staff members can arrive and depart at will. The studio-based experience is also offered throughout the medical center by means of transporting studio materials to patient rooms. Referrals for this service can be made through doctors, nurses, family members, or the patients themselves. The materials available to each patient are restricted by isolation and infection control protocols. Each floor of the hospital has its own procedures; some floors have made special arrangements for art therapy staff and interns to make regular visits to patients' rooms, introducing services. Oncology, rehabilitation, abdominal transplant, and acute care for older adults are examples of floors that use art therapy services regularly.

The studio experience is also made mobile to waiting areas of the hospital, including intensive care and same-day surgery family waiting areas. The featured process of the waiting room cart is primarily that of expressive card making. It is not uncommon for family members and friends of patients to spend significant amounts of time in these waiting areas. The art cart brings distraction, personal investment, and anxiety reduction. Infusion clinics are another area where the art studio cart is welcome. Restrictions in space and mobility limit material access. Small projects such as origami and polymer clay work easily in the confined space. Individual and group situations occur in the infusion clinics. Through her work in an infusion clinic, Cassidy (2010) found an opportunity to create a supportive community among the patients participating in open studio via the art cart. Efforts were made to create community works of art such as that seen in Figure 19.1. Cassidy built a supportive group culture by encouraging patient participants to engage together, responding to the collective image in paint and imagination.

Group art processes are also available within the open studio art space. Participation in community is available though joint efforts on the same base or compilation of individual works, as in a tile structure. One community process available at every open studio session evolved naturally through attention to circumstances. Throughout the evolution of the studio, it was noticed that a considerable amount of paint was being

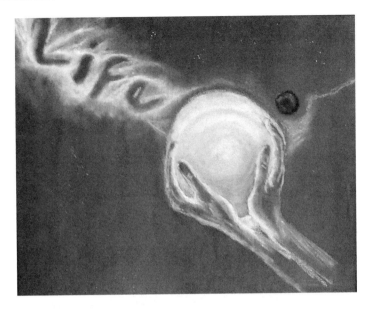

FIGURE 19.1. "Life."

thrown into the garbage. In the interest of conservation, a "green" painting process was developed, in which leftover paint is added to a collective painting canvas. An example of a green painting is shown in Figure 19.2. The 48″ square artist canvas was fashioned, then offered to studio artists as a disposal method for paint. The work, completed over a period of 4 months, involves a layering process and includes the efforts of over 60 artist participants. The completed painting is now displayed in the hospital, with a description about the healing properties of art making and art studio.

OUTREACH

Among the most important roles of the expressive arts program is outreach and education. Art therapy is a new effort within the health care system. It is not enough to assume that others know what art therapists do or what art therapy has to offer patients, family members, or the staff. Art therapy and art studio processes are relatively unknown within the medical setting. The importance of outreach cannot be overstated. The Expressive Arts for Healing program has grown since its inception largely due to outreach efforts designed to reach the most people, with as much impact as possible. Sharing stories of healing, group exhibitions, and display of collective processes and publication in local media are effective ways to invite the community into the creative paradigm of the open studio space. Other outreach forms include up-to-date studio flyers with studio dates for 3 months posted on every hospital bulletin board, guest appearances with experiential components at various support groups and staff meetings, participation in the form of booths at staff events, fundraising walks, and survivorship picnics.

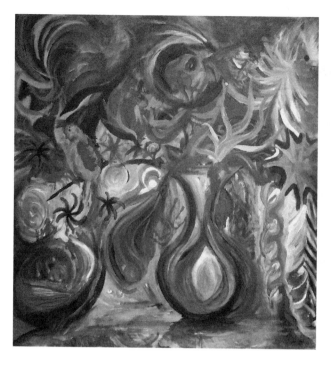

FIGURE 19.2. "Green Painting I."

An effective method has involved interactive presentations at every new staff orientation. New employees are given a brief introduction to the art therapy services available hospitalwide. A poll of the audience of new employees asks which persons consider themselves to be creative. Most often, only a few people raise their hands and share their affinity for drawing, playing music, scrapbooking, and so forth. Many are surprised when the definition of creativity is expanded beyond the fine arts and most are able to find ways that they have been creative in the week prior. A review of how to find services, an invitation to open art studio, and the referral process follows.

Goals of art therapy services are broken down into the three general areas of relaxation and distraction, introspection and self-learning, and transformation and reframing. The audience of health care professionals is educated to recognize ways that relaxation and distraction aid hospitalized patients, including reduction of anxiety, stress, pain, and boredom. Examples of wet-on-wet watercolor tiles and mandalas are shared as examples. Introspection and self-learning are explained. Examples of collage and a series of body shapes are designed to have the patient artist reflect on the body and begin a communication between the mind and body. The collages shared demonstrate artists' insights and reflection on image size, position, and strength. The body forms are representative of a mind–body intervention in which patients are asked to select the body form that best represents their current selves. Choices include figures that are praying, walking a balance beam, dancing, rushing with a briefcase, or meditating. Patients are then asked to listen to their bodies and fill in the body form with colors, lines, and shapes. This intervention was designed to help patients start a communication between the mind and body. Finally, transformation and reframing are shared through examples of polymer clay–covered medicine bottles and scribble drawings. The importance of reframing and opening to possibility is described. In this short introduction to art therapy and its benefits, it is important to simplify the essence in order to translate these services to the health care market.

An experiential group scribble drawing is incorporated into each orientation session. Each table of three to five people is given an 18″ × 18″ sheet of paper, with an oil pastel for each person at the table. The group is given 10 seconds to scribble all over the paper. Participants are then instructed to turn the paper 90° and are given 10 more seconds to scribble; this is repeated three times. When the scribbles are completed, the papers are rotated between tables. Group members at the second table who work on the paper are asked to look at the scribble as if it were clouds and find the image(s) that emerge. They are asked to use their oil pastels to draw out that image so that it is recognizable. The pages are rotated to the next table, and participants are asked to add a title to the work. The pages are then passed to the final table, where participants are given instructions to create a three- to five-sentence story about the work and elect one person to share the table's contribution.

Finally, the images and stories are shared with the larger group. The stories are generally humorous, reflect health care language, and are light in nature. The group is polled after the experience as to how the room changed during the art-making experience. Feedback often includes reports of laughter, engagement, teamwork, communication, freedom, and fun. The nature of art participation including all of these components is among the reasons that art therapy and art process should be available throughout the hospital setting. Two final questions asked of the orientation group: (1) to whom do the created artworks belong and (2) to whom does the patient experience belong? The answer that comes is inevitably "everyone," because all participated in the art and know that all hospital staff members have an effect on patient care.

CONCLUSION

Since its inception the open studio has grown in capacity and attendance. This open studio model upholds the ideals of treating the whole person and/or system. The program upholds art therapy as an essential component that is accepted as integral to patient-centered health care.

REFERENCES

Allen, P. B. (2005). *Art is a spiritual path*. Boston: Shambhala.
Art Therapy Studio. (2012). About the art therapy studio. Retrieved January 27, 2012, from *www.arttherapystudio.org/aboutus.html*.

Cassidy, M. (2010). *A shared experience with outpatient cancer patients*. Unpublished master's thesis, Mount Mary College, Milwaukee, WI.

Collie, K., & Kante, A. (2010). Art groups for marginalized women with breast cancer. *Qualitative Health Research, 21*(5), 652–661.

Hill, A. (1945). *Art versus illness*. London: Allen & Unwin.

Hill, A. (1951). *Painting out illness*. London: Williams & Norgate.

Jones, D. (1983). An art therapist's personal record. *Art Therapy: Journal of the American Art Therapy Association, 1*(1), 22–25.

Kahn, K., McGraw, M., & Myers, L. (1977). A pioneering art therapy program at Highland View. *Cuyuga County Hospital Foundation Quarterly, 2*, 17–20.

Kaye, C., & Blee, T. (1997). *The arts in health care: A palette of possibilities*. London: Jessica Kingsley.

Malchiodi, C. A. (1999). Art therapy and medicine: Powerful partners in healing. In C. A. Malchiodi (Ed.), *Medical art therapy with adults* (pp. 13–23). London: Jessica Kingsley.

McGraw, M. (1999). Studio-based art therapy for medically ill and physically disabled persons. In C. A. Malchiodi (Ed.), *Medical art therapy with adults* (pp. 243–261). London: Jessica Kingsley.

McNiff, S. A. (2004). *Art heals: How creativity cures the soul*. Boston: Shambhala.

Moon, C. H. (2002). *Studio art therapy: Cultivating the artist identity in the art therapist*. Philadelphia: Jessica Kingsley.

State of the Field Committee. (2009). *State of the field report: Arts in health care 2009*. Washington, DC: Society for the Arts in Healthcare. Retrieved August 18, 2009, from *http://thesah. org/doc/reports/fieldreport2%206.pdf*.

Stuckey, H. L., & Nobel, J. (2010). The connection between art, healing and public health: A review of current literature. *American Journal of Public Health, 100*(2), 254–263.

Warren, B. (2008). *Using the creative arts in therapy and health care*. New York: Routledge.

CHAPTER 20

Young Adult Bereavement Art Group

Hannah K. Hunter
Donald Lewis
Catherine Donovan

Art therapy has long been seen as a valid means of addressing the bereavement needs of children and teens. Numerous articles describe the success of an art therapy bereavement group model for children. After a thorough literature search, we discovered that art therapy bereavement groups existed for youth ages 4–16, and discussion-based groups for adults of all ages were available, but there were no art therapy bereavement groups for young adults (Community Bereavement Resource Directory, 2011). Intuitively and professionally, we knew there was a gap: a developmental age group between children and adults, whose bereavement needs were not being served. We also knew that loss and grief damage the transition from childhood to adulthood, and we wanted to help repair that damage. In this chapter, we explore a unique collaboration within the UC Davis (University of California–Davis) Health System between the UC Davis Children's Hospital and UC Davis Hospice Program that led to the formation of an innovative and successful art therapy bereavement model for young adults, ages 17–24. This chapter describes the implementation of this new art therapy model into the health care delivery system.

In order to understand better the specific needs of this developmental stage, and how to deliver an art therapy model effectively, some neurological background is necessary. Until the early 21st century, neuroscientists assumed that brain development ceased following puberty. Contrary to previous thought, new findings from a National Institute of Mental Health (NIMH)-sponsored longitudinal study show that the brain continues to mature well into the 20s (Henig, 2010). Current delivery of care models assume that bereavement needs for children and adults are two *separate and distinct* categories. The NIMH findings demonstrate the need for a *new* category, one that addresses the developmental tasks of individuals *between* these two life phases, a newly identified life stage referred to by Jeffrey Jensen Arnett, a psychology professor at Clark University, as "emerging adulthood." Arnett notes that emerging adulthood has its own unique psychological profile, including identity exploration, instability, self-focus, and a sense of feeling in-between (Arnett, 2004).

Qualitative research studies indicate that emotional responses to death and grief in emerging adults are similar to those experienced by adults. These include feelings of shock, numbness, confusion, anger, guilt, sadness, despair, loneliness, and depression. However, while the range of emotions experienced is similar, the emerging adult's process of grieving is different (Mearns, 2000). The failure to appreciate these differences is a common source of misunderstanding between young adults, parents, and professionals (Christ, Siegel, & Christ, 2002).

From a neurobiological standpoint, significant changes occur in the prefrontal cortex and cerebellum of emerging adults, areas involved in the ability to control emotions and higher-order cognitive functioning. NIMH research has shown that the limbic system, where emotions originate, is highly active during puberty. On the other hand, the prefrontal cortex continues to mature for another 10 years. During this maturation period, emotions can outweigh rationality. When emerging adults, who are still developing the ability to rationalize and express their emotions, are confronted with the trauma of the death of a loved one, they need specific tools adapted for their level of development in order to express those difficult emotions and continue on a healthy path of development (Henig, 2010).

During this period of life, young adults need older adults to be stable and consistent, receptive and accepting of who they are. Paradoxically, often the person who died is the very person from whom they drew that support. The experience of a significant loss magnifies the psychological turmoil already created by the developmental changes of emerging adulthood (Mearns, 2000). While independence and separation are the goals for many of their peers (Henig, 2010), death generates apprehensions in young adults about attaining the goal of adulthood. For the young adult, the death of someone close is often followed by multiple losses. Losing jobs, losing sight of previous goals, such as completion of school, and loss of interest in virtually everything meaningful are all possible consequences when this age group's grief issues are ignored. Employers and teachers are often intolerant of emerging adults' behaviors with regard to declining attendance and motivation, rather than recognizing these behaviors as part of the grief reaction and providing appropriate support and understanding (Christ et al., 2002).

As health professionals, we have both an opportunity and a moral obligation to have a positive influence in the lives of these vulnerable young adults, and to provide the care, healing, and attention they so desperately need. This support can enable them to rejoin their peers and continue a healthy transition to adulthood.

"From the earliest markings found in the caves of Lascaux to yesterday's graffiti still wet on the sides of subways, visual art has powerful ways of evoking thought and emotion in the viewer, holding within it joy, pain, love, hate . . . or a person's hope to speak in ways he or she could not manage otherwise" (Boldt & Paul, 2010, p. 41). Art therapy is an obvious modality for this group. As creative and rational brain development continue at an uneven pace, art can bridge the gap in communicating difficult emotions and, when used within a bereavement support group, it becomes a powerful tool for healing (Finn, 2003; Talwar, 2006).

CURRICULUM DEVELOPMENT

UC Davis Hospice has long offered a traditional grief support group based upon Worden's (1982, 2002) four tasks of mourning. Although open to all adults, over the past 20 years, members of this group have ranged in age from 25 to 90, with a mean age of 55. Participants report benefiting from this modality due to the safety provided by a closed group, education regarding grief reactions, normalization of those reactions, and peer support. Typically, the teen and young adult population—ages 17–24—has not been denied access to teen or adult groups, but there has been little encouragement for them to attend. In addition, young people are busy with work, school, extracurricular activities, transportation needs, and caring for other family members.

Our goal was to provide a model that would address these challenges. Art therapy is a natural vehicle for opening doors to nonverbal communication when facilitating a group in which initial discussion is difficult (Ferstz, Heineman, Ferstz, & Romano, 1998). Art promotes the expression of emotions and bypasses the need for participants to edit their thoughts and feelings. "Art indeed, offers us another way of seeking the truth—through the inner-realities of our feelings, experiences, beliefs, sensations, and perceptions" (Malchiodi, 2002, p. 31). Once expressed in the physical form of an object, grief becomes easier to talk about with others. When participants share their art projects with each other and the facilitators, the therapeutic benefits are multiplied (Boldt & Paul 2003). With an art-centered focus for the group discussion, peer connection is made as members identify with others' grief reactions. Art projects also become the tangible objects of memorial and remembrance.

Adapting an art therapy format used with children and teens,[1] we created a curriculum of developmentally appropriate art therapy directives for this age group, integrating these modalities with discussion and education directives based on Worden's (2002) four tasks of mourning. This task-oriented model provides an excellent road map for grief work. Our curriculum comprises an 8-week program in which we identify weekly goals, and match them with the most effective art and discussion/education tools. The combination of these approaches is effective in helping participants bridge the world between adolescence and young adulthood. It is our intent as facilitators to create a group in which successful facilitation leads to group members supporting each other, and to encourage them to develop community and closeness.

Two main constants in all of the projects are ongoing assessment and creating a safe and supportive space. "Making art is not only therapeutic for the creator, it also provides diagnostic information for the treatment team" (Malchiodi, 1999, p. 10). The continual

---

[1] The Children's Bereavement Art Group, implemented in Sacramento in 1985, by Peggy Gulshen, MFT, ATR.

assessment of what we see and hear from group members allows us as facilitators to make adjustments to the curriculum, providing the art projects earlier or later, as needed, depending on the needs of the group.

As we begin the group, we establish ground rules to initiate the building of a safe and supportive space. We continue to build on these initial boundaries and guidelines, because the need for safety, trust, and support cannot be overemphasized. Members need to feel they can safely share any and all feelings without judgment. For that reason, there is a therapeutic arc to the design of the curriculum. As the level of safety and trust develops, we are able to offer the members more in-depth art projects that require greater risk taking and allow greater insight and change. Of course, this is up to the individual, and no one is asked to go deeper into sharing than he or she is comfortable doing. As we near Week 8, we prepare the members for closure. Art projects return to a level of safety, allowing individuals to feel contained as they prepare to leave the group. The final project is literally and metaphorically a container for members. The Memory Box, described on pages 297–298, functions as a container for memories of both loved ones and the group, that the person can take home and return to as needed.

CURRICULUM CONTENT

The following outline of our 8-week curriculum includes an art project and discussion for each week, focusing on one or more relevant tasks of mourning (see Table 20.1).

TABLE 20.1. The Four Tasks of Mourning

Task 1: To accept the reality of the loss. To come full face with the reality that the person is dead, that the person is gone and will not return; that reunion is impossible in this life.

Task 2: To experience the pain of grief. Allowing yourself to experience and express your feelings, difficult though it may be. Many feelings and experiences are normal: anger, guilt, loneliness, anxiety, depression.

Task 3: To adjust to an environment in which the deceased is missing. There may be many practical daily affairs you need help and advice with, but there will be a great sense of pride in being able to master these challenges. The emotions involved in letting go may be painful but, again, necessary to experience.

Task 4: To emotionally relocate the deceased and move forward with life. To effect an emotional withdrawal from the deceased person so that this emotional energy can be used in continuing a productive life. Rebuilding your own ways of satisfying your social, emotional, and practical needs by developing new or changed activities or relationships.

Note. Based on Worden (2002).

Week 1/Task 1: Educational Overview and Introductions

Facilitators' roles are established as we lay the groundwork, introducing the group to Worden's (2002) tasks of mourning, the framework of the eight-week curriculum, as well as normalizing many of the grief reactions the group members may be experiencing. The first week can be awkward for everyone. Participants often arrive with feelings of anger, sadness, betrayal, and isolation, coupled with the anxiety of the unknown. We provide guidelines, request commitment from group members, and stress confidentiality and mutual respect. All of these details are intimately connected to the task of accepting the death of a loved one and establishing safety in the group. In addition, they provide the necessary foundation for the art therapy projects to follow. We close each week by asking everyone to say one word that best describes where they are.

Week 2/Tasks 1 and 2: SoulCollage®; Expression of Grief-Related Feelings

The 5″ × 8″ cards for the SoulCollage (an expressive arts process designed by therapist Seena Frost) help to set limits, providing containment for what could be overwhelming feelings of grief. The use of magazine images in this process is not intimidating, and it removes the pressure to "be artistic." The process of making a SoulCollage card creates a tangible product: a safe container for feelings, allowing group members to be at one remove from their grief for a short period of time. This outward expression of grief facilitates discussion of difficult feelings. At the end of each art project, we allow time for sharing and discussion. Jessica's card depicts the experience of being a stranger in a strange land. At the time of her loved one's death, they were living in another country. She depicts her reactions (see Figure 20.1) to her loved one's sudden death with a picture of someone jumping off a cliff, surrounded by turbulent waters—a powerful expression of emotions.

Week 3/Task 2: Feelings Word Inventory and Body Outline; Continuation of Grief-Related Feelings

The Feelings Word Inventory (a list of 70 different loss-related emotions) is nonthreatening due to its cognitive nature. We ask participants to use colored, felt-tip markers, to circle all the words that apply to their loss, then to circle the five most relevant words. Using a standard body outline, the exercise leads naturally to mapping those feelings in the body outline, complete with a color–emotion symbol key. Once again, the body outline acts as a safe container for feelings that are often volatile. The sharing that follows this directive can be very lively. Once feelings are identified, participants are often surprised by their strength and complexity. This sharing also helps participants identify the physical aspects of grief (exhaustion, headaches, stomachaches, loss of appetite, sleep disorders, etc.).

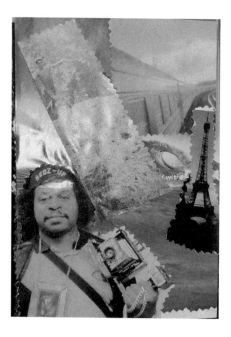

FIGURE 20.1. Jessica's SoulCollage. Week 2.

Week 4/Task 2: Making a Clay Grief Mask; Exploring Grief's Character

Having identified predominant feelings within grief, we carry it one step further and ask participants to create a clay mask that expresses the most powerful of these feelings. Our goal is to create a vehicle that allows for the expression of these most difficult emotional reactions. Each person is given a ball of clay. The evening starts with a warm-up. We pound, poke, tear, rip, and shred the clay, finally forming it back into a ball. After giving some brief explanation of technique, we ask participants to remember the Feelings Word Inventory from the previous week. Then we ask, "What is the strongest feeling you are experiencing now? Make a mask expressing that feeling." After the cathartic warm-up, the mask making is most often quiet and very focused, with little discussion. We allow virtually the whole evening for this one activity, leaving enough time at the end for sharing and cleanup.

Week 5/Tasks 2 and 3: Narrative Therapy; Sharing of Pictures and Mementos

We wait until Week 5 to share the stories of the people who died, because trust and safety need to be established before sharing at this level. This week we ask participants to bring pictures and mementos, which give form to feelings, to help make the loss more concrete. These objects are also another tool to help group members externalize their feelings of grief and loss, individuating them from the deceased (White & Epson 1990). Telling the story facilitates the adjustment to life without their loved one. The tangible objects—photos, eyeglasses case, wallet, fishing hat, diplomas, awards, obituaries—are at once proof of the loved one's existence and acknowledgment of his or her death.

Week 6/Tasks 3 and 4: Reinvesting in Life

As we continue through Worden's tasks of mourning, we incorporate into this session gentle yoga designed specifically for grieving individuals to explore the physical nature of grief and to introduce the importance of self-care in healing. The yoga is introduced as one means by which participants may identify and let go of the physical manifestations of grief. We review the body outline project from Week 3 as we become aware of the feelings the body is holding.

Week 7/Tasks 3 and 4: Painting the Grief Mask; Adjusting to Loss

Three weeks have transpired since the creation of the clay grief masks. In that time, thoughts and feelings about the deceased have changed. We provide a large array of acrylic paint colors and a wide assortment of paintbrushes, and note that the painted feelings may look different than the sculpted feelings. This time lag gives participants an opportunity to reflect upon and discover those changes. By this time, the whole mood of the group is different. No longer is it rocked with the intensity of anger, sadness, betrayal, and isolation that often characterizes the earlier weeks. Participants chat with each other as they mix colors—dabbing, splashing, and brushing on the layers of paint. A willingness to move on and a sense of completion envelopes the room (see Figure 20.2).

Week 8/Task 4: Creating Memory Boxes; Moving On and Saying Goodbye to the Group

We provide wooden boxes with sliding lids and a variety of materials, including magazines, paint, tchotchkes, glitter, and glue sticks. We ask participants to use the materials

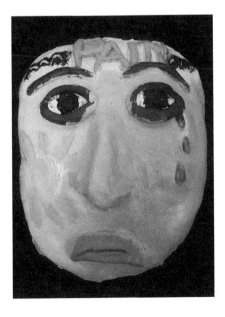

FIGURE 20.2. Sean's painted grief mask. Weeks 4 and 7.

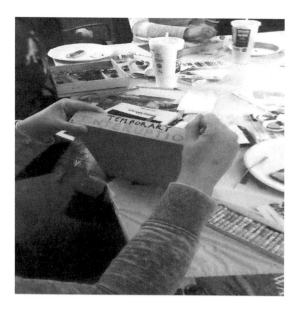

FIGURE 20.3. Making memory boxes. Week 8.

to create a Memory Box in which to store memories of their loved ones. The Memory Box allows for containment of feelings about the death and the end of the group. It gives members a tangible place they can revisit following the group (Malchiodi, 2002). It also gives them a living project they can continue to add to long after the group has disbanded, with pictures, mementos, and written thoughts (see Figure 20.3).

LOCATION

Although our facilitators are both medical team members, it is important to remove the participants from the hospital setting, associated as it is with negative images and memories for many who may attend the group (Christ et al., 2002). As a result of our collaboration with hospice, we were able to utilize their conference room, in an office park location removed from the hospital campus. The unassuming one-story building, complete with adjacent kitchen (very advantageous for art projects) and surrounded by trees and mature landscaping, is an inviting and safe setting (Steiner, 2006). This allows participants to feel safe sharing their grief experiences, while engaging in the various art therapy directives (Chapman, 2010).

FACILITATION

We developed a two-person facilitation team, an art therapist and a social worker. Having at least one person trained in art therapy is essential. In our research, we noted several times that other professionals did not see the importance of this training, but our own experience underscores the necessity for it. Having expertise in both art therapy and grief counseling is crucial to executing the group curriculum (Steiner, 2006). Although art therapy is a perfect modality for this population, we still meet with resistance (e.g., "I can't do this, I'm not an artist"). The art therapist has both the therapeutic and the technical art skills to guide participants through that resistance, enabling them to utilize the art project as a means of expressing their grief.

We developed training for facilitators for two reasons. One, to familiarize them with the curriculum and, two, for the non–art therapists to experience the art therapy component of the group. The hands-on experience changed the perception of the non–art therapists. Facilitators discovered they could not have understood the power of working with art without this training, which also gave them a better understanding of participants' experiences when exposed to these projects in the group.

SCREENING TOOLS AND ASSESSMENT

Participants are required to complete a screening tool via telephone or in person with one of the facilitators. To determine an individual's appropriateness for the group, and to assist in finding the right support, it is important to learn about his or her support system, as well as mental health issues, suicidality, and alcohol and other drug use. None of the individual's responses will exclude him or her from attending, but it's important to look at the combination of these factors to understand whether the group experience will be beneficial to both the individual and the group (Henig, 2010). We have been continually amazed at how honest the young people have been when divulging sensitive information, and how often they expressed appreciation for having been asked what was really going on in their lives.

CASE EXAMPLES[2]

The art was great because it didn't have to look nice. I could just be fingerpaint messy and focus on the messy imperfection of grief as normal.
—A GROUP MEMBER

Sean started the group depressed, jobless, and without goals. While working on the East Coast, Sean returned to his apartment one night to find that his roommate had mysteriously died. At 19, it was his task to contact his friend's parents and to make arrangements for the body to travel home to California, difficult for anyone. Sean completed the tasks at hand and returned home to live with his parents, giving up his apartment, career, and boyfriend. Describing weeks spent on the sofa watching television, Sean seemed lost. He

---

[2] All the details of the following case studies have been modified to protect the confidentiality of the individuals involved.

shared that without his father's prompting he would not have come to the group at all. However, once in the group he was pleasant and conversational. Drawn in by the art projects, he said that he enjoyed them, and spent time outside the group engaged in art activities. At the same time, it was difficult to gauge whether he was making any changes in regard to his apparent depression and grief. We didn't realize that the seeds of change were being planted by the art group. At a bereavement support group reunion, we discovered that Sean had gained employment and planned to apply to a local university.

A few months later, we received the following e-mail from Sean:

Dear Hannah and Don,

I just wanted to let you know how much the bereavement group was a positive influence in my life. The group meetings provided me with all the tools and all the things I needed to think about. I did get accepted into school. I received a partial scholarship that will pay for one-fourth of the tuition. I feel I am moving forward with my life and it feels good. Thank you again for all the good work that you do.

Thanks again,

Sean

Chris had lost a sibling to suicide. Chris and her sister, less than a year apart in age, both had a history of depression. They had supported each other throughout their struggles in childhood and young adulthood. Chris initially presented wearing dark clothing, dark eye makeup, and had gained weight and was unhappy about it. Pairing off with a group partner to discuss the loss, Chris immediately disclosed provocative personal information. Listening, we wondered whether she was indeed appropriate for the group. As the group progressed, however, Chris was able to pick up on the social cues of the group, and she began to change both outwardly and inwardly. By the end of the eight weeks, she expressed greater self-confidence and self-esteem. She emerged as a leader in the young adult bereavement art group, ended a negative relationship, and participated in an additional depression support group; Chris also began a walking program and lost the weight she had recently gained.

RESULTS

In order to evaluate the group, we created and used an evaluation tool that allowed participants to rate their experience with various aspects of the group: the art therapy directives, the discussions, the facilitators, and so forth. Initial results show that participation in the art therapy directives, and guidance and support of the facilitators were equally and highly important to group members. Also high on their list were peer support and the ability to talk about the person who had died. Overall, results reflect that the young adult bereavement art support group is a life-changing experience for the individuals enrolled. Based on these results, we continue to evaluate and update our curriculum.

We also are using this data to strengthen conclusions at a quantitative level and have received Institutional Review Board (IRB) approval for study of this group.

WHAT WE HAVE LEARNED

We began this journey with an observation and a premise. The observation was that in our community no groups existed to support members of this vulnerable age group at such a pivotal point in their lives. While experiencing the death of a loved one, the very nature of which is transitional, these young adults are also facing societal pressure to achieve goals that include finishing school, holding down a job, caring for siblings or other family members, living alone without parental support or presence, and so forth, and with little or no peer support for their grief process (Henig, 2010).

Our premise was that if we created an art therapy group to support these young adults, we could effect an intervention that would allow them both to grieve the loss of their loved one successfully and continue their journey to adulthood in a healthy manner.

Our community was identified as one of the most racially and culturally diverse in the nation (Stodghill & Bower, 2002) and our group membership is a reflection of that diversity. We found that understanding and awareness of the varying cultural approaches to grief and loss are absolutely necessary in providing support to those attending the group. We also observe that group members have an enormous capacity for understanding as they learn about each other's differences and recognize how much they truly have in common.

We discovered that unlike the traditional adult groups, young adult groups need greater flexibility in the timing of discussions and the use of art therapy directives, based on the personality of the individuals and the growing personality of each group.

Conversely, we discovered the importance of consistency. Based on a discussion with art therapist and youth group specialist Linda Chapman (2010), we learned that when there is an interruption caused by loss in an emerging adult's development, his or her need for consistency becomes similar to that of younger children. We conducted our first groups based on the common practice of arranging the room according to the night's activities. And, of course, as normal adult human beings, we wore different clothes every week. Linda pointed out that we would achieve better results by increasing the consistency of all aspects of the environment, the curriculum, and the facilitators' appearance. We incorporated her suggestions, setting up the room identically each week, agreeing to dress in the same outfits each week, and providing as much similarity in the environment as possible. Prior to applying this strategy, there was a sense of obvious resistance, including late arrivals and absences, best demonstrated the second week of a group when one member who noticed additional art supplies in the otherwise identical room visibly bristled and asked warily, "What's going on tonight?" After implementing these changes, there was a noticeable difference. Employing Chapman's approach, we noted a change in behaviors that included a tangible sense of confidence and desire to be present and participate in the group. Attendance was dramatically improved, and attendees arrived early and stayed late. We believe that consistency in environment and appearance accounted for these improvements.

We can all relate to experiences of feeling safe and comfortable when we can trust our surroundings, both the environment and the people in it. This simple adjustment increased the level of safety that is so important for participants to develop trust and to feel they can share and be heard.

CONCLUSION

As we hoped, our original program, a mixture of art modalities and discussions, proved successful in both engaging this group, and providing the verbal and art therapeutic tools necessary for members to express their emotions in a safe way. At this age, individuals often feel misunderstood. The safety created in the group setting, the peer support, and the dynamic approaches to communicating feelings allowed group members to feel understood and supported. The outcomes of the art directives, coupled with the feedback from peers and facilitators, gave the participants tangible reminders of their progress (Ferstz et al., 1998). The art directives offer participants an opportunity to express and to discharge painful and difficult emotions, *and* to experience a renewed sense of self-control and accomplishment. Although they had suffered enormous losses and pain, the group gave them the support and tools they needed to grieve those losses fully and to recognize that they could move forward in their lives, employing the tools they learned.

The combination of art therapy and discussion provides a balance between the heaviness of emotions in discussion and the pure joy in manipulating sensory materials such as clay and paints. Participants gain support to strengthen their existing roles in the world, as well as the support they need to develop new roles.

The experience of creating and facilitating a successful group for these vulnerable young people on the brink of adulthood is exhilarating and rewarding. We watch these young adults grow and change before our very eyes, seeing and hearing the changes in real time. Examples include a transition to independent study to complete high school; celebrating holidays with new friends; starting a new relationship after the death of a fiancé; moving into a first apartment; and starting college. It is proof to us that combining discussion therapy and art therapy has a synergistic effect, providing much greater results than the sum of the two separate therapies. We work in a hospital setting, where death is seen as an endpoint to medical care. Our goal was to extend the continuity of care past the death of a loved one, in order to support the grief process of the emerging adult population, so often forgotten. We sought to provide a healing atmosphere and to support a natural emerging adult bereavement process through therapeutic means, employing art as the primary tool for expression. Not only have we created and implemented this model, but our health system also has proudly embraced it as a vital component of the health care system's delivery of services. To us, the true success remains in the stories and the outcomes of the young adults who continue to attend these groups.

REFERENCES

Arnett, J. J. (2004). *Emerging adulthood: The winding road from late teens through the twenties.* New York: Oxford University Press.

Boldt, R., & Paul, S. (2010). Building a creative-arts therapy group at a university counseling center. *Journal of College Student Psychotherapy, 25*(1), 39–52.

Chapman, L. (2010, June 16 & 17). *Family assistance: Ways to provide support and assistance to and for families experiencing a loss of a child.* UC Davis Children's Hospital Bereavement Conference, Davis, CA.

Christ, G. H., Siegel, K., & Christ, A. E. (2002). Adolescent grief: "It never really hit me . . . until it actually happened." *Journal of the American Medical Association, 288*(10), 1269–1278.

Community Bereavement Resource Directory. (2011). Bereavement Network Resources of Sacramento. Retrieved from *www.griefhelpsacramento.com.*

Ferstz, G. G., Heineman, L., Ferstz, E. J., & Romano, S. (1998). Transformation through grieving: Art and the bereaved. *Holistic Nursing Practice, 13*(1), 68–75.

Finn, C. A. (2003). Helping students cope with loss: Incorporating art into group counseling. *Journal for Specialists in Group Work, 28*(2), 155–165.

Frost, S. (2010). *SoulCollage evolving: An intuitive collage process for self-discovery and community.* Santa Cruz, CA: Hanford Mead.

Henig, R. M. (2010, August 22). What is it about 20-somethings? *New York Times Magazine,* p. 28.

Malchiodi, C. A. (1999). *Medical art therapy with children.* Philadelphia: Jessica Kingsley.

Malchiodi, C. A. (2002). *The Soul's Palette: Drawing on art's transformative powers for health and wellbeing.* Boston: Shambhala.

Mearns, S. J. (2000). The impact of loss on adolescents: Developing appropriate support. *International Journal of Palliative Nursing, 6*(1), 12–17.

Steiner, C. S. (2006). Grief support groups used by few—are bereavement needs being met? *Journal of Social Work In End-of-Life and Palliative Care, 2*(1), 29–53.

Stodghill, R., & Bower, A. (2002, September 2). Sacramento: Where everyone's a minority. *Time Magazine,* pp. 26–31.

Talwar, S. (2006). Neuropsychology of art: Neurological, cognitive and evolutionary perspectives—A review. *Art Therapy: Journal of the American Art Therapy Association, 23*(4), 200–202.

White, M., & Epson, D. (1990). *Narrative means to therapeutic ends.* New York: Norton.

Worden, J. W. (1982). *Grief counseling and grief therapy: A handbook for the mental health practitioner.* New York: Springer.

Worden, J. W. (2002). *Grief counseling and grief therapy: A handbook for the mental health practitioner* (3rd ed.). New York: Springer.

CHAPTER 21

Bringing the Family into Medical Art Therapy

Elizabeth Sanders Martin

When providing medical art therapy, art therapists must recognize the impact that illness, trauma, and hospitalization have on the family unit. After defining the family and gathering valuable information about its strengths and coping styles, practitioners can then determine the needs of each family member and the family as a whole. With this information, therapists can then support the family by sharing pertinent information with the medical staff and empower the family through advocacy. They can also offer many activities that allow for expression and communication, which can unite and aid the family.

This chapter offers a framework for how to include family members within young patients' medical art therapy experience. The hospital setting is designed for treating the patient but does not necessarily include and support the family, which may not understand what is happening to the child. The medical art therapist can provide much needed services to support, educate, and comfort a patient's family members. Interventions and strategies are explained.

THE IMPORTANCE OF WORKING WITH THE FAMILY

"No man is an island, entire of itself; every man is a piece of the continent, a part of the main" (Donne, 2008, p. 152) is an ideal phrase to describe working with children in the hospital setting. Each child comes with a father and a mother, and sometimes siblings and extended family members, such as grandparents or other relative. This traditional family unit becomes the center of the child's world prior to birth. However, not every child has the traditional family unit. Some parents are absent or lose custody of their children, while others may be deployed overseas because of military assignments or even deceased. So defining a family becomes important in determining how to work with children who are hospitalized. According to the *Merriam-Webster Dictionary* (2011), a family is "a group of individuals living under one roof and usually under one head; a household" or "a group of persons of common ancestry; clan." Some family members may consider themselves a unit even if one member lives elsewhere, such as in a residential treatment center, jail, or the military. Grandparents or cousins may live with the child and be defined as immediate family.

When a child is hospitalized, the entire family feels the impact (Landolt, Vollrath, Ribi, Gnehm, & Sennhauser, 2003; Melnyk, Feinstein, & Fairbanks, 2006; O'Haver et al., 2010; Packman et al., 2005; Walsh, Radcliffe, Castillo, Kumar, & Broschara, 2007). The parents feel the need to be at the hospital with the patient but worry about the other children at home. The financial stress increases with acute and chronic illness. Employment may become jeopardized. The siblings struggle with fears and possible guilt, added responsibilities, and change in family routines. Stevens, Rytmeister, Proctor, and Bolster (2010) note that the quality of the family's first few weeks after diagnosis of a chronic or serious illness can set the stage for how family members cope with their new situation.

Riley and Malchiodi (1994) describe the family as a system or organized structure that strives to maintain a steadiness despite external factors such as births, illnesses, and deaths. They add that feedback within the system allows a stimulus to cause a response, which then influences a second response, while still acting on the first response and, subsequent responses. Feedback is not linear but circular, in that the stimulus is constantly impacting all members at one time while they impact each other. Each of these responses works toward a balance to maintain the family system, or homeostasis. Having a child with an acute, chronic, or terminal illness changes this homeostasis for all family members.

COMMON ISSUES FOR PARENTS/CAREGIVERS AND SIBLINGS

In order to design art therapy for families, it is important to understand some of the common issues parents/caretakers and siblings experience when a child is hospitalized. Parents/caregivers of a chronically or terminally ill child struggle with feelings of isolation, symptoms of stress, lack of self-care, and lack of understanding from extended family and friends. They may begin to lose their identities and become absorbed in being the caregiver (Barlow, Swaby, & Turner, 2008). If the child is admitted due to a traumatic injury, the parents may feel guilt and become vicariously traumatized by both having witnessed the harmful event and watching their child's reactions to medical treatment (Landolt et al., 2003). Some parents lack the medical knowledge needed to help with the care of their child. Many parents worry about the future of their child and whether he or she will ever become healthy again. When a child is hospitalized, the parents may be split between home and the patient's hospital room. The need for extra help makes single parents feel very dependent on others, an emotion that is not acceptable to some. If that single parent is employed, he or she may not be present with the child until after the work shift is complete. Often the medical staff is not present in the evenings, so the parent feels less informed. These complications only mean more stress for the parents and children.

Landolt et al. (2003), who measured posttraumatic stress symptoms (PTSS) of pediatric patients and parents, found that parents had a higher rate of PTSS than their children. They found that single mothers and mothers who had undergone previous traumatic life events reported even more symptoms. When parents were physically involved in the accident, they reported higher rates of PTSS. O'Haver et al. (2010) found that increased parental distress and decreased social support led to decreased adaptation in well siblings.

Packman et al. (2005) conducted research on the quality of life of siblings of pediatric cancer patients. They found that siblings' emotional needs were met at a much lower rate than the rest of the family. Siblings have their list of concerns, such as isolation because friends are not able to come over to play; internalized emotions that cause increased somatic complaints; a loss of parental attention due to demands of medical care on ill child; guilt for fear that they may have caused the illness; and anger over the lack of attention, then shame for having these emotions (Gammer, 2009; Hashemi & Shokrpour, 2010; O'Haver et al., 2010; Packman et al., 2005). Children need their own time to feel special and wanted, but when a sibling is hospitalized, parental time with well siblings is limited. Many times these well siblings refrain from openly telling their parents how they feel, knowing that this may add more stress on the parents. To ease the strain on the family, they keep their feelings hidden, only to silently suffer or become apparent through acting-out behaviors.

FAMILY ART THERAPY VERSUS FAMILY MEDICAL ART THERAPY

This section differentiates family art therapy and medical art therapy with the family. While many patients and their families could benefit from family art therapy, many professionals find the application of medical art therapy approaches with the family and patient much more practical.

FAMILY ART THERAPY

Riley and Malchiodi (2003) note that family art therapy is a valuable approach due to the equality among all members of the family in sharing their perspective of the relationships through the art making process. By using group art activities, members of the family unit can share simultaneously. Family art therapy encourages communication and provides a visual record of family patterns and dynamics. New patterns of behaviors can be learned through family members' creative strengths and visual communications. Family art therapy provides an opportunity for insight in the individual client session as well. Through drawing, clients can open the door for discussion of family patterns, roles and interactions. Family art therapy uses many family therapy approaches, such humanistic, solution-focused, systems theory, psychodynamic, Adlerian, and narrative approaches. Riley and Malchiodi (2003) note that family art therapy's contributions include art-based assessments of family systems; art interventions for families; art therapy for couples and child–parent dyads; and narrative, solution-focused, and integrative approaches.

In contrast, providing family art therapy in the medical setting may be ideal in some situations, but in actuality it is rather unrealistic. Most sessions conducted in the hospital include the patient and possibly one family member. Usually the siblings are in school and staying with extended family or friends. One parent may be working or trading off with the other parent in taking care of the rest of the family. In the pediatric intensive care unit, the patient may be sedated and not able to participate, or may be undergoing a procedure or asleep. Sometimes, parents choose to not bring the siblings to see the patient admitted to the pediatric intensive care unit due to fear of their reaction. The therapist may get to visit a patient once or twice when an admission lasts only a few days. Consequently, working with the entire family together is extremely difficult.

With these limitation, the goal is to include any family members in the therapeutic session as much as possible. Encouraging creation of therapeutic art together has multiple benefits for the patient and family, including but not limited to the following:

- The patient can see how the family is concerned and cares for him or her. For example, family members can discuss their emotions openly with each other about changes within their family unit; through art activities, therapists can learn the family dynamics and coping styles.
- The process of art making can model improved communication about the patient, the family separation, trauma, and stressors. The patient who is physically or emotionally unable to speak may choose to use art as a voice.
- Siblings can learn more about the patient's condition/treatment, express emotions, and clarify any misunderstandings through the art process. Parents can also assess the siblings' understanding of the trauma/illness/hospitalization.
- The therapist can learn the bereavement history of the family and offer ways for members to grieve together.

MAJOR GOALS OF MEDICAL ART THERAPY WITH FAMILIES

This section presents an overview of art therapy with families and strategies for working with families and siblings. The following aspects are discussed: (1) evaluating the family; (2) working with a patient's siblings; (3) helping family members express feelings and trauma stories; (4) addressing medical crises; and (5) addressing grief and loss.

Evaluating the Family

As an art therapist working in a pediatric hospital, I have found that introductions are essential in meeting the patient within the context of the family. By asking directly about each person in the room, I learn how this patient is connected and supported by his or her family and community. During the critical moments, my focus may shift from the patient to the family members and/or friends. By understanding each person's role and relationship to the child, I can then design appropriate interventions for the patient and family to use their strengths to cope with the pain, diagnosis, and treatment involved.

In order to learn more about complex family relationships, art therapists may have the family co-create a genogram or family tree to gain a better understanding of the connections. A "genogram" is a diagram delineating the pattern of behaviors within a family over several generations. This information can be valuable for all medical staff members who treat the patient and family. Patients may also be able to provide information about their families and their role within the family unit through photographs. When photographs are not available, art therapists can ask patients to substitute magazine images resembling family members or friends, or patients can draw figures or portraits to place on the family tree. Displaying the family tree on the wall in the patient's hospital room provides a visual reminder of love and support; it also can provide the art therapist a greater understanding of the family system.

Mask making may not only be a positive and creative activity for families, but it also may help them to express identity, feelings, and perceptions of each other and the hospitalized individual. Driessnack (2004) describes mask making as a form of self-identity. Masks focus on the face, which we use to communicate our emotions. In the hospital setting, therapists have access to casting materials, gauze, ace bandages, and other medical supplies. By using medical supplies in the art-making process, the artist can gain a new perspective and mastery over the medical equipment.

Masks can be used as a safe role-playing technique within the family context, because the masks provide some distance from reality. This technique also encourages the projection of emotions that siblings may have difficulty expressing directly. I use masks with patients, parents, and siblings in all units of the hospital. Family members and patients can decorate the outside of the mask as desired. The art therapist asks each person to name the mask, to share what it likes and does not like, and to share what his or her mask would say. This stimulates a dialogue between the artist and his or her mask or other masks within the family. The art therapist also may direct family members to decorate the inside of the mask with symbols of thoughts, feelings, wishes, concerns, and dreams that their masks may have.

Working with Siblings

Working with siblings, in addition to the entire family, is an important part of family medical art therapy. For example, when a brother or sister comes to visit a patient in the pediatric intensive care unit (PICU), the child life specialist and art therapist often work as a team to offer some preparation about what to expect. Many times the patient is on a ventilator and has intravenous (IV) fluids and medications. Sometimes the patient may have an arm bandaged or a shaved head due to surgery. All of these strange and unusual visuals can alarm siblings. To ease adjustment, art therapists can take photographs of the patient to show the sibling and explain each aspect of the patient's care. Education about the patient's condition or injuries and the treatment is critical to ease siblings' fears and help them understand the patient's treatment (Hashemi & Shokrpour, 2010). Parents are often not sure how much information to give and how best to phrase what they share with the children; child life specialists and art therapists can work with parents/caregivers on how to best explain the patient's condition to siblings.

After an educational visit from the art therapist, siblings may need some debriefing and can be asked to express in a drawing their feelings about what has been presented. The therapist can then also ask siblings to draw what makes them feel better or strong and safe; it is important not to leave siblings with only their feelings of fear or anxiety, but to give them an experience to support resilience and adaptive coping skills. Parents can benefit from what siblings express through this process, too, in order to gain insight into how much the siblings understand and how much detailed description they want to hear about the patient. Additionally, the art therapist can offer suggestions for self-care and self-soothing activities if the patient's condition is critical or uncertain.

The sibling of an oncology patient created this book with the oncology art therapist (see Figure 21.1). By choosing characters of the opposite sex to represent himself and his sister, he developed the distance he needed to safely tell his story. He described the patient as "Super Bob," showing his admiration of his sister as she courageously went through treatment. The content of the story lets his parents and medical staff know that he understands all that is happening with his sister as well as what he is experiencing as the observant sibling. To create the ending for the story, the art therapist helped empower the sibling by asking him to share with others what helped him the most during his sister's treatment.

Helping Families Express Feelings and Trauma Stories

Many pediatric patients experience injuries that their family members or friends have actually witnessed. Siblings also can be vicariously traumatized even if they did not see the accident occur. Everyone in the family system is vulnerable to trauma reactions and may potentially suffer posttraumatic stress reactions. Steele and Raider (2001) found that children who witness or physically experience a traumatic event benefit from using sensory integrative therapies such as art, play, and music to slowly release the emotions stored within the brain.

Narrative therapy is one way that art therapists can help children work through trauma. If family members are emotionally ready, asking parents and siblings to draw

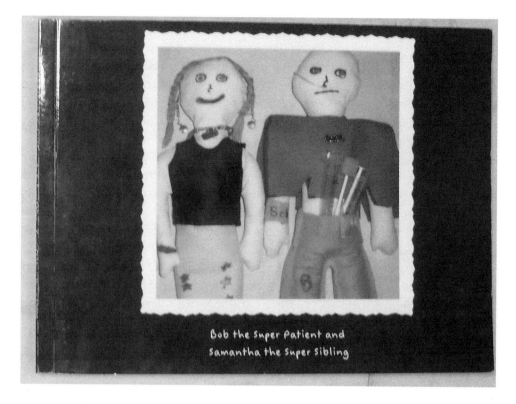

Bob the Super Patient and
Samantha the Super Sibling

FIGURE 21.1. Sibling art activity.

what happened to the patient validates their experiences and, with the help of the therapist, can clarify the event, allowing them visually to work through any gaps in their
memory. It is important to underscore that some family members will not be ready to
talk about traumatic events and may actually become more anxious and avoidant if
asked to draw and talk about painful memories too soon. If this occurs, the art therapist
can intervene by introducing activities that help parents and siblings feel better at that
moment. I like to give siblings some clay, because handling it allows soothing tactile
qualities and still encourages creativity; others may benefit from learning an arts-and-
crafts activity or simply practicing relaxation strategies, with or without art expression.

In working with a young male involved in a motor vehicle accident, I introduced the
idea of creating a book about his trauma story. We began discussing what he was doing
prior to the accident. He became very quiet and refused to make eye contact. He would
not answer any questions, and he moved his body away from me, into a more fetal position in the bed. At this point, I realized he was not ready to talk about what happened
to him. So I opened some Crayola Model Magic® and began playing with it, showing
him how I could squeeze it. He turned to watch what I was doing and took some. Once
he started playing with it, he began spontaneously talking about the accident. His family
members noticed the difference and began playing with the clay themselves.

Addressing Family Separations

Hospitalizations, for various reasons, can cause family members and patients to become separated and disrupt normal routines of family life. Diane, a 10-year-old African American female with a new diagnosis of a chronic illness, was admitted to the hospital with breathing difficulties. Unfortunately, her family had to leave to visit her grandmother in the critical care unit at a nearby hospital. It became important to find ways to connect Diane to her family members, especially during the day, when her mother could not be with her.

In order to develop an appropriate intervention, the art therapist asked Diane to participate in making art by offering her a list of possible activities; she chose to make a "wish doll." Dolls provide children with socialization of nurturing, exploration of relationships and reenactment of experiences, and companionship (Feen-Calligan, McIntyre, & Sands-Goldstein, 2009). Dolls have been used in cultures all over the world, so they can be adapted with all populations. In the hospital setting, dolls mainly adopt the role of patient, so the child can practice nursing care and gain mastery over medical equipment. They are also used in teaching about upcoming procedures and surgeries. Feen-Calligan et al. documented how art therapist Gerity's work explores the transformative nature of doll making in healing the human body. While the doll holds the child's pain, the child can alter the doll to create healing. Making wish dolls gives the art therapist insight into patients' or siblings' hopes and dreams, and keeps those hopes and dreams connected safely to the owner of the doll.

As Diane was physically weak, she worked with the art therapist to co-create her wish doll (Figure 21.2). Diane chose the yarn color and all of the design elements. She

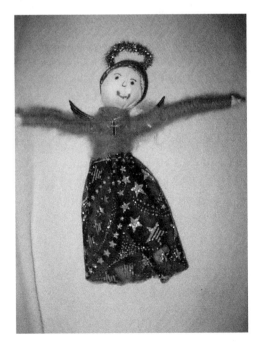

FIGURE 21.2. Wish doll.

talked with the therapist during the process, sharing about her grandmother's condition. She also shared about her love of her uncle's cooking and the special times that the family came together. In making her wishes, she wrote "for me and my grandmother to get better." She decided to make the doll into an angel by adding a halo and wings. She asked her family members to take the doll to her grandmother; it was placed on her shoulder and remained there until her death a few days later. This doll kept Diane connected to her grandmother and her family members when they were physically separated. When the therapist saw Diane on a later admission, they discussed the doll and her grandmother's death. Diane felt she had been able to express adequately her grief about her grandmother.

Addressing Grief and Loss

Whether a child recovers or dies as the result of an illness or injury, therapists inevitably deal with issues of grief and loss in medical settings. Helping families to find ways to develop resilience when they confront uncertainty is a major part of intervention, and includes preparing them for death of a child or helping them mourn losses and changes associated with hospitalizations. Art therapy may focus on grief work or be directed to help family members create images of strength, faith, and hope, including prayer, scriptures, inspirational quotes, or symbols for recovery and wellness, if appropriate.

Scrapbooking may also be introduced as a way for family members to put together images and words about memories or events important for themselves and the patient. Even though scrapbooking began back during the Renaissance (McCarthy & Sebaugh, 2011), it has recently gained popularity as a method for people to archive their memories. Studies show the value of using scrapbooking therapeutically, especially in the medical setting (Davidson & Robison, 2008; McCarthy & Sebaugh, 2011; Schwarz, Fatzinger, & Meier, 2004). Scrapbooking programs have been used in many neonatal intensive care units (NICUs), pediatric hematology/oncology units, and PICUs around the country. These scrapbooks are created uniquely; each is personalized according to the designer of each page, allowing for individual projection of emotions and insight.

Aspects of therapeutic scrapbooking include therapeutic photography, journaling, and preserving keepsakes (Schwarz et al., 2004). Therapeutic photography involves capturing moments of a child's medical treatment that may be considered difficult to see, witness, or experience in the present. These are life-changing moments in many cases for the patient as well as the parents and family. According to Judy Weiser, the photographs become "natural bridges for accessing, exploring and communicating about feelings and memories" (in Schwarz et al., 2004, p. 356). Some family members may not be able to articulate their emotions about the photograph taken until after the child's condition has improved. Later, the parents or caregivers are able to look at the photograph and express how they felt at the time; they may even show gratitude for having the importance of the moment saved and commemorated.

Journaling has long been considered a therapeutic intervention for processing emotions in a safe, confidential manner. During scrapbooking, parents or caregivers are encouraged to comment about the photographs of their child's hospitalization. By writing about each photograph, the parent is creating the child's trauma story (Davidson & Robison, 2008). This adds the narrative technique that many practitioners use to help patients work through trauma and reduce PTSS.

The preservation of mementos helps caregivers to hold tangibly onto aspects of the patient's life. In the NICU, many parents keep patient identification bracelets, a piece of medical equipment used, a small diaper, or a handprint. Each of these items reminds them that their child is alive, especially when the patient's condition is critical. Schwarz et al. (2004) note that parents of premature or sick newborns are also grieving the loss of the healthy, full-term infant for which they had hoped.

In the PICU, many patients are admitted for critical injuries related to trauma. For example, a mother stayed in the PICU with her son, who sustained a major closed head injury in a motor vehicle accident that required a lengthy hospital admission for recovery. Upon meeting the mother, the art therapist encouraged her to keep documentation of his treatment, because he would not remember the next few weeks due to the sedation given. The mother photographed her son every few days, including images of each staff member who provided care for her child. This mother also attended each weekly scrapbooking session offered to all parents and caregivers of PICU patients. She filled two books with photographs and journaling about each accomplishment her son made in his recovery (Figure 21.3); she added medical supplies as well. Her son later enjoyed looking

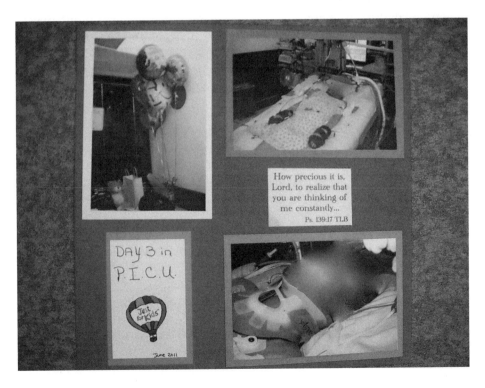

FIGURE 21.3. Scrapbook as memory of patient.

at each page she created. It allowed him to discover what he had experienced but missed because of sedation. His mother's scrapbooking encourage the son's continued progress toward recovery. The mother repeatedly shared her gratitude for the opportunity and support that gave her an emotional outlet during this difficult time.

While working in the PICU, unfortunately, I have also had many experiences with the loss of a patient. During these critical times, the parents are mostly focused on the patient and the moment of death, whether that means turning off life-supportive measures or watching the child during a "code" situation, which occurs when a patient experiences sudden respiratory and/or cardiac arrest requiring resuscitation. So much activity is happening around the patient that the parents are consumed with questions, multiple levels of decision making, and often shock. If death is anticipated, the art therapist may get the opportunity to provide parents and siblings with art experiences that center on memory making or emotional release prior to the patient's death. Additionally, self-soothing activities, such as coloring pre-printed mandala designs, journaling, or photography, are the most popular choices of art making in the PICU.

CONCLUSION

In conclusion, pediatric hospitals across the country are progressing in inclusion of families in all aspects of the patient's care. Medical art therapists can lead the way by involving the families and siblings in self-expression and stress reduction through creative activities. By offering art therapy services to the family, medical art therapists are providing better family-centered care for their patients.

REFERENCES

Barlow, J., Swaby, L., & Turner, A. (2008). Perspectives of parents and tutors on a self-management program for parents/guardians of children with long-term and life-limiting conditions: "A life raft we can sail along with." *Journal of Community Psychology, 36*(7), 871–884.

Davidson, J., & Robison, B. (2008). Scrapbooking and journaling interventions for chronic illness: A triangulated investigation of approaches in the treatment of PTSD. *Kansas Nurse, 83*(3), 6–11.

Donne, J. (2008). *Devotions upon emergent occasions.* Charleston, SC: BiblioBazaar.

Driessnack, M. (2004). Remember me: Mask making with chronically and terminally ill children. *Holistic Nursing Practice, 18*(4), 211–214.

Feen-Calligan, H., McIntyre, B., & Sands-Goldstein, M. (2009). Art therapy applications of dolls in grief recovery, identity, and community service. *Art Therapy: Journal of the American Art Therapy Association, 26*(4), 167–173.

Gammer, C. (2009). *The child's voice in family therapy: A systemic perspective.* New York: Norton.

Hashemi, F., & Shokrpour, N. (2010). The impact of education regarding the needs of pediatric leukemia patients' siblings on the parents' knowledge and practice. *Health Care Manager, 29*(1), 75–79.

Landolt, M., Vollrath, M., Ribi, K., Gnehm, H., & Sennhauser, F. (2003). Incidence and associations of parental and child posttraumatic stress symptoms in pediatric patients. *Journal of Child Psychology and Psychiatry, 44*(8), 1199–1207.

McCarthy, P., & Sebaugh, J. G. (2011). Therapeutic scrapbooking: A technique to promote positive coping and emotional strength in parents of pediatric oncology patients. *Journal of Psychosocial Oncology, 29*(2), 215–230.

Melnyk, B., Feinstein, N., & Fairbanks, E. (2006). Two decades of evidence to support implementation of the COPE program as standard practice with parents of young unexpected hospitalized/critically ill children and premature infants. *Pediatric Nursing, 32*(5), 475–481.

Merriam-Webster Dictionary online. (2011). Retrieved October 3, 2011, from *www.merriam-webster.com/dictionary/family.*

O'Haver, J., Moore, I., Insel, K., Reed, P., Melnyk, B., & Lavoie, M. (2010). Parental perceptions of risk and protective factors associated with the adaptation of siblings of children with cystic fibrosis. *Pediatric Nursing, 36*(6), 284–291.

Packman, W., Greenhalgh, J., Chesterman, B., Shaffer, T., Fine, J., VanZutphen, K., et al. (2005). Siblings of pediatric cancer patients: The quantitative and qualitative nature of quality of life. *Journal of Psychosocial Oncology, 23*(1), 87–108.

Riley, S., & Malchiodi, C. A. (1994). *Integrative approaches to family art therapy.* Chicago: Magnolia Street.

Riley, S., & Malchiodi, C. A. (2003). Family art therapy. In C. A. Malchiodi (Ed.), *The handbook of art therapy* (pp. 362–374). New York: Guilford Press.

Schwarz, B., Fatzinger, C., & Meier, P. P. (2004). Rush SpecialKare Keepsakes. *MCN: The American Journal of Maternal/Child Nursing, 29*(6), 354–361.

Steele, W., & Raider, M. (2001). *Structured sensory intervention for traumatized children, adolescents and parents: Strategies to alleviate trauma.* Lewiston, NY: Edwin Mellen Press.

Stevens, M., Rytmeister, R., Proctor, M., & Bolster, P. (2010). Children living with life-threatening or life-limited illnesses: A dispatch from the front lines. In C. A. Corr & D. E. Balk (Eds.), *Children's encounters with death, bereavement, and coping* (pp. 147–166). New York: Springer.

Walsh, S., Radcliffe, R., Castillo, L., Kumar, A., & Broschard, D. (2007). A pilot study to test the effects of art-making classes for family caregivers of patients with cancer. *Oncology Nursing Forum, 34*(1), 1–8.

CHAPTER 22

Beyond the Patient

Art and Creativity for Staff, Management, Executives, and Organizational Change

Deborah Koff-Chapin

When I first came upon the simple yet profound process of touch drawing (Koff-Chapin, 1996) in 1974, I was completing my years as an art student in New York City. Something deep had been stirring in me—a longing to find a more natural way to create and to tap the authentic roots and purpose of art. On the last day of my final year in school, I received a response to this subliminal search. I was helping a friend clean an ink plate in the print shop. Before wiping it with a paper towel, I playfully moved my fingertips upon it. As I lifted the towel off the inked plate, I saw lines that had been transferred to the underside by my touch. It was as if these marks had come directly from my fingertips onto the page. Amidst bursts of laughter, I created one drawing after another. They were a natural extension of my being, a record of each moment as it passed. (See Figure 22.1.)

Although this experience had the appearance of child-like play, under the surface was something profound and powerful. Though I am sure that others have made marks on paper this way before, there was more to the experience that the physical act. I opened to something larger in those moments; with that opening came a sense that this simple process had a greater purpose than my personal use; it felt like I was receiving an impulse from a level of consciousness that was outside of time. I had a sense that this simple way of drawing could become a significant form of human expression in the future. I was receiving a gift that came with a responsibility. Somehow, I would have to share this process with the world (Hobson, 2005). (See Figure 22.2.)

That commitment to share touch drawing has continued deepen over the years. My approach has been like that of "Johnny Appleseed"—introducing the process, and encouraging and supporting others to cultivate its application within their unique field of expertise. (Koff-Chapin, 2001). The unique qualities of touch drawing lend themselves

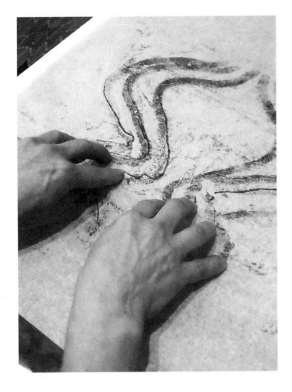

FIGURE 22.1. Touch drawing is a simple yet powerful process. Roll paint onto a smooth surface. Place paper on top and move your fingertips. Everywhere you touch an impression is formed on the underside of the paper. With thin paper you can see it as you draw. Copyright 2010 by Deborah Koff-Chapin. Used with permission.

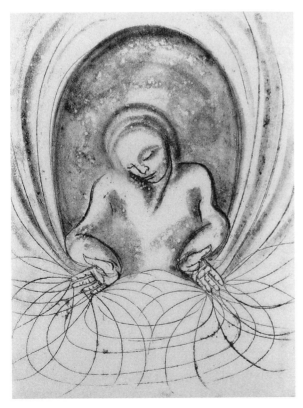

FIGURE 22.2. A touch drawing that expresses the feeling of doing touch drawing. Copyright 2010 by Deborah Koff-Chapin. Used with permission.

to a great range of applications. The ease, directness, and speed with which images can be created inspires people who otherwise would be afraid to draw. I could have written a chapter for this book on the many ways touch drawing is being used with patients in health care settings: people with Parkinson's disease and their caregivers; patients rehabilitating from stroke, in treatment for cancer and AIDS, in pain management, in pregnancy education (Koff-Chapin, 2001; *www.touchdrawing.com/2touchdrawing/tdstories1.html*); and people in grief counseling (Rogers, 2007). I even did touch drawing in the hospital myself, during contractions in my 32-hour labor. My experience of the pain was entirely different while drawing. Those were the easiest contractions of the whole birth!

But touch drawing has also found its way beyond the patient into every level of the hospital organization: from executives to clinical and nonclinical staff, middle management, and community outreach. This dynamic development has unfolded out of a collaborative relationship with the Kaiser Institute, a team of visionary medical consultants who work with hospitals around the United States. Through their potentiating work at executive levels, they have developed a vital network of people bringing transformative processes into every level of health care organizations. This chapter focuses on two ways touch drawing is being integrated into this work to help shape organizational culture: the process of creative expression and the power of visual images.

CREATIVE EXPRESSION FOR STRESS RELIEF, RENEWAL, CREATIVITY, AND INTUITION

There is widespread agreement that medical and support personnel who work in hospitals and health care organizations are often affected by stress (Fisher & Anderson, 2002). The variety of approaches used includes mindfulness practice (Cohen-Katz, Wiley, Capuano, Baker, & Shapiro, 2005), interventions for compassion fatigue (Figley, 1995), and positive psychology techniques (Seligman, Steen, Park, & Peterson, 2005). Art therapy and the arts in health care have also been applied with health care workers and staff (Italia, Favara-Scacco, DiCataldo, & Russo, 2008; Repar & Patton, 2007).

This section offer examples of how the process of touch drawing is being used with clinical and nonclinical staff, middle management, medical school faculty, and executive leadership. Combined with other creative processes and a sense of the sacred, these experiences are helping professionals cope with the inevitable stresses of any large organization. Participants gain a sense of renewed possibilities and access deeper capacities in their work. Through collegial collaborations, touch drawing has found its way into every level of the health care organization.

STRESS RELIEF AND RENEWAL FOR CLINICAL STAFF

Many professionals in health care work with people facing the most vulnerable and significant times in their lives. A close and open-hearted dynamic must occur in order for patients and family members to trust these professionals and allow a collaborative "we" to occur. This is the precious part of the work. It is also what makes clinical staff members vulnerable to burnout and compassion fatigue. The rising prevalence of fatigue in health care creates an imperative to intentionally resource strategies and practices that build caregiver resiliency, and develop the capacity to work from the heart. Resilient, renewed, and compassionate caregivers evoke healing potentials in the patient and their family.

Sandy Johnson[1] is the Executive Director of Mission and Culture at a faith-based community hospital. The hospital policy acknowledges that caregivers in every department create the healing environment. They can do that only to the degree that they embody personal wholeness. Sandy has developed a program of monthly "staff renewal retreats" meant to reconnect staff members to the heart of their work, and enlarge their connection to their own sense of life purpose and their work as a spiritual path. She designed the entire day to promote a sense of well-being, through the organic and colorful way the space is created; the use of music and other sound healing modalities; and activities that center around storytelling, generous listening, relaxation, creating a personal vision, and a closing blessing ceremony.

The visual art modality that she has chosen to use is touch drawing. Sandy describes what she witnesses as participants draw:

> "The employees get completely immersed in the creative expression of their joys, sorrows, and dreams through touch; drawing with their fingers, hands, and at times even feet. Often, someone experiences tears as deep feelings are evoked, or an awareness surfaces that was unconscious. One employee got in touch with deep-seated grief over an estranged relationship with a sibling that she said was impacting her at work. Within a week, she was able to create healing in that relationship. Another, who had considered quitting his job, found the courage to approach a coworker and work out differences. This resulted in the employee choosing to stay at his job. Participants feel renewed and connected to their sense of calling and purpose."

Sandy also uses this retreat modality with her hospital's leadership team and is currently planning to open it up for physicians and the community. (See Figure 22.3.)

The next step toward integration of any therapeutic creative process is to use it at the moment it is most directly needed. Shemaya Blauer[2] is a social worker who has personally practiced of touch drawing for many years. When she began working as a hospice professional, she discovered how vital this form of expression was in helping her to integrate and release the intensity she found herself experiencing. She describes one experience here:

> "I was asked to be with a woman who was crying out to be held. I sat with her and entered a space somewhere between my body and hers. Afterwards, I needed to

---

[1] Sandy Johnson, RN, BS, is Executive Director of Mission and Culture at San Joaquin Community Hospital in Bakersfield, California.

[2] Shemaya Blauer, LCSW, is a medical social worker at Providence ElderPlace in Portland, Oregon.

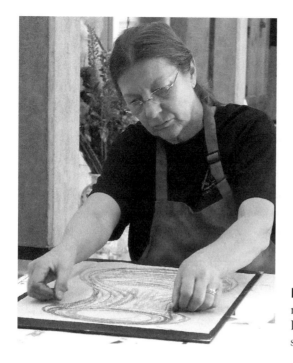

FIGURE 22.3. Touch drawing is so natu-ral and releases stress. Copyright 2006 by Deborah Koff-Chapin. Used with permis-sion.

release the experience and find a way to return to myself. Even more important was to honor and explore what it touched within my soul. Those words that she spoke and cried were the same words that were my secret longing for years as a child and young adult. When I went home that night, I created a series of 12 touch drawings and titled them 'Hold Me.' The drawings told the story of our sacred time together as she cried out the yearning that I had, and allowed me to hold her in my heart, and find peace."

Imagine what it would be like if every hospital had a creative studio available for staff breaks. Rather than a having a coffee, sugary snack or cigarette, a nurse might cre-ate a drawing, move, or write a poem. Soulful creative expression allows one to touch the sacred aspect of the work, and explore and integrate the deeper personal impact. This also provides a buoyancy and resiliency, something more than the typical form of self-care might provide.

Healing the Clinical Leaders

Janet Nix[3] is Director of Learning in a faith-based regional health care system. One of the hospitals in this system had just gone through the second round of layoffs in less than 2 years; the majority of layoffs were at managerial and directorial levels, leaving

---

[3]Janet Nix, EdD, is System Director of Learning at Hospital Sisters Health System in Illinois and Wiscon-sin.

the middle management team demoralized. Janet offered a touch drawing workshop as a vehicle for healing. Every leader at the hospital was required to attend. They started out with a discussion about how to stay connected to the system's mission despite all the chaos. A Sister from the community that sponsors the hospital co-led the discussion with Janet. They facilitated a meditation that connected everyone at the heart, followed by the touch drawing experience.

Janet described what she witnessed that day:

"I was impressed with how much everyone enjoyed touch drawing and the deep insights that came out. The Chief Nursing Officer remarked that no matter how hard she tried to change her color to a brighter one, it kept coming out black and gray, just like she was feeling. She knew she had to keep going to clear out that darkness before she could get to the color. One manager commented on how this process was a waste of her time and that she was too busy to be playing. This manager tended to be very negative on a day-to-day basis so I took the criticism with an open mind. In the afternoon session, this manager's boss came up to me and said, 'I don't know what happened here this morning but Betty [the manager] is like a new person. She actually came up to me and asked if there was something she could do to help me! She has never done that in the 5 years we have worked together.'"

The evaluations of the process were excellent, reflecting the fact that participants felt refreshed after the experience.

Let's Not Forget Nonclinical Staff

In addition to the previously mentioned clinical challenges, layoffs that occurred at the hospital where Janet Nix was employed dramatically affected the Information Management Department. Word had spread about the positive impact of touch drawing when Janet used it with the clinical staff. Subsequently, she was asked if she could provide it for the department staff that had survived the cuts. When she brought touch drawing to the group, participants were very open to the experience. Some were somber and went deep into their hearts as they drew; others found it to be a playful experience and a welcome release from their day-to-day pressures. They had fun with colors and found symbols emerging from the touch of their fingertips on paper. All came through the experience feeling uplifted and joyful. Many took their drawings back to their desks and hung them up. This experience served to support the staff members as they regrouped and entered their next phase of challenges.

College of Nursing Faculty Access Their Creativity

The same hospital's College of Nursing was going through a transition of leadership. An outside consultant was brought in to be the interim chancellor, and many faculty members were experiencing anxiety over the forthcoming changes. The interim leader wanted the faculty to be part of the change and contribute ideas; in contrast, the previous leadership was perceived as controlling. Innovation had not been used for so long that it was hard to motivate the team to be creative. Through the touch drawing process and Janet Nix's facilitation, the faculty members found that the freedom of the process stimulated their creative juices. This sense of possibility and creativity unleashed much joy and fun. They decided to take a drawing from each person and make a collage to hang in their faculty lounge area. As participants brought their drawings out from the personal realm to the community space, they were also able to share a vision for the future.

Executives and Physicians Cultivate Intuitive Abilities

Kaiser Institute has developed many innovative programs that challenge convention for hospital executives, upper management and physicians. One of these is the "Program in Intuition," designed and directed by Kevin Kaiser.[4] It is based on the premise that intuition is an innate human capacity. Development of intuitive awareness can help anyone function more effectively in his or her personal and professional life. Imagine an emergency room physician, faced with the urgent need to make a decision that impacts the life of a patient. The ability to follow subtle cues and draw upon deeper resources could make the difference between life and death.

I was invited to join the faculty of this program, both as intuitive artist and facilitator of the drawing process. I suggested that we take a chance and introduce an application of touch drawing that I call "Inner Portraits." In this process, individuals are paired up and do a series of drawings for each other. They do not draw what they see with their physical eyes; rather, they draw from a felt sense or images that arise from within. When we met for our session, I set people up in pairs. As they stood facing each other I guided them through an attunement to one another's presence. After a time of mutual openness, I suggested they let go of their judging mind, relax, and create a series of touch drawings for their partners. If a symbolic image rose to awareness, they should put it down on paper without trying to understand its connection to their partner or worrying about how well it was drawn. This was not a test of their drawing skill, but an opportunity to practice trusting their intuition. (See Figure 22.4.)

They sat across the tables from each other, hands moving upon the paper, lifting one sheet off the board and laying a new one down, until each had completed a series of drawings. They then looked through the drawings, exploring the associations the images might have for their partners. When participants shared their experience, there were many stories with surprising connections. One man had thought of a bear but didn't want to draw it, because he didn't know how. But he just couldn't get it out of his mind, so he finally scribbled it on the page to get it out of his system. When looking through the drawings, his partner immediately recognized it, saying, "That is a bear. It's my power animal!" The experience of having another person find deep recognition in something

---

[4]Kevin Kaiser is Cofounder of the Kaiser Institute in Brighton, Colorado.

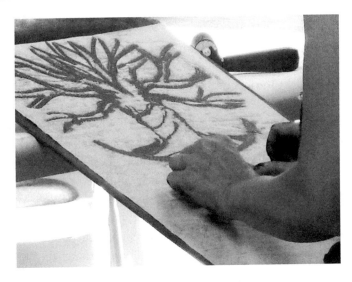

FIGURE 22.4. Accessing intuitive images through touch drawing. Copyright 2010 by Deborah Koff-Chapin. Used with permission.

one has created for him or her is a graphic and hard-to-deny affirmation of the access we each have to something more than linear knowledge. Coming at the end of their yearlong "Program in Intuition," this drawing experience provided undeniable confirmation and helped participants internalize this ability as part of their identity. This affirming experience of insight and connection could then be applied to understanding and awareness of others within the workplace.

THE POWER OF VISUAL IMAGES IN THE SHAPING OF ORGANIZATIONAL CULTURE

As Leanne Kaiser Carlson[5] traverses the continent in her capacity as consultant to hospitals and health care organizations, she finds that the health care setting at best has the look of a destination hotel or spa. She sees beautiful pictures, soothing colors, and gorgeous sculptures. Yet little speaks to the spiritual essence of the people in the place and how they are growing and transforming. Leanne notes:

> "The purpose of art is more than decorative beauty. Art has the power to remind us who we are and draw us toward our potentials. The highest dimension of art is mythic. Myths are stories that explain the world and tell us who we are in relationship to it. They convey meaning and often provide the inspiration to step beyond our small lives and apparent limitations. It is through myths that people have understood the world since the beginning of time."

[5]Leanne Kaiser Carlson, MSHA, is a Futurist with the Kaiser Institute in Brighton, Colorado.

Leanne focuses on harnessing the mythic power of art to move health care organizations toward their vision and mission. This is especially important now, with so many clinicians, executives, and staff members feeling disconnected from why they entered their profession and adrift in the chaos of change.

> "Art has the potential to help people become more whole when it speaks to what lies beyond the tasks and mechanics of medicine. It has the power to hold an image of what people or an organization can be in their highest expression. Art drawn from deeper levels enables patients to touch into the soul of the organization and viscerally feel the passion and purpose of those who work within it. An artist working from 'soul levels' can give form to potentials that people cannot articulate themselves. When a vision takes form in an artistic image, it becomes real in a way that is both evocative and concrete. The image creates a container that holds an originating impulse over time. Art contains a potency that can uniquely energize a vision and draw together executives, clinicians, staff members, board members, donors, and the people they serve."

Kaiser Institute's work with health care organizations across the country is harnessing the power of art to help heal their culture and create the future.

One Image, Many Places

Another project of the Kaiser Institute in which I have taken part is their "Program in Philanthropy." It brings together working teams from hospital foundations to expand understanding of their foundation's role is fostering philanthropy. This program encourages the development of projects that inspire generosity and enrich the hospital's relationship to the greater community. My role at these working retreats is to act as a visual scribe. I call the process "interpretive touch drawing." I sit at the sidelines, listening to the heartfelt stories of generosity that have emerged from these hospitals. I internalize the thoughts, feelings, and images, and translate them into form on the page through the touch of my fingertips. The speed of touch drawing allows me to keep pace with the stories, moving swiftly from one drawing to another during each session. Select drawings are later enhanced with color and made available for use by hospital foundation projects. The following is an example of how one of the drawings I created during a "Program in Philanthropy" retreat found its way to full integration into the life of a hospital and community.

Barbara Fulton[6] is Director of Development at a nonprofit critical access community hospital. She notes:

---

[6] Barbara Fulton, PhD, is Director of Community and Organizational Development at Hayes Green Beach Memorial Hospital in Charlotte, Michigan.

"When we began our work several years ago with Leanne Kaiser Carlson, our community envisioned a future as the 'most generous community.' Leanne also introduced us to Deborah's art and we immediately connected with the image entitled 'Abundance' as a meaningful symbol of the generosity we wanted to foster. The energy of this particular image became very important to our team. We adopted it as the official symbol of our work. Deborah had an enlarged version produced for us in a beautiful silk wall hanging. When we would travel to community gatherings or presentations, we often brought along the silk version. As such, 'Abundance' has inspired countless people along the way. One powerful image can go so much further than an abstract discussion in reaching people's emotion and releasing both ideas and the desire to act on them. [See Figure 22.5.]

"Our generosity initiatives have sparked many new projects: our 'charitable assets pillar' group, a time bank, exciting (and moving) connections between youth groups and various think tanks and strategic economic groups, the beginnings of communitywide 'power of one' initiatives, and many other results. The image has helped keep our 'possibility thinking' flowing. It is the central image linking our many projects. We currently have the poster version of 'Abundance' at our new experience-based destination health park called AL!VE. And the silk version is hanging in the lobby of our Administration office suite at the hospital. All employees, as well as visitors who come to meet with our executives, and members of the

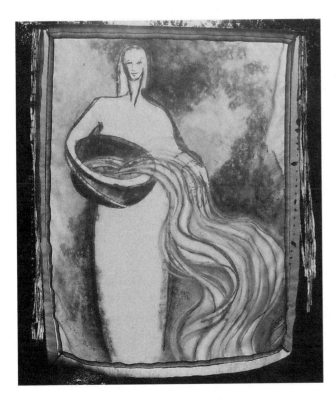

FIGURE 22.5. Abundance: Silk wall hanging created to inspire generosity. Copyright 2008 by Deborah Koff-Chapin. Used with permission.

marketing department and development office have the opportunity to see 'Abundance' and be inspired by the image."

Integrating Art into Executive Visioning and Strategic Planning

As a nurse, health care consultant and executive coach, Eileen Zorn[7] often partners with leaders from health care organizations that are in the midst of crisis, chaos, and transition. In many of the situations there is a sense of restriction, turbulence, scarcity, and a less than desirable future. Executives look to the visioning and strategic planning processes as means to navigate into a better place. Traditional strategic planning approaches are linear and analytical. Numbers and data drive the process. They do not allow for the expansiveness, creativity, and innovation that a "whole-brain" attitude allows. Art can be a bridge between a traditional approach and one that holds deeper meaning and possibility (Zorn, 2006).

Eileen was working with a faith-based community hospital in the midst of major challenges related to quality, service, and commitment to values and mission. They truly wanted to renew the original intentions of the founders. Eileen's coaching role was to help them identify an approach that would evoke a more heart-based, innovative response. Based on the new CEO's strong commitment to positive transformation, Eileen encouraged him to form a partnership with the Kaiser Institute to create a "Visioning Retreat." The intention was to launch a values-based organization that more consistently reflected their mission. I was invited to join Leanne Kaiser Carlson and Kevin Kaiser to help them set the stage for this transformation.

The executive team came together in a circle designed to foster collaboration, conversation, and deep listening. I was sitting in the center of the circle, ready to draw. My board was rolled with fresh ink and a large stack of paper was by my side. After an introduction to the "intention" of the session, the facilitators suggested that the executive leaders close their eyes and project forward 3 to 5 years, imagining the best-case scenario for their organization. They were asked to imagine what this would look and feel like. They were guided in connecting these images with the mission and the original intention of the founders, which was "service to the community." The leaders were given a period of silence to allow their minds to generate the possibility of a future filled with well-being and abundance for their organization. They imagined the form that the organization might take if it fully embraced its values. Then they were asked to open their eyes.

One by one, they described their visions. I listened intently, internalizing their images and translating them into form on paper. Each leader watched in awe as drawings reflecting their own hopes and dreams emerged from my fingertips. Visioning supported by artistic expression removed obstacles and released limitation, opening doors that launched a new phase for this hospital. The executives who collaborated in this

---

[7]Eileen Zorn, MS, RN, is President and CEO of Zorn Consulting Network (consultant to St. Mary's Medical Center in Apple Valley, California).

experience were transformed through connecting with the deeper meaning of their work and their own personal mission for health care. They rediscovered and reaffirmed who they were as leaders and as human beings. Janet Nix, Director of Organizational Development at the time, shared her view of the experience and its impact:

> "It brought us together at a different level of consciousness—not only at the verbal level but also at the soul level. This experience connected us more deeply than any other time together. It was the foundation of the next 2 years of success and growth."

From the group of images created that day, five primary focus pieces were chosen. I developed the drawings with additional color, to be used in a booklet given to all staff members. In this way, the leadership team was able to convey, with pictures and words, how it had chosen to recommit to mission and meaning, and "reframe" the future. Many of the managers chose to use individual images as part of their inspirations/devotions at the beginning of their meetings in an effort to keep the original core message of the vision alive. Many staff members hung prints of the images in their offices as a reminder of the values and possibilities they represented. The staff members discussed ways in which the images could become potent reminders for all when printed on cubicle curtains, scrubs, or banners in the waiting rooms. From the initial visioning process emerged a new focus on serving the community, partnering with other providers, supporting staff, and creating healing environments for patients. The drawings played an essential role as touchstones to the possible future, holding the signature of what gave each person meaning within the context of their professional lives. (See Figure 22.6.)

Universal Images, Personal Meaning

Over the years, as I continued to draw in the studio, the images evolved into more refined forms that express mythic and transpersonal levels. A selection of these images entered the lives of many people when I published them in the form of SoulCards® (Koff-Chapin, 1995, 2000) (see Figure 22.7). Without written meanings, people are encouraged to trust their own response to a chosen card and explore what it evokes in them. SoulCards have found their way into a range of health care settings: with patients as part of post-acute services, with chaplains as they assist people diagnosed with life-threatening illnesses, and with participants in management team meetings (Koff-Chapin, 1995; *www.touchdrawing.com/3soulcards/scstories.html*). Cynda Rushton[8] is a professor of nursing and pediatrics at a major university hospital. As co-chair of the hospital's Ethics Service Committee, she was responsible for designing a daylong retreat. At the opening, she invited members to select a SoulCard that represented healing for them. After some initial resistance, members chose diverse images from the array of cards. They then divided into pairs to share about themselves, their work, and the meaning of healing through an

---

[8]Cynda Rushton, PhD, RN, FAAN, is Professor of Nursing and Pediatrics at Johns Hopkins University and a core faculty member at Berman Institute of Bioethics in Baltimore, Maryland.

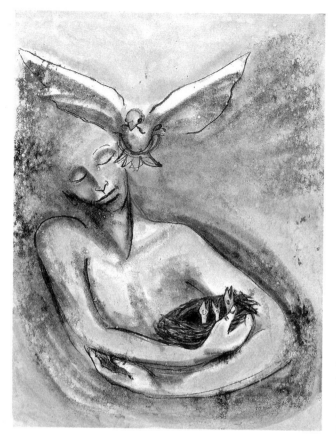

FIGURE 22.6. Nurturing the innovators: A touch drawing created during the executive retreat at St. Mary's Hospital. Copyright 2005 by Deborah Koff-Chapin. Used with permission.

exploration of their chosen cards. Following this, each person in the pair introduced the other to the entire group. The introductions were deeply meaningful, going beyond the usual data disclosed in professional settings. At the closing of the retreat, several participants mentioned the impact of knowing each other differently and asked to keep their cards as a reminder of their work. The experience helped to add depth to the retreat and to shift their interactions beyond mind to soul and heart.

A COMMON THREAD

What is the common thread in all these stories? It is the power of soul-level art, both process and product, to help access a fuller range of our human capacities: communication, compassion, creativity, intuition, generosity, authenticity, and a sense of wholeness and love. The potent emergence of the arts in health care in recent years may be somewhat surprising. But hospitals are places of birth, suffering, healing, and death. No wonder these large, technologically sophisticated institutions are now so attracted to the timeless, primal, mysterious human impulse for art. Creativity fosters life.

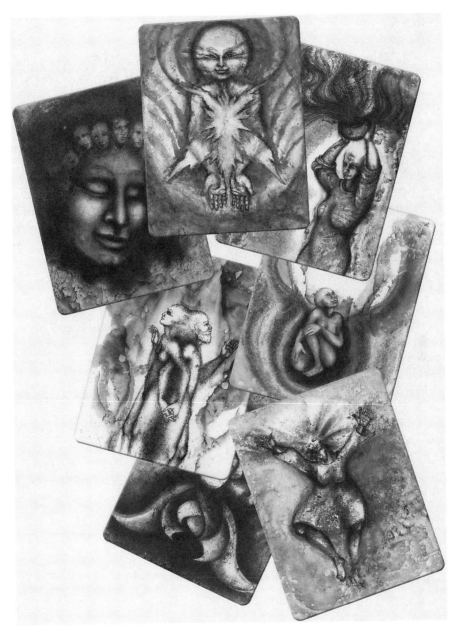

FIGURE 22.7. A deck of images intended to evoke personal insight and interpersonal communication. Copyright 1995 by Deborah Koff-Chapin. Used with permission.

REFERENCES

Cohen-Katz, J., Wiley, S., Capuano, T., Baker, D., & Shapiro, S. (2005). The effects of mindfulness-based stress reduction on nurse stress and burnout: Part II. A quantitative and qualitative study. *Holistic Nursing Practice, 19*(1), 26–35.

Figley, C. R. (Ed.). (1995). *Compassion fatigue: Coping with secondary traumatic stress disorder in those who treat the traumatized.* New York: Brunner/Mazel.

Fisher, P., & Anderson, K. (2002). *When working hurts: Stress, burnout and trauma in human, emergency, and health services.* Victoria, BC: Spectrum Press.

Hobson, D. (2005). AHN INTERVIEW: Deborah Koff-Chapin Arts and Healing Network News. Retrieved from *http://tinyurl.com/ahninterview.*

Italia, S., Favara-Scacco, C., DiCataldo, A., & Russo, G. (2008). Evaluation and art therapy treatment of the burnout syndrome in oncology units. *Psycho-Oncology, 17,* 676–680.

Koff-Chapin, D. (1995). *SoulCards® 2: SoulCards stories and uses.* Langley, WA: Center for Touch Drawing.

Koff-Chapin, D. (1996). *Drawing out your soul: The touch drawing handbook.* Langley, WA: Center for Touch Drawing.

Koff-Chapin, D. (2000). *SoulCards® 1.* Langley, WA: Center for Touch Drawing.

Koff-Chapin, D. (2001). Touch drawing facilitator workbook. In *Touch drawing stories and uses.* Langley, WA: Center for Touch Drawing.

Repar, P., & Patton, D. (2007). Stress reduction for nurses through arts-in-medicine at the University of New Mexico Hospitals. *Holistic Nursing Practice, 21*(4), 182–186.

Rogers, J. E. (2007). *The art of grief: The use of expressive arts in a grief support group* (pp. 153–176). New York: Routledge Press.

Seligman, M. E. P., Steen, T. A., Park, N., & Peterson, C. (2005). Positive psychology progress: Empirical validation of interventions. *American Psychologist, 60*(5), 410–421.

Zorn, E. (2006). Building the bridge: Helping nurse leaders find a vision though art. *American Holistic Nursing Association Beginnings, 26*(3), 28–29. Available at *www.touchdrawing.com/4deborah/zorn_summer06_final.pdf.*

PART IV

PROFESSIONAL ISSUES IN ART THERAPY AND HEALTH CARE

INTRODUCTION

This final section addresses three areas important to the practice of art therapy in health care settings: (1) patient art expressions, (2) supervision, and (3) research. There are many other professional issues involved in best practices of art therapy with individuals coping with medical illness or disability; these are reviewed in the Appendix of this volume and provide basic information about art materials and patient safety; challenges of confidentiality in hospital settings; and cultural aspects that impact medical art therapy with children, adults, and families.

Any exhibition of patient artwork requires art therapists and health care professionals involved in the treatment of a patient to consider ethical and legal aspects of making public a patient's creative work. While these issues are not insurmountable, art therapists in particular are required by their ethical code (Art Therapy Credentials Board, 2011) to work with the patient and the health care facility to insure that exhibition of art expressions is in the patient's and family's best interests and in concert with best practices.

Because art expression often becomes a way for patients and families to communicate experiences with illness, many individuals want to share their creative work with others, including viewers outside the hospital or clinic. For some patients, artwork becomes a way of not only telling their stories about treatment or recovery, it also empowers them to use images to increase public awareness about illnesses, such as cancer, and reach a wider audience. In this sense, patient artwork provides education on the prevalence of a particular disease, its psychosocial impact on the individual and family, and the challenges encountered during treatment. For example, Chapter 23 explains the relevance of art, photography, and creative writing for one cancer survivor, Jennifer Brunner, who decided to share her body of work in a gallery open to the public. This type of exhibition served another purpose in addition to self-empowerment and public information; it became a visual testament of one person's experience with serious illness that inevitably symbolized hope and possibility for recovery for all cancer survivors.

For all mental health and health care professionals, supervision is expected to help practitioners stay current in best practices and to assure that they provide optimal services to patients. Because providing psychosocial care in hospitals and other health care settings has unique aspects, as compared to strictly mental health or community agencies, Chapter 24 explores and explains clinical supervision in hospital settings, with an emphasis on pediatric work.

As mentioned throughout this book, research on the effectiveness of art therapy with various medical populations is growing; in fact, of any area of art therapy research, the most randomized clinical trials and measurable data have emerged, underscoring a growing understanding and acceptance of art-based approaches in the treatment and rehabilitation of patients with cancer, chronic illnesses, and disorders such as asthma or epilepsy, and conditions such as traumatic brain injury, Alzheimer's disease, and dementia. Chapter 25 presents an approach to evaluating art therapy via physiological measures, also known as "biomarkers." This approach is applicable to many populations and medical populations in particular because the possibility for measuring pre- and postassessments of respiration rate, blood pressure, factors related to immunity, and cortisol and other stress-related hormones can be evaluated or are regularly measured in patients. Because art therapy is believed to be an intervention that reduces perceptions of pain and fatigue (Nainis, Paice, & Ratner, 2006) and stress and anxiety, physiological measures offer exciting pathways to evaluation of the body's responses to art-based approaches used by medical art therapists.

Professional issues in the practice of art therapy in health care settings will undoubtedly emerge in coming decades. Within the continuum of art therapy services, medical art therapy is one that is experiencing increased recognition and program development at hospitals and related settings. Changes in health care practices and the growing understanding of the connections between art expression and mind–body interventions are only a couple of the areas that impact practice, programming, and research. As art therapy continues to become an integrated part of patients' treatment, it will be exciting to witness the profession's impact as an effective, established, and sophisticated approach to health and well-being.

REFERENCES

Art Therapy Credentials Board. (2011). *Code of professional practice.* Retrieved May 2, 2012, from *www.atcb.org/code_of_professional_practice.*

Nainis, N., Paice, J., & Ratner, J. (2006). Relieving symptoms in cancer: Innovative use of art therapy. *Journal of Pain and Symptom Management, 31*(2), 162–169.

CHAPTER 23

Patient Art Exhibitions in Health Care Settings

Emily R. Johnson

An art exhibition can be a powerful therapeutic tool when used by art therapists in a health care setting. Historically, the art products created within the framework of counseling or art therapy are seen as private and even as a confidential part of medical records. Practitioners must take into consideration the ethics and challenges of showing client artwork. However, exhibiting client artwork can also open doors to personal empowerment, identity, and self-efficacy.

Spaniol (1994) calls for art therapists to "respect the right of the clients by negotiating the conditions of use with them. In doing so, art therapists will treat the clients as collaborators rather than as cases to be cured or as subjects to be studied" (p. 69). Exhibitions in medical settings can be designed and implemented in various ways. Both community and in-house exhibitions can provide an outlet for patients and families to contribute to something greater and can empower them to share their stories with viewers. In this chapter I discuss how art therapists can use exhibitions with patients in medical settings, underscoring therapeutic goals, challenges, ethical considerations, and technical aspects.

BRIEF HISTORY OF THE USE OF EXHIBITIONS IN ART THERAPY

The term "exhibition" can be defined as "a public display of works of art or items of interest, held in an art gallery or museum or at a trade fair" (Oxford English Dictionary, 2011). With regard to patient art, public exhibitions of art may also take place in hallways, lobbies, and cafeterias in hospitals and clinics, including any place where artwork can formally be presented and shared with others who may not otherwise be exposed to it. Community spaces outside of the medical setting may include galleries, museums, restaurants and coffee shops. In brief, these may include spaces that the art therapist deems suitable for the safety and presentation of artwork.

Inherent to the use of exhibitions is that individuals who create the art are considered to be *artists*. In other words, they are no longer clients, patients, or people with diagnoses (Spaniol, 1990). Vick (2000) says "By stepping into the gallery, clients could step out of their role as health care recipients and be seen—by their family, the intern and agency staff, and themselves—in a new light" (p. 218). This shift in roles can expand one's identity, thus empowering the creator of the artwork (Thompson, 2009; Vick, 2000).

Exhibitions have been used for years in different art therapy settings. Mary Huntoon was one of the first art therapists to write about the therapeutic use of exhibitions. Huntoon, an art therapy pioneer whose approach is based on creative process and intuition (Wix, 2000), highlighted art expressions by people with mental illness, both in and outside of psychiatric settings. She developed the Museum Project and Little Gallery that showed her students' and patients' work at the Winter's Veterans Administration Hospital in Topeka, Kansas. Huntoon asserted that having their artwork hanging in their environment makes patients "feel in contact with the world around them" (1953, p. 29); this is an early example of an art therapist recognizing the therapeutic value of decreased isolation for patients participating in exhibitions.

Spaniol has written extensively on the therapeutic advantages and ethical considerations of exhibiting the work of people with mental illness within the context of art therapy. In 1990, she summarized three key issues that should be addressed in exhibiting work by artists with mental illness or disabilities: (1) the opportunity to exhibit; (2) safeguards to protect artists' rights; and (3) potential empowerment that can come through public exhibition of artwork. Spaniol (1995) also developed the manual, *Organizing Exhibitions of Art by People with Mental Illness*, which addresses many technical considerations of how to put on an art exhibition and special considerations for the artists with mental illness. In a third publication, Spaniol (1994) highlights ethical issues and problems of exhibition and proposes a shift in how art therapists obtain consent for use of artwork by their clients or artists.

Thompson (2009) shared his endeavor of creating a permanent gallery within a psychiatric institution and how it interfaces with a studio art therapy approach. Others describe a variety of art therapy exhibitions including art therapy student and client artworks, and integration of exhibitions into treatment plans (Alter-Muri, 1994). Many of the principles noted by these and other art therapists are universal and can be applied to exhibition as a therapeutic tool for psychosocial goals and personal growth in the medical setting.

ETHICAL CHALLENGES OF PATIENT ART EXHIBITIONS

There are inherent ethical challenges in using exhibition as a therapeutic tool in the context of art therapy in the health care setting. Art therapists working in a health care setting have two sets of guidelines they must follow in order to maintain ethical practice. The Art Therapy Credentials Board (ATCB; 2011) provides a code of professional practice; relevant sections of this code are included in the Appendix at the end of this book. Additionally, the Health Insurance Portability and Accountability Act (HIPAA) regulates use and disclosure of protected health information (PHI; U.S. Department of Health and Human Services, 2011). It is possible both to share client artwork and information through exhibitions, and to abide by these important rules. In brief, major ethical challenges for exhibition of patient art include but are not limited to the following: (1) permission to share artwork; (2) confidentiality; and (3) ownership.

Permission to Share Artwork

The ATCB Code of Professional Practice (2011) provides specific guidelines for what art therapists are mandated to consider regarding release of art products and information from their work with clients. The ATCB document states, "3.2.4 Art therapists shall obtain written, informed consent from a client or, when appropriate, the client's parent or legal guardian, before displaying the client's art in galleries, health care facilities, schools, the Internet or other public places." The ATCB ethical code also states that signed consent must be obtained for use of imagery or information from sessions, and this consent must indicate the specific formats for release of imagery and information (e.g., audio recording, video, artwork, and/or personal identification). Additionally, patients much have the right to revoke permission for display of images at any time (see the Appendix at the end of this book for pertinent sections of the ATCB ethical code).

Most mental health professionals agree that child assent must be also taken into consideration. A child assent form explaining display of artwork in a developmentally appropriate language should be offered to pediatric patients. As long as the parent or legal guardian consents, it is recommended that children also be given a choice about displaying their artwork in exhibitions. This is not only important for the trust relationship between therapists and child clients, but it also provides a sense of control to those who are hospitalized. Therapists may also use this as an opportunity to explain the importance of children's self-efficacy and trust to parents/guardians.

Confidentiality

In the field of art therapy, it is widely accepted that artworks are part of the client or patient medical record. Like all mental health and health care professionals, art therapists are required to abide by ethics and legal requirements for confidentiality of patients' disclosure, including those made through art. If permission is given to exhibit patient artwork, many aspects must be considered in order to assist patients and families in making informed decisions about sharing art expressions with others, including the public.

HIPAA, enacted by the U.S. Congress in 1996, regulates use and disclosure of PHI. All employees working within hospital settings in the United States must abide by HIPAA regulations. PHI can include medical information, treatment, diagnosis, prognosis, photographs, tapes, video, and artwork (U.S. Department of Health and Human Services, 2011). Because of the HIPAA, ethical codes, and legal guidelines, many hospitals now provide more than one consent form when acquiring patient or guardian permission for involvement in art exhibitions. For example, an "Authorization to Release Protected Health Information" includes consent to release PHI to the general public, Internet, media, and a third party designated by the patient and/or guardian and therapist. It provides options for patients and/or guardians to specify the purpose of the disclosure and to release the name of the artist. It is also preferable to identify how individuals giving consent would want their names to be shared (e.g., first and/or last names, nicknames, or pseudonyms).

Specific consent and child assent forms are also recommended for authorization to photograph, videotape, and/or record an interview with patients and/or family members. This is also important in discussions with patients about the possibility of artwork in exhibition being photographed, and with clients and families attending opening receptions where media may be present. In using either authorization form, patients and caregivers may choose not to consent with the clear understanding that their refusal would not affect medical intervention or eligibility for treatment. Spaniol (1994) adds that if therapists are negotiating terms of use of the artwork and other information with clients, they must use very specific questions and statements on releases that allow clients to write in information or decline very specific possible disclosures.

In terms of exhibition of patient art, how much information is provided about exhibited artwork must be extensively considered because of the impact it will have on both the artist and audience. In some cases, artists or families feel it is important to provide the context for artwork (e.g., the hospital where it was created, age of the individual, or patient's diagnosis), and personal information may be shared with this therapeutic goal in mind (Spaniol, 1994). Spaniol (1990) suggests that safeguards should be built into the process, and that one option for protection is limiting the "dissemination of information to statements written and signed by the artists" (p. 78), which allows them to be in more direct control of exactly what they wanted to communicate. Therapists may ask the artist or guardian to write a few lines to go along with the artwork if doing so supports both therapeutic goals and limits of confidentiality. As an alternative, therapists may interview the person or guardian, write about the context for the work, and have the patient or guardian approve the description.

Because art exhibitions can reveal a great deal about patients, therapists should discuss with patients and families how sharing their story or creative expressions may affect them. All parties must be fully informed that putting these often very private and personal things out for the public to see has the potential to bring about feelings of vulnerability or overexposure. Henley (2004) warns that showing art "may evoke feelings of anxiety and even intimidation. Once shown to an audience, the artist not only displays his or her level of skill, but also discloses content that may be highly personal, thus heightening feelings of vulnerability" (p. 79). It is suggested that art therapists discuss this directly with clients before showing artwork to provide clarity about audiences that would be privy to the show or information about the show.

Spaniol (1994) provides another perspective and emphasizes the need to look closely at how therapists approach confidentiality with clients to best "ensure we are working from current values rather than past assumptions" (p. 74). The client's right to privacy, or nondisclosure of case material, must be considered independently for each artist. Anonymity, which is a part of confidentiality, offers clients the possibility to remain unidentified by name. Spaniol notes that therapists must look at these two issues separately: whether the use of a patient's name or case material is in the best interest of the client. She also underscores the need to empower patients in this decision-making process. Additionally, anyone showing patient artwork in the public setting must take care not to present artwork as synonymous with a diagnosis or illness or describe products as representative of pathologies. This would in turn negate any therapeutic objectives of empowerment or identity shift for the client when using exhibitions in art therapy.

Finally, the Internet as a venue for exhibition of patient artwork presents both exciting possibilities and new ethical concerns, particularly in the areas of confidentiality and ownership (see below). Website galleries and photo-sharing platforms such as Flickr and Facebook provide opportunities for artists to share their artwork with a limitless audience; for artists who are hospital- or homebound, these platforms can decrease a sense of isolation, and exhibits can reach other patients and the public in ways that traditional brick and mortar galleries cannot. However, exhibition of patient artwork on the Internet leaves images unprotected; anything displayed on a website or photo-sharing platform can be copied, altered, and used by anyone without permission. The multidimensional issues regarding display of artwork through electronic means are still being explored in the field of art therapy (Sabados, 2009), and art therapists and other professionals are advised to discuss fully the possible ramifications of electronic art exhibition with patients.

Ownership

Who owns artwork a patient creates while at a hospital or other medical setting? It is possible that some hospitals or agencies may believe the artwork belongs to them or to the treatment team, just like medical samples or patient records discussed in sessions. Art therapists generally agree that there is an intrinsic value in the art product as an extension of the client's identity, and that artists ultimately own their artwork. Although the artistic expressions may be used therapeutically, art therapists recognize patients as artists, therefore giving them ultimate ownership of their art to enhance personal growth and empowerment (Spaniol, 1995).

Additionally, if artworks are the property of patients, returning artworks after an exhibition in a timely manner is of utmost importance. This can also provide a therapeutic avenue to review work with the therapist and wrap up the sessions. Although most situations would require that the artist be given complete ownership of artwork, one possible dilemma occurs when the artwork is deemed unsafe for the artist to retain. This may occur for a number of reasons, including materials used or content of the artwork (e.g., disclosure of abuse or intent to harm others). In all cases, the disposition or retention of artwork should be discussed, and an agreement between therapist and artist should determine what is to be done with the artwork. Some possible solutions include disposing of the product in a specific way or recording the work through photographs to be retained by the artist.

To sell or not to sell artwork is also part of ownership issues that therapists should discuss with patients. Spaniol (1990) suggests including artists in the decision-making process each step of the way. In many exhibitions, artwork was not for sale, although donations to the children's hospital in support of the art therapy program were accepted. Many studio art therapy programs do sell client artwork in exhibitions, and the client themselves may benefit directly from this, profiting from a standard percentage, often set by the gallery. Involving the artists in the decision of selling or not is yet another way to offer control in the process (Spaniol, 1990). In my experience of working with children and families in the medical setting, I have observed that the majority of artists want their original work returned. There are other ways of selling artwork without using the original, such as reproduction prints. Of course, whether selling the original or making reproductions, these elements need to be carefully considered and specified in the signed consent forms.

Finally, is art exhibition always in the best interest of all patients? Clearly, many medical patients of all ages can greatly benefit from showing their art. However, there may be situations in which public exhibition does not have a patient's best interests in mind. For example, Malchiodi (1999) warns that art shows may not always contribute to the wellness of patients, particularly children: "Because children's art expressions, especially those made by children in distress, are so visually compelling hospital and clinics often want to exhibit them to draw attention to the needs and issues of hospitalized children. Although these public exhibitions of children's work may have the best intentions, this practice may not be in the best interest of the children" (p. 29).

GOALS FOR ART THERAPY EXHIBITIONS IN MEDICAL SETTINGS

Alter-Muri (1994) calls for "the art therapy community to consider integrating exhibition of artwork within the treatment plan. This can be an important expansion of the intrapsychic and interpersonal course of development, healing, and growth for clients" (p. 224). To these ends, art therapy goals for art exhibition include, but are not limited to the following:

1. *Increasing control and self-efficacy.* In hospital settings, helping patients and families to regain control as much as possible is very vital to their overall well-being (Pollin, 1995). Malchiodi (1999) identified one of the three main sources of stress in pediatric patients as "loss of independence and control" (p. 15). One of the primary goals of an art therapist working in the medical setting is to help the patient to regain control. Giving the person in the medical setting the choice to share artwork publicly can be extremely

valuable. Regardless of the patient's choice, the art therapist is able to give the patient the control and autonomy to make this decision at a time when they do not have many choices due to hospitalization or medical diagnosis.

2. *Reducing isolation and increasing social interaction.* Being in the hospital can often be very isolating. Whether due to long hospital stays, or a diagnosis that does not allow patients to return to school or normal activity, patients often feel alone (Pollin, 1995). Friends or family may not be able to visit them in the hospital, or patients may not be able to come out of their room due to possible spread of infections. Being a part of an exhibition in which other patients show their work and perspectives can reduce these feelings of isolation in two ways: (1) by seeing that others are undergoing similar treatments and experiences in the medical setting, and (2) by aiding in expression and communication with friends, family, and the community. Spaniol (1990) noted, "For many, it was their first awareness of belonging to a community of artists who shared similar issues and concerns. For others it was an opportunity to begin to network and establish a support system" (p. 76). As previously mentioned, a website gallery may be another possible venue for exhibiting artwork, providing a sense of communication with others and accomplishment.

3. *Creating purpose.* Facing a medical diagnosis or trauma may suddenly change a person's purpose for living and the meaning of life. For example, if a young adult who is actively working on a career or school suddenly is faced with a life-threatening illness or trauma, he or she may feel like life has been thrown off course. An exhibition, whether group or individual, can give a patient the opportunity to work toward something greater (Henley, 2004). Malchiodi (1999) notes, "Art therapy is one of few therapies where the individual becomes actively involved in treatment through the process of art making and through the creation of a tangible product" (p. 16). Involvement in art therapy and exhibitions requires that one become an active participant in one's own health care and overall wellness, providing purpose and meaning.

4. *Developing a sense of empowerment.* Medical conditions can rob a person of his or her identity (Pollin, 1995). Exhibiting artwork allows for a shift in self-perception, therefore enhancing a feeling of empowerment. Patients are no longer people with diagnoses but have instead become artists. It can be affirming to see efforts and art product on display (Franklin, 1992). The ability to give to others is also a common need for people who deal with severe medical illnesses or traumas. Many patients feel that they want to bring more awareness to the community about illness or related issues through art expression. They may want to share their stories in the hope of inspiring others to find healing, and ultimately bring meaning and wholeness to their own lives.

Finally, there may be stigma, discrimination, and fear when dealing with hospitalization or medical treatments (Pollin, 1995). Confronting these labels and addressing the community in a public setting through exhibiting artwork can be reparative and empowering for not only patients but also viewers. This can ultimately affect society's knowledge of the psychosocial aspects of illness, therefore bringing more financial support for programs and research, and increasing understanding of survivors of the disease.

5. *Normalizing the hospital experience.* Life-changing illnesses and medical traumas can have a major impact on the developmental and emotional growth of both children and young adults (Malchiodi, 1999). School-age children may be missing opportunities to share artwork in school. Young adults may have additional needs to interact with peers. Giving children and adolescents the opportunity to share artwork with others outside the medical setting may help to normalize their hospital experience and keep them connected to their peers.

6. *Increasing motivation and involvement.* Exhibitions help to engage a greater number of patients in art therapy by motivating their involvement. If offered art therapy services for the purpose of making art for oneself, a person may decline. But if offered art therapy services for the purpose of helping with a project that could be a part of public display, one may feel more excited to help. This incentive of being part of something greater may be reinforcement for patients to engage in art making when they might not have done so otherwise. Additionally, having an exhibition to work toward can provide a goal and something to look forward to, especially during days of debilitation or exhausting medical treatment.

7. *Sharing a visual legacy.* Exhibitions provide an opportunity for clients to make a tangible product that in the future may serve as "visual legacy" (Malchiodi, 1999, p. 17). This artwork not only communicates feelings but, as Malchiodi describes, also can become a "visible and external record of the self" (p. 17). For example, the artwork of someone who has died may be presented with permission of the family and a memorial statement from family members or friends. This can provide parents a way to retell the story of their children and honor their experiences.

EXAMPLES OF EXHIBITIONS IN MEDICAL SETTINGS

Art exhibitions to enhance patients' psychosocial growth can go in many different directions and take place in various locations. Artwork created by patients in hospitals may be displayed in hallways, lobbies, or conference rooms. It may be shown in more formal galleries outside the facility or informal community spaces, such as coffee shops or restaurants. These exhibitions may involve individual artists, groups, or collaborative works. The Internet is also an expanding venue for exhibiting artwork.

"A Bone Fractured Fairytale: My Year Lost in Cancer Land," an example from a solo exhibition in a community gallery space, included original artwork, photography, and writing by patient/artist Jennifer Brunner (see Figure 23.1). Jennifer was a young adult being treated for Ewing sarcoma at a pediatric hospital when I first met her and offered art therapy services. She confided that she had always wanted to have an art show, to be an artist and writer, and she introduced me her blog entitled "I Won the Crap Lotto." Over the following year, she created drawings, collages, paintings, photography, and writings for the purpose of exhibition in a local gallery. Jennifer had over 50 works of art in this show, which told her story of being diagnosed with a rare bone cancer through

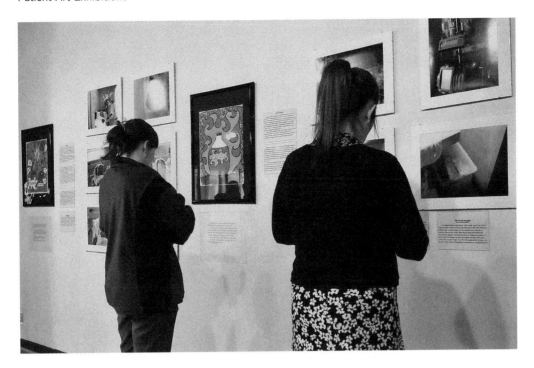

FIGURE 23.1. "A Bone Fractured Fairytale" artwork in the gallery space during opening reception.

photographs of her actual treatment, and a corresponding allegorical fairytale of her creation through writing and mixed-media artworks.

The "Wall of Hope," an example of a group show, was a project located on the oncology unit of a children's hospital (see Figure 23.2). It comprised over 100 paintings in various sizes in response to patients or family members being asked to illustrate the meaning of hope. Patients were specifically asked the think about "what gives me hope, what I hope for, or what I think hope looks like." The paintings were then put together in a patchwork style on the wall, where everyone could share in viewing these images, colors, and shapes of "hope."

TECHNICAL ELEMENTS OF EXHIBITIONS

A number of pragmatic considerations in planning and arranging patient art exhibitions include the following:

1. *Creating a timeline.* A timeline is important when considering how long it takes to plan and implement and exhibition. As a general estimate, 1 year or longer is recommended to put together an exhibition effectively. When gathering artwork and resources involved in promoting an exhibition, 1 year goes by quickly.

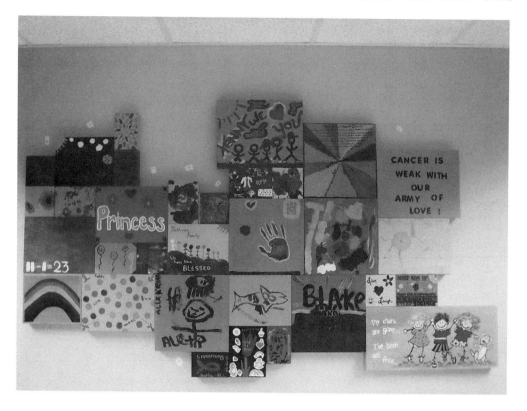

FIGURE 23.2. "Wall of Hope" installed on a pediatric oncology unit.

2. *Developing resources and partnerships.* Funding sources and partners in the exhibition must be considered early on in the planning stage. Donors of materials, framing, space, food, and so forth, may be motivated by the recognition of their services in collateral materials. Therefore, it is important to have these partnerships, sponsorships, or supporters confirmed in the beginning of developing an exhibition.

3. *Writing press releases.* Creating excitement and an audience for the exhibition is important, especially if there is a goal of raising community awareness. Consider sending press releases to newspapers, radio stations, TV stations, an online event calendar, magazines, and local publications. Write articles for internal publications, too. Include print postcards, if appropriate, providing them to each artist who is able to give an address list to send as bulk mail. In addition to traditional forms of advertisement, social media are also great places to promote exhibitions and events.

4. *Framing, printing, and mounting.* Materials involved in preparing the artwork to be exhibited properly and respectfully must also be considered. Artwork may need to be framed or mounted so it is ready to be hung in the gallery. Photographs of artwork may need to printed and may require mounting. Framing and mounting styles are endless and should be based on what one is trying to achieve when presenting the artwork. For example, if the work needs to be presented directly and without distraction, a simple

foam core mounting or pinning to the wall may be best. Some artwork may be best presented if framed or put under glass for safety. The materials used in presenting the artwork can greatly affect how one perceives the artwork in a gallery setting and must be considered with care.

5. *Organizing and hanging.* Artwork can be organized in a gallery or community space in many ways. Pieces may be in chronological order, portray a story from beginning to end, or be arranged to best balance the space based on size and media. Some gallery or museum spaces have curators or other staff members in charge of hanging and addressing technical elements of an exhibition, while others may require the artist or organizer of the show to hang the work. The owners of the space may also have some considerations for how artwork should be hung, depending upon wall material and ability to repair damage. Communication with the staff of the exhibition space early in the planning stages is key to understanding the best approaches.

6. *Creating labels and signage.* Labeling of artwork should take place at the very beginning of the exhibition process, and artists should be involved. Artists may be asked the title of their work or any additional information they would like to add to their artwork label. As a general rule, labeling artwork in gallery spaces includes the artist's name, title of work, and the medium. Dates and other information may also be added if they are pertinent to the audience's understanding and respectful of the artists' and/ or guardians' consent and wishes. Signage involved in an exhibition can include the title of the exhibit and possibly artists' names, biographies, artist statements, and further information about a program or the context of the artwork.

7. *Planning opening receptions.* Many exhibitions include an opening or closing reception, because it is a great way to honor the artists involved in the exhibit. A reception can be open and attended by the general public or by invitation only. Some may arrange a specific viewing for artists and friends/family of artists only, and another viewing that is open to the community. If the artists attend the reception, then preparing them for what to expect and possible community response is important. Elements of an opening reception often include practical aspects, such as refreshments and music. Print materials and brochures can inform audience members about the exhibit and artists' work, and a guest book provides important feedback from people who view the exhibition and gives them the opportunity to share their experiences at the show. Nametags may be used for artists interested in sharing their personal story with the audience, or artists may choose to not be identified.

8. *Involving the audience.* An interactive project or activity may also be an exciting element for participants of an exhibition, if space allows. For example, participants were given the opportunity to create printed fabric flags, also called "message flags," for exhibition. The gallery space was located next to a classroom area in a local museum. The viewers attending the opening reception could print their message on their piece of fabric, then hang it on a line in the gallery (see Figure 23.3). This way through this installation piece that expanded over time, they too were able to contribute to the evolution of the exhibit.

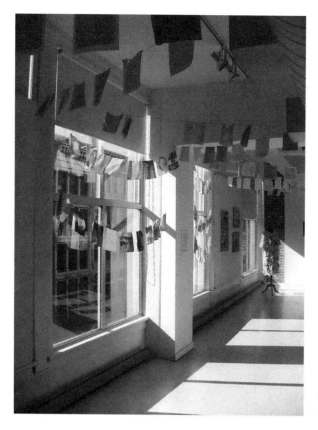

FIGURE 23.3. Message flags created by the audience during the opening reception.

MAINTAINING THERAPEUTIC OBJECTIVES WHILE COLLABORATING WITH OTHERS

Art therapists implementing an exhibition must always keep in mind their therapeutic goals and objectives during the process of working with others. Necessary collaborators in the exhibition process, such as marketing and public relations departments or funding sources, may have different perspectives on how to approach the exhibition. Practitioners must maintain the best interests of patients at all times and use any challenge as a chance to advocate for patients.

For example, Jennifer Brunner's original choice of image for her postcard was a medical scan in black and white. The hospital's marketing department was concerned that this would not entice people to look further into the show or see the other side of the postcard for more information. They suggested using another photo of her shaving her head. The art therapist discussed this with Jennifer, providing her with the feedback from the marketing department, and was candid about it being her choice, so she could make her decision. This initiated an opportunity to discuss the possible stereotyping of the typical "bald cancer patient." The art therapist gave Jennifer full control to make the final decision on the image to be used. Jennifer was then able to take into consideration the marketing perspective and to synthesize her own approach. She chose another photo and a drawing of her face in color (see Figure 23.4).[1] The art therapist made it clear that maintaining her voice and perspective for the exhibition was of primary importance. Collaboration with other departments is vital in making exhibition successful, while maintaining the therapeutic value in the process.

CONCLUSION

Exhibitions can be a valuable therapeutic component of art therapy in a health care setting. Whether in the hallways of the hospital, as with the "Wall of Hope," or at a museum or community gallery space, such as Jennifer Brunner's solo show (2009), these exhibitions provide multiple therapeutic benefits for patients and families facing medical illness. Sharing artwork can increase a sense of control and self-efficacy, decrease isolation, increase social interactions, create purpose, normalize the hospital experience, increase motivation and involvement, and provide the opportunity to share visual legacies. Exhibiting patients' artwork also brings up many possible ethical challenges. Fortunately, art therapists' contribution to therapeutic applications of an art exhibition, and codes of professional practice and other guidelines, assists both themselves and other medical professionals in helping patients make appropriate decisions when it comes to exhibiting art created in medical settings. Ultimately, art therapists must approach the possibility of sharing their patients' and families' artwork in the public arena mindfully, and with utmost regard for their clients' well-being.

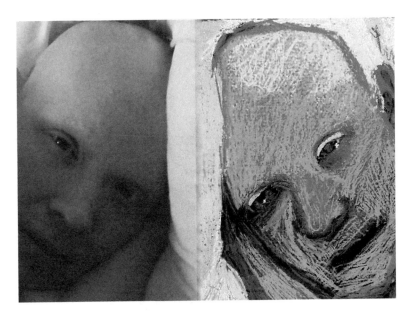

FIGURE 23.4. Artist Jennifer Brunner's final choice for exhibition postcard.

---

[1]Original artwork in this chapter was in color. It is reproduced here in black and white.

REFERENCES

Alter-Muri, S. (1994). Psychopathology of expression and the therapeutic value of exhibiting chronic clients' art: A case study. *Art Therapy: Journal of the American Art Therapy Association, 11*(3), 219–224.

Art Therapy Credentials Board. (2011). Code of Professional Practice [Data file]. Retrieved from *www.atcb.org/code_of_professional_practice*.

Brunner, J. (Artist). (2009). "A bone fractured fairytale": My year lost in cancer land [Art exhibit]. Louisville, KY: Kosair Children's Hospital Foundation.

Franklin, M. (1992). Art therapy and self-esteem. *Art Therapy: Journal of the American Art Therapy Association, 9*(2), 78–84.

Henley, D. (2004). Meaningful critique: Responding to art from preschool to postmodernism. *Art Therapy: Journal of the American Art Therapy Association, 21*(2), 79–87.

Huntoon, M. (1953). Art therapy for patients in acute section of Winter VA Hospital. *VA Department of Medicine and Surgery Information Bulletin, 10,* 29–32.

Malchiodi, C. A. (Ed.). (1999). *Medical art therapy with children.* London: Jessica Kingsley.

Oxford English Dictionary (Online). (2011). Exhibition. Retrieved from *http://oxforddictionaries.com/definition/exhibition*.

Pollin, I. (1995). *Medical crisis counseling.* New York: Norton.

Sabados, D. (2009, November). *Art therapy and technology: Ethical considerations for use of the Internet, social networking, and electronic media.* PowerPoint presentation at the American Art Therapy Association Conference, Dallas, TX.

Spaniol, S. E. (1990). Exhibiting art by people with mental illness: Issues, process and principle. *Art Therapy: Journal of the American Art Therapy Association, 7*(2), 70–78.

Spaniol, S. (1994). Confidentiality reexamined: Negotiating use of client art. *American Journal of Art Therapy, 32*(3), 69–74.

Spaniol, S. E. (1995). *Organizing exhibitions of art by people with mental illness: A step-by-step manual.* Boston: Boston University Center for Psychiatric Rehabilitation.

Thompson, G. (2009). Artistic sensibility in the studio and gallery model: Revisiting process and product. *Art Therapy: Journal of the American Art Therapy Association, 26*(4), 159–166.

U.S. Department of Health and Human Services. (2011). Centers for Medicare and Medicaid Services [Data file]. Retrieved from *www.cms.gov/hipaageninfo*.

Vick, R. (2000). Creative dialogue: A shared will to create. *Art Therapy: Journal of the American Art Therapy Association, 17,* 216–219.

Wix, L. (2000). Looking for what's lost: The artistic roots of art therapy—Mary Huntoon. *Art Therapy: Journal of the American Art Therapy Association, 17*(3), 168–176.

CHAPTER 24

Art Therapy Interventions with Clinical Supervision Groups in a Pediatric Health Care Setting

Shari L. Racut

It is essential for helping professionals to develop a regular and healthy practice of self-care so that we are equipped to serve and take care of others with empathy and compassion. For psychosocial professionals providing services to pediatric patients and their families, it can be easy to get caught up in work with others and forget about oneself in the process. Clouder and Sellars (2004) confirm that "staff appeared to attend to patients' needs ahead of their own when time was short" (p. 267) an attitude typical in current health care culture. Clinical supervision is one way to engage in self-care and reflective practice within the workplace. Cutcliffe and Hyrkas (2006) suggest that clinical supervision for the variety of disciplines involved in providing health care in the 21st century is critical, particularly in times of uncertainty, low morale, high stress, and high burnout rates. At the same time, they recognize that clinical supervision within a multidisciplinary context remains underexamined.

Topics and issues that arise in pediatric medical settings are unique when compared to other health and human services settings, and therefore deserving of special attention. This chapter examines the topics of clinical supervision in health care and the use of art therapy interventions in clinical supervision in pediatric care. The importance and uniqueness of clinical supervision in a pediatric health care setting is demonstrated, using outcomes of a survey and an example of one health care institution's programming for group clinical supervision, including case material from art therapy interventions used.

CLINICAL SUPERVISION IN HEALTH CARE

"Clinical supervision" may be defined as an exchange between practicing professionals to enable the development of professional skills (Lakeman & Glasgow, 2009). It is a practice-focused professional relationship that enables one to reflect on one's practice with the support of a skilled supervisor, and through reflection further develop skills, knowledge, and an enhanced understanding of one's own work (Jones, 2006). Walsh et al. (2003) reiterate that clinical supervision "involves a process of reflection upon practice, the aim of which is to improve clinical practices and hence improve patient outcomes" (p. 33).

In addressing the often demanding and stressful work environments of pediatric medical settings, Jones (2008a) suggests that "work discussions that take place in clinical supervision can help by providing a consistent holding environment to bridge gaps between what can realistically be achieved in human service and the frequently destabilizing demands of health-care provision" (p. 379). Stress often goes unrecognized in many areas by clinicians and managers; clinical supervision has been found to help employees deal with feelings of stress and change the circumstances that lead to stress (Williamson & Dodds, 1999).

Hawkins and Shohet (2000) discuss the primary areas of focus for clinical supervision, ranging from supportive, educational, and managerial categories. The supportive functions of clinical supervision include validating and supporting employees both as persons and professionals, preventing employees from feeling overburdened or isolated in carrying their workloads, offering personal and professional resources, fostering proactive rather than reactive behavior, and providing space for employees to explore and express personal distress and reactions that may be brought up by their work. Clinical supervision also includes educational functions for employees, such as space for reflecting on the content and process of their work, feedback about the content and process, aid in development of understanding and skills within their work, and information and other perspectives concerning their work. While many of these functions can be considered managerial, as well as supportive or educational, a managerial focus involves ensuring the quality of employees' work (Hawkins & Shohet, 2000).

Clouder and Sellars (2004) note that "clinical supervision provides a practical and economical means of building on experience to ensure quality and optimal standards of care" (p. 265). Often employees with different levels of professional and life experience, as well as years of service within a particular institution, can enrich a clinical supervision process through their participation. When the clinical supervision process involves professionals in different disciplines, the process is enriched even further. A rapidly changing health care environment requires changing outdated ways of working, and exploring and utilizing common skills in teamwork, while still valuing the unique skills and qualities of each of the different professions (Clouder & Sellars, 2004).

Clinical supervision can also foster self-reflective practice, provide a collegial support system, and offer a safe space for feedback and growth (Clouder & Sellars, 2004; Lakeman & Glasgow, 2009). One group of mental health nurses developed its own model for clinical supervision in order to meet the needs of varying degrees of expertise and experience among the nurses. The aims of this clinical supervision model were to develop knowledge and skills, monitor quality of care, identify solutions to problems, improve nursing care, increase understanding of professional issues, and give support to fellow clinicians. After implementing and evaluating the model during a 6-month pilot group, the group also identified the need to incorporate reflective practice and a higher degree of critique and challenge into the process (Walsh et al., 2003).

In a medical or health care setting, clinical supervision has been found to be beneficial in the role development of nurses (Lakeman & Glasgow, 2009) and general medical practitioners (Launer, 2007; Meadows, 2007), but it seems to be more widely accepted among the psychosocial and mental health professions. Mental health professions have had longer traditions of clinical supervision practice, whereas "other disciplines have lacked a framework for professional development around the powerful emotions and complex interactions that relational work engenders" (Koivu, Saarinen, & Hyrkas, 2011, p. 645). According to Malchiodi and Riley (1996), supervision in both the training and continuing education of art therapists is considered to be essential to professionalism. This is true for many of the helping professionals who may also be part of a pediatric health care team, including music therapists, child life specialists, social workers, counselors, and psychologists.

ART THERAPY IN CLINICAL SUPERVISION

There is little literature on the use of art therapy interventions in clinical supervision, particularly in pediatric medical settings. The majority of literature discusses the use of art interventions in art therapy clinical supervision. Moon (2000) defines "clinical supervision" as "a metaphoric journey in which the mentor serves the supervisee as both a guide and a fellow traveler" (p. 111). The word "metaphoric" in this definition might suggest that an experiential or expressive component be part of clinical supervision, such as the use of art therapy interventions.

A way to incorporate art therapy into clinical supervision is through responsive art making. Moon (2000) describes "responsive art making" in supervision as "a process that involves the art therapy mentor and supervisee in creating art works in reaction to images, ideas, or feelings that are the subject of supervision" (p. 113). The three benefits of responsive art making in supervision include establishing empathy between the mentor and supervisee; providing an expressive outlet for feelings that can often come up in the supervisory context; and serving as a starting place for dialogue between mentor and supervisee (Moon, 2000). All three of these benefits exist through art therapy interventions used in multidisciplinary clinical supervision groups in a pediatric health care setting, as illustrated later in the case examples in the chapter.

Malchiodi and Riley (1996) state that "art making is a potent modality through which one can sort out reactions to new situations, new identities, new clients or new ways of thinking" (p. 97). They suggest that making art in supervision can aid the supervisee in expressing complex feelings about clinical work that may be difficult to verbalize and problem-solving through visual exploration of complex issues. Although Malchiodi and Riley discuss the benefits of art in supervision, they also caution that art making can elicit emotional content of the supervisee, and care must be taken not to confuse what could be perceived as personal therapy with the purpose of clinical supervision. "Talking about patients and one's therapeutic work, in preference to oneself and one's personal issues, is the cornerstone of supervision" (Yegdich, 1999, p. 1272). Jones (2008b) emphasizes that a competent supervisor (or facilitator) should create an environment for group supervision that keeps emotional issues in check, and when required, directs participants to appropriate methods of personal and professional support outside of the group.

SUPERVISION IN PEDIATRIC MEDICAL SETTINGS

Clinical supervision for art therapists and other psychosocial professionals in a pediatric medical setting is unique compared to clinical supervision in nonmedical settings. In order to gather information specifically about clinical supervision, I informally surveyed other professionals in pediatric settings (see Appendix 24.1). The pediatric health care institutions of those who participated in the survey ranged in size from 45 to 500 beds and included inpatient and outpatient facilities. In brief, the majority of respondents had opportunities to engage in clinical supervision at their respective health care institutions; both individual and group opportunities were available to them. The two most popular types of clinical supervision available were art therapy supervision and multidisciplinary supervision with professionals from different disciplines. Also, a majority of health care institutions supported clinical supervision during work time, and the most common types of clinical supervision supported by institutions were onsite individual and group clinical supervision.

The results of a rating question on the survey revealed the four most common topics and issues that surfaced during clinical supervision sessions: (1) compassion fatigue/ burnout of those working with critically or terminally ill patients, or patients who have experienced trauma (e.g., emergency departments and intensive care units); (2) death of patients/issues of loss, grief, and bereavement; (3) spiritual and diversity issues that come up in artwork/art therapy interventions; and (4) multidisciplinary communication, sharing patient/family information with colleagues/medical team. Another common topic noted by several of the survey respondents is worth mentioning—coping with change in the health care setting (e.g., health care climate change, hospital change, and department change).

The majority of respondents indicated their clinical supervision group(s) met "every other week" and for "1–2 hours per session"; most groups met for 6 to 10 sessions. Most also participated in "multidiscipline" as opposed to "single-discipline" groups; in "closed groups" rather than "open, drop-in groups"; and in "process-oriented groups" rather than "structured groups." A "closed group" is one that, once begun, accepts no new members and meets for a predetermined number of sessions. An "open group" continues indefinitely, maintaining a consistent size by replacing members as they leave the group (Yalom, 1995, p. 267). A "process-centered" or "process-oriented" approach to group supervision is rooted in interpersonal theory (Bransford, 2009) and refers to groups of individuals who meet to learn more about themselves through interacting with others (Yalom, 1995). A process-oriented group is not focused primarily on verbal content itself, but on the "how" and "why" of the verbal content, or the motivation behind the verbal statement and how it impacts interpersonal relationships with others. Process-oriented groups also focus on and explore what is happening at the present moment in the group (Yalom, 1995).

ART THERAPY AND MULTIDISCIPLINARY CLINICAL SUPERVISION GROUPS

The following case examples illustrate the use of art therapy interventions in multidisciplinary clinical supervision groups in a 250-bed pediatric hospital. The two different groups comprised five psychosocial staff members each, and included child life specialists, child life assistants, art therapists, a consumer health librarian, and a coordinator for a pediatric patient fitness program. The closed groups met every other week for 90 minutes, for a total of 10 sessions per module. A process-oriented approach was utilized for the groups, as well as structured beginning and ending of each group session. Group guidelines were established by the facilitator in advance and introduced during the first group session; subsequent groups continued after all the members agreed to the guidelines and committed to them by signing.

For the first group module, the bulk of the group time was left open for members to bring up current issues or topics for discussion; in the second group module, the members brainstormed to determine topics in advance. In fact, there were always current topics determined by members, and often, at the beginning of a group session, members would bring up an issue or topic that could then be used for discussion.

The facilitator of the group was an art therapist who provided art materials (markers, oil pastels, glue, scissors, and magazine images for collage) for group members to use at the start of each group session. The first 15–30 minutes of the session were dedicated to art making. Sheets of 8½″ × 11″ paper, with and without pretraced circles, were also available. The facilitator explained the potential benefits of creating art within a circle, or mandala, including the calming and relaxing effect on the mind and body, and as an expression of the self. Most group members chose to use the circles for their check-in images. The check-in activity provided members an opportunity to share how they were doing or feeling as they came into the group on that particular day. It also allowed members to introduce topics or issues and helped them to transition from a fast-paced, busy day in the hospital to a safe, calm space for discussion, debriefing, processing, and self-reflection. The first two case examples illustrate how two different group members used the art to check-in with the rest of the group, and how this impacted their experience of clinical supervision.

"SWIRLS OF BUREAUCRACY"

The first example highlights artwork created by Member A, a coordinator for a pediatric patient fitness program. After hearing about the visual check-in option, Member A made a conscious decision to create a series so she "didn't have to think as much" about what she was going to do for her art check-in at the start of each group session. She chose to work within the pretraced circles and stated that having a framework helped her to express herself and her feelings. Her art always included swirly lines; however, the patterns, colors, and media changed from session to session.

One particular image (Figure 24.1) stood out for Member A. Using shades of blue and white oil pastel, Member A created a branch with protruding swirls that moved from the left of the circle to the right, with another, shorter branch emerging from the bottom of the circle. The swirls themselves were all white in the center and moved from light to dark blue on the outside edges, with the darkest blue color filling in the background of the circle.[1]

As Member A spoke about her finished image, she noted that the larger branch of swirls represented the "strong forward motion of projects she was working on," while the shorter jutting branch represented obstacles "working against all the forward motion." The visual image helped to facilitate insight for Member A as she made a connection

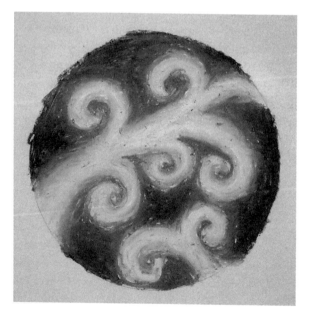

FIGURE 24.1. Member A's check-in image of swirls.

---

[1]Original artwork in this chapter was in color. It is reproduced here in black and white.

between her image and what she had been experiencing in her work at the time the image was created. She had been productively working on a project and gaining momentum until things were slowed down by bureaucracy and red tape. Other group members related to Member A's experience and added that within a health care setting, obstacles can impede getting work done efficiently (e.g., space constraints, vying for time, and competing responsibilities). If the art materials had not been available as an option for the group check-in process, this member would not have produced a visual image to help encourage insight and communication, and the group discussion that followed might not have occurred.

When asked about her overall experience of group clinical supervision, Member A explained how "special" it was to have designated time to be creative during the workday. Much of Member A's role involved developing and organizing fitness events in the community, and spending time with patients and families in community environments outside of the hospital. According to Clouder and Sellars (2004), having protected time to meet colleagues for clinical supervision made those working alone in community environments feel less isolated professionally. Member A also valued the "shared experiences and feelings of everyone in the group, even though all were in different professions and roles." Finally, Member A appreciated the check-in at the start of each group, particularly "having time to sit down, assess, and take stock of the day," as well as checking in with herself. This was one of the more valuable and memorable parts of the experience of group clinical supervision for her.

"ROLLERCOASTER OF CHANGE"

Member B shared similar thoughts about the benefits of the group clinical supervision experience. She stated, "Even though we're all in different disciplines and our paths don't always cross, we're all working with the same people and facing the same sorts of struggles; it was helpful to get ideas from each other." Member B also enjoyed getting to know people in the department she did not often have the opportunity to work with or see. One of the challenges for her, as a consumer health librarian, was understanding the term "clinical supervision" and what it means to those who routinely practice it.

Being a health librarian in a hospital setting presented a unique experience for Member B, very different than that of a librarian in a library. A "consumer health librarian" is someone who has a subject specialty in consumer health and expertise in the identification, selection, organization, and dissemination of evidence-based information for education of patients and people with health and health care information needs (Rees et al., 1996). Terminology and topics common to clinical supervision, such as "clinical responsibilities" and "therapeutic boundaries," were new concepts for Member B, but engaging in the group clinical supervision experience with other psychosocial professionals helped to foster a better understanding for her.

Member B also liked starting the groups with art and said she looked forward to that experience at the start of each group session. She shared, "It was a nice way to check in

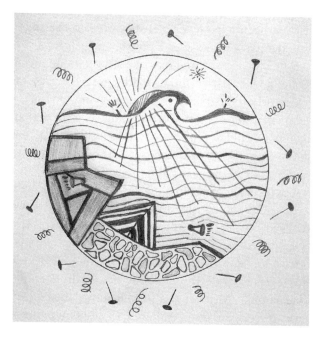

FIGURE 24.2. Member B's check-in image in pencil.

and helped me to figure out where I was with things." As Member B reviewed all of her art during the last group session, she chose two pieces that stood out for her. The first image (Figure 24.2) was done in pencil; Member B recalled choosing pencil because she wanted the art to be simple on that given day. The drawing itself turned out to be complicated, though, as were her life and work at the time.

When the drawing was done, Member B was recovering from a serious ankle sprain and walking with a boot on her injured foot. She noticed that the footprints in her drawing, one near the bottom right and the other near the middle left, were going in different directions; she attributed this to what actually happened to her feet when she was injured. The wave near the top of the circle, with what looked like the head of a bird in the wave, represented turmoil for Member B. The hand-like images reaching up from the wave were her hands, reaching out above the wave since she felt as though she was drowning in life and work. The springs and nails represented everything else coming at her, but she recognized that the circle served as a barrier of protection, and those springs and nails were not getting in.

Even more significant for Member B was a check-in image she created after learning unsettling news at work about a transition in leadership for the department—just one of many changes that seemed to be taking place in the health care environment at the time of this writing. At the same time, one of Member B's own children was having some medical concerns. She chose collage materials for this particular visual check-in and found herself drawn to a blurred photo of a rollercoaster. When Member B saw the rollercoaster she related to it and shared with the group that her "life was like a rollercoaster." She glued the photo in the middle of the predrawn circle on her paper, and her image evolved from there (Figure 24.3).

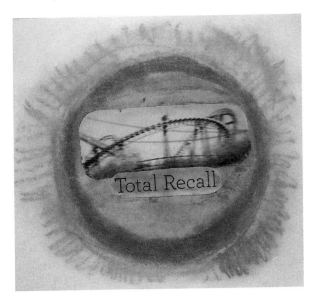

FIGURE 24.3. Member B's check-in image of a rollercoaster.

Next, Member B found the phrase "Total Recall" among the magazine pages. The phrase made her realize that she had been in situations like this before. She had been on the rollercoaster before, and she had gotten off it before, too. She glued the phrase under the photo and began filling in the surrounding space with oil pastel. She chose colors such as light brown and yellow ochre, because she wanted the image to be more relaxed. As she worked on her image, she thought the colors quieted the image and helped to illustrate that it was actually not chaotic at all. She smoothed the pastels with her finger to give the colors and the image a muted effect. She did the same to the lines coming out from the edges of the circle, softening the lines to represent life's "fuzzy edges."

Member B discovered something during the process of creating this image. She came in to the group session feeling disjointed and chaotic, but not knowing how to express it; creating the image helped her transition from disjointed and chaotic to "I've been here before, this is not new, and I'll get through it just as I have before." As she reflected further, she realized from her own past experiences that the rollercoaster would not be as scary as she thought. During times of change, which are common and frequent in the world of health care, this type of insight can be efficacious in managing the stress of change and preventing it from escalating.

"POWER OF APPRECIATION"

The last case example is not a check-in image but art done by a group member after discussion of a discouraging topic in one of the group sessions. The topic was brought to the group by Member C, a child life specialist, on a day that she was feeling misunderstood and underappreciated by other medical professionals in the hospital. At the institution where these clinical supervision groups took place, psychosocial professionals, including child life specialists, art therapists, music therapists, librarians, schoolteachers, child life assistants, and a fitness program coordinator, were all part of the health care team. However, as in many health care settings, their psychosocial services were ancillary and occasionally viewed by other medical professionals as less essential aspects of patients' medical care. For this reason, their roles were at times misunderstood and their services underutilized. Although these professionals appreciated and respected one another, at times they found themselves justifying those roles to other medical professionals and educating others about their professions, services, and practice.

During this particular session, the discussion focused on how to manage this dilemma to prevent it from negatively impacting morale. In order to capitalize on the respect and appreciation the group members already had for one another, the facilitator of the group introduced an intervention near the end of the session. The facilitator asked the group members to do some homework before the next session: to write down one positive thing they appreciated about each of the other members and to bring their lists back to the next session.

During the subsequent session, the facilitator demonstrated how to make a simple accordion-folded book that would hold the appreciative thoughts shared between the group members. These small books could be revisited anytime the group members needed a reminder of what others appreciated about them. The materials for the books included pieces of mat board and decorative papers for the book covers; drawing paper for the folded pages; and ribbon, cording, yarn, and beads for decorative closures. Member C's book (Figure 24.4) is highlighted, since she initiated the aforementioned group discussion that prompted the art intervention just described.

Some of the thoughts shared between group members were typed or handwritten; others were a few words in length, and still others were longer paragraphs. Figure 24.4

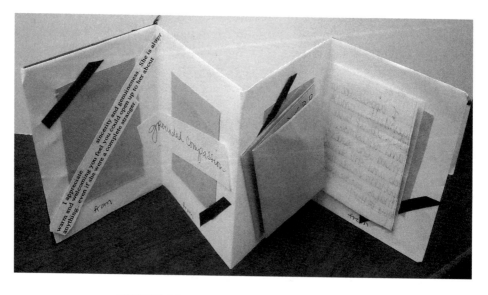

FIGURE 24.4. Member C's appreciation book.

illustrates how Member C chose to place her words of appreciation from the other group members into her accordion-folded book. The two pages on the left included phrases like "sincerity and genuineness" and "grounded compassion." The two pages on the right included lengthier writings on pieces of paper that were folded to fit, then glued onto the pages of the book. When the book was closed, it could be wrapped with ribbon and fastened to a wooden bead on one cover to keep it from popping open. After reflecting on this intervention, Member C shared, "It's always nice to hear what other people appreciate about you." She also mentioned that this type of positive feedback and praise is not always offered spontaneously and is not something one would necessarily think about oneself. She described experience as "a nice pick-me-up, a nice boost," even though it was a bit stressful to think of meaningful, uplifting, and "the right" things to say about each person in the group. Whatever she was experiencing in her work, it was nice to know that others were experiencing similar things, too; it helped her to feel less isolated. The mixture of disciplines in the group provided the opportunity to share and receive new perspectives and ideas, and Member C felt as though she gained something from everyone's contributions during each group session.

Discussion

In reviewing these case examples, it is apparent that each fits well into one of the three benefits of responsive art making described by Moon (2000). Each case example also addresses at least one of the common clinical supervision topics discussed in the survey outcomes. And, in all three case examples, the members whose art is highlighted spoke about how the artwork helped them to slow down, check in with themselves, and savor the time and space of clinical supervision group to focus on taking care of themselves. This is testimony to the infrequent opportunities for intentional self-reflection and designated time to focus on oneself in the midst of helping others in a pediatric health care setting, and how important it is to do so.

In the first case example, Member A's check-in image encouraged insight through talking about the meaning of the image; this served as a stepping-stone to a group discussion about bureaucracy and obstacles to efficiency in the workplace. This particular case example also addressed two of the common clinical supervision topics— multidisciplinary communication and coping with change in health care.

For Member B in the second case example, the check-in images served as outlets for expression about feelings that combined the professional and the personal. Although the feelings were not directly related to the clinical supervision process, the process of creating art in the context of a clinical supervision group enabled Member B to see a new perspective through her artwork. She gained insight about how better to manage what she called "life's rollercoaster," both at work and at home. Once again, the common topic from the survey of coping with change in the health care setting presented itself.

In the final case example, engaging in reflective, appreciative writing about one another and creating appreciation books established greater empathy among all the members of the group. This case example also demonstrated some of the benefits of clinical supervision as discussed in the literature; it provided opportunity for colleagues to share feedback and support for one another, and to gain new perspectives and ideas from one another. The discussion about managing the dilemma of misunderstood roles is often a common clinical supervision topic in multidisciplinary communication with professionals on the health care team who do not have a psychosocial role. Constantly having to justify roles and educate others is a factor that can contribute to compassion fatigue, a form of secondary stress from work with patients.

The literature and the case examples in this chapter underscore the importance of clinical supervision in health care. Art therapy interventions in clinical supervision serve as a creative tool for self-reflection that can enhance and enrich the supervision process, as the case examples have illustrated. Facilitating clinical supervision groups, particularly in a pediatric health care setting, offers an efficient way to provide the necessary time and space to examine clinical work and engage in self-care. Clouder and Sellars (2004, p. 267) ask, "How, if not through encouraging reflective practice, might we promote introspection, analysis, discussion and enhanced understanding of the complexities of practice?"

CONCLUSION

Wicks (2003) states, "Keeping an eye out for the oases in our lives and expanding their presence and use are just common sense. Once again, we should not only do this for ourselves but for those who count on us to be a healing presence in their lives. We can't share what we don't have. It is as simple as that" (pp. 51–52). If we consider tools for self-care as oases in the middle of a barren desert of health care, then one of these oases can and ought to be regular and consistent clinical supervision that includes the use of art therapy interventions. Our work in the helping professions requires compassionate care, and we need these oases to replenish our wells of compassion before they run dry.

Group clinical supervision that includes art therapy interventions provides a safe and designated oasis in which to explore the impact of our work on ourselves as human beings, and to express ourselves verbally and creatively. It offers a space to enhance our interpersonal skills and communication, to learn from and about one another, and to recognize the value of different perspectives. It creates a place to share best practices, and to develop and grow professionally and personally. Finally, it affords us an opportunity to slow down and catch up with ourselves, so we can be fully present in our service to others.

REFERENCES

Bransford, C. L. (2009). Process-centered group supervision. *Clinical Social Work Journal, 37,* 119–127.

Clouder, L., & Sellars, J. (2004). Reflective practice and clinical supervision: An interprofessional perspective. *Journal of Advanced Nursing, 46*(3), 262–269.

Cutcliffe, J. R., & Hyrkas, K. (2006). Multidisciplinary attitudinal positions regarding clinical supervision: A cross-sectional study. *Journal of Nursing Management, 14,* 617–627.

Hawkins, P., & Shohet, R. (2000). *Supervision in the helping professions* (2nd ed.). New York: Open University Press.

Jones, A. (2006). Group-format clinical supervision for hospice nurses. *European Journal of Cancer Care, 15,* 155–162.

Jones, A. (2008a). Clinical supervision is important to the quality of health-care provision. *International Journal of Mental Health Nursing, 17,* 379–380.

Jones, A. (2008b). Towards a common purpose: Group-format clinical supervision can benefit palliative care. *European Journal of Cancer Care, 17,* 105–106.

Koivu, A., Saarinen, P. I., & Hyrkas, K. (2011). Stress relief or practice development: Varied reasons for attending clinical supervision. *Journal of Nursing Management, 19,* 644–654.

Lakeman, R., & Glasgow, C. (2009). Introducing peer-group clinical supervision: An action research project. *International Journal of Mental Health Nursing, 18,* 204–210.

Launer, J. (2007). Moving on from Balint: Embracing clinical supervision. *British Journal of General Practice, 57*(536), 182–183.

Malchiodi, C. A., & Riley, S. (1996). *Supervision and related issues: A handbook for professionals.* Chicago: Magnolia Street.

Meadows, J. (2007, May). Embracing clinical supervision. *British Journal of General Practice,* p. 412.

Moon, B. L. (2000). *Ethical issues in art therapy.* Springfield, IL: Thomas.

Rees, A., Marshall, J., Bandy, M., Lindner, K., McCormick, L., & Schneider, J. (1996). The librarian's role in the provision of consumer health information and patient education. *Bulletin of the Medical Library Association, 84*(2), 238–239. Retrieved from *http://caphis.mlanet.org/chis/librarian.html.*

Walsh, K., Nicholson, J., Keough, C., Pridham, R., Kramer, M., & Jeffrey, J. (2003). Development of a group model of clinical supervision to meet the needs of a community mental health nursing team. *International Journal of Nursing Practice, 9,* 33–39.

Wicks, R. J. (2003). *Riding the dragon: 10 lessons for inner strength in challenging times.* Notre Dame, IN: Sorin Books.

Williamson, G. R., & Dodds, S. (1999). The effectiveness of a group approach to clinical supervision in reducing stress: A review of the literature. *Journal of Clinical Nursing, 8,* 338–344.

Yalom, I. D. (1995). *The theory and practice of group psychotherapy* (4th ed.). New York: Basic Books.

Yegdich, T. (1999). Lost in the crucible of supportive clinical supervision: Supervision is not therapy. *Journal of Advanced Nursing, 29*(5), 1265–1275.

APPENDIX 24.1. Survey Questions about Clinical Supervision in Pediatric Medical Settings

1. Do you have opportunities to engage in clinical supervision at your healthcare institution?
   Yes
   No
   Not applicable
   Other (please specify)

2. If you DO have opportunities for clinical supervision at your healthcare institution, what format/s are offered? Select all that apply; you may choose multiple answers.
   Individual clinical supervision on-site
   Individual clinical supervision off-site
   Group clinical supervision on-site
   Group clinical supervision off-site
   Not applicable
   Other (please specify)

3. What type of clinical supervision is available to you? Select all that apply; you may choose multiple answers.
   Art therapy clinical supervision
   Counseling clinical supervision
   Social work clinical supervision
   Child life specialist clinical supervision
   Multi-disciplinary/joint clinical supervision with professionals from different disciplines
   Not applicable
   Other (please specify)

4. Does your healthcare institution support clinical supervision during worktime?
   Yes
   No
   Not applicable
   Other (please specify)

5. If your institution DOES support clinical supervision, what types of supervision are supported? Select all that apply; you can choose multiple answers.
   On-site individual clinical supervision during worktime
   On-site individual clinical supervision off worktime
   Off-site individual clinical supervision on worktime
   Off-site individual clinical supervision on own time
   On-site group clinical supervision during worktime
   On-site group clinical supervision off worktime
   Off-site group clinical supervision on worktime
   Off-site group clinical supervision on own time
   Not applicable
   Other (please specify)

(cont.)

APPENDIX 24.1. *(cont.)*

6. What is the size of your pediatric medical setting? If it's an INPATIENT setting, how many BEDS? If it's an OUTPATIENT setting, how many PATIENTS are served DAILY?

7. Please rate the following clinical supervision issues/topics from most common to least common (rating scale included "Most common," "Very common," "Somewhat common," "Least common").

Professional boundaries with patients and families

Confidentiality/privacy of health information

Multi-disciplinary communication; sharing patient/family information with colleagues/ medical team

Patient/family artwork as medical records

Ethics of patient/family artwork created in public areas (waiting rooms, common areas, hospital rooms)

Displaying/exhibiting/photographing patient/family artwork

Dealing with infection control and related issues with art materials

Death of patients; issues of loss, grief, and bereavement

Spiritual and diversity issues that come up in artwork/art therapy interventions

Compassion fatigue/burnout of those working with critically or terminally ill patients, or patients who have experienced trauma (ED, ICU's)

Child abuse/neglect issues and mandated reporting

8. If you have experienced an issue/topic in clinical supervision that was not listed in the question above, please describe it briefly below.

The following questions are to be answered by those who have opportunities to participate in group clinical supervision:

9. How many people are in your clinical supervision group(s)?

0–5

6–10

11–15

>15

Other (please specify)

10. How often does your clinical supervision group meet?

More than once a week

Once a week

Every other week

Once a month

Other (please specify)

(cont.)

APPENDIX 24.1. *(cont.)*

11. How long does your clinical supervision group meet?

      < 1 hour per session

      1–2 hours per session

      > 2 hours per session

12. Is your clinical supervision group single discipline or multi-discipline?

      Single discipline

      Multi-discipline

      Other: please indicate which discipline(s)

13. Is your clinical supervision group an open or closed group?

      Open, drop-in group

      Closed group

      Other (please specify)

14. Is your clinical supervision group structured (agenda/topic-focused) or process-oriented (open forum/discussion, focus on whatever comes up in the moment)?

      Structured

      Process-oriented

      Other (please specify)

15. What is the overall duration/length of your clinical supervision group?

      Ongoing (open, drop-in group)

      Modules of 1–5 sessions each

      Modules of 6–10 sessions each

      Modules of 11–15 sessions each

      > 15 sessions per module

      Other (please specify)

This appendix is a direct reprint of the online survey questionnaire used by the author to gather information regarding clinical supervision in pediatric medical settings.

CHAPTER 25

Physiological Measures in Evidence-Based Art Therapy Research

Elizabeth Warson
John Lorance

With the necessity for evidence-based art therapy research in health care, the inclusion of physiological measures may provide valuable information regarding the effects of art therapy. Surprisingly, physiological measurements are seldom used in art therapy research, even though such measurements do not always require direct involvement from a medical professional. Obtaining a physiological measurement can be as simple as providing participants with a cotton swab to chew on. Although, art making has been found to play a role in physical, emotional, and mental healing, there has been no published empirical research involving biomarkers to support a correlation between art making and stress reduction. In contrast, music therapy has conducted the most evidence-based research examining the physiological effects of music, measured through biomarkers such as cortisol, heart rate variability, and finger surface temperature (Leardi et al., 2007; McKinney, Antoni, Kumar, Tims, & McCabe, 1997).

The field of art therapy is rich with opportunities for research that can enhance and validate what is already common knowledge to most art therapists and their clients: that art is life enhancing. What is not known is that the act of making art can have a positive impact on physiology. This type of research involves the collection of "biomarkers":

> A biological molecule found in blood, other body fluids, or tissues that is a sign of a normal or abnormal process, or of a condition or disease. A biomarker may be used to see how well the body responds to a treatment for a disease or condition. Also called molecular marker and signature molecule. (National Cancer Institute, n.d.)

Designing research protocols around physiological measurements and their interpretations may be a challenge for those already familiar with psychological assessments, measures, and tests, because the inclusion of physiological measurements requires additional information and training. However, it is not an either–or question: Determining specific psychological measurements and their associated physiological counterparts is a necessary step in designing an effective evidence-based study. Likewise, it is important that the research team understand the physiological and psychological implications of the medical diagnoses of research participants. In our particular study, we focused on the cancer population because of the prolific research on mind–body interaction.

Our aim in this chapter is to introduce the reader to the physiology of stress and immunity, and how specific physiological measures were included in our art-based research with cancer patients. We chose to concentrate on stress because of the role of stress in the diagnosis of cancer, the stress related to determining treatment options, and the effect of stress on the immune system. Another reason to focus on physiological measures is that stress is a common experience related to many medical diagnoses and procedures. Therefore, information regarding physiological measures related to stress has further implications for the field of art therapy, beyond the scope of our research.

STRESS

Cannon spoke of stress as early as 1914; however, the term "stress" was not popularized until the 1950s by Selye (McEwen, 2004; Sapolsky, 2004; Selye, 1956), in his experiments with rats. Selye noticed that the thymus gland, which plays an important role in immunity, would shrink when a rat was injured or placed under extreme circumstances. He named these extreme circumstances "stressors," and defined "stress" as the organism's nonspecific response to the stressor. Selye called this response to a stressor the general adaptation syndrome (GAS) and identified three subsequent stages associated with this adaptation process.

The first stage of the GAS is the alarm reaction that activates the response to a stressor by the release of hormones from the adrenal cortex into the bloodstream. The second stage is the stage of resistance, denoted by an opposite effect and a restoration of the hormones. These first two stages represent successful adaptation and resilience, whereas the third stage of exhaustion indicates failure to adapt to the stressor. Selye's (1956) findings marked an important development in the history of stress research and provided a basis for extending stress research to the human population.

Therefore, not all stress is bad, and Selye's research indicated a resiliency factor in the role of stress. Some experiences in life are positive, and these positive adaptations represent a type of stress known as "eustress" (Kabat-Zinn, 1990). Examples of eustress are exercise, life events (e.g., getting married, going on vacation, changing jobs, moving to a new location), and other similar adaptations. Failure to adapt successfully to changes may result in distress.

ALLOSTASIS AND ALLOSTATIC LOAD

The role of adaptation in stress management implies the existence of a "set point," or a level of homeostasis within the body in relationship to stress. "Allostasis" describes the body's process for maintaining homeostasis through change and adaptation (McEwen, 1998, 2004). When an experience is perceived as stressful, both physical and psychological responses that are engaged lead to allostasis and adaptation. Over time, these physiological responses may lead to strain on the various bodily systems and result in the condition of allostatic load. Therefore, allostasis parallels the first two stages of Seyle's GAS, whereas the third stage is represented by allostatic load. This trajectory of stress management also considers individual responses that may exist when adapting to stressors, including genetic and early life experiences that may predispose an individual to overreact physiologically or behaviorally. In addition, the recurrence and frequency of stressful situations are considered, in addition to adverse life choices that may have impact on allostatic load, such as smoking, drinking, and unhealthy diet.

STRESS CATEGORIES

In a meta-analysis of psychological stress and the human immune system research spanning 30 years, the five categories of identified stressors were based on duration and course (Segerstrom & Miller, 2004). These categories included acute, time-limited stressors; brief, naturalistic stressors; stressful event sequences; chronic stressors; and distant stressors. Acute stressors and brief, naturalistic stressors are both short-lived. In a stressful event sequence, such as a natural event or loss of a spouse, there is a sense that, in the future, the event will have an ending. Chronic stressors, in contrast to acute stressors, force one to restructure one's life, and there is no indication of when, or whether the stressor will end. "Distant stressors" are defined as experiences, usually traumatic, that happened in the past and continue to impact the immune system. The results of this meta-analysis revealed that acute stressors enhance the immune system, whereas chronic stressors suppress the immune system. Stress impacts the various systems of the human body: the immune system, the nervous system, and the endocrine system. The following overview of these systems helps us understand their interrelations.

The Immune System

The immune system comprises cells and molecules that function as a defense against infectious microbes (Abbas & Lichtman, 2005). There are two types of immunity: innate immunity and adaptive immunity. "Innate immunity," sometimes referred to as "natural immunity," is the first line of defense in the immune system and comprises cells and biochemicals that are readily available in the body and enable a fast response to infections (Abbas & Lichtman, 2005; Sompayrac, 2003). Innate immunity comprises epithelial barriers, granulocytes, blood proteins, and cytokines that coordinate the activities of cells involved in immunity. "Adaptive immunity," sometimes referred to as "specific immunity," is slower to respond than natural immunity and has more diverse specialization (Abbas & Lichtman, 2005). As its name suggests, specific immunity adapts to respond to infection and has the ability to remember the invader. Components of adaptive immunity are lymphocytes, antibodies, and T cells.

The Nervous System

The nervous system is divided into two parts: the brain and spinal cord comprising the central nervous system (CNS); and the peripheral nervous system (PNS), which comprises the nerves of the body (Tortora & Grabowski, 2000; Vedhara & Wetherell, 2005). The PNS is further divided into the somatic nervous system and the autonomic nervous system (ANS). The ANS controls the body's involuntary activities, outside of conscious control. The ANS comprises two branches: the sympathetic branch and the parasympathetic branch. Whereas the sympathetic branch of the ANS responds to a stimulus by increasing heart rate and blood pressure, dilating the airways and the pupils, increasing sweat production, and playing a role in "fight or flight" responses, the parasympathetic branch plays a role in "rest or digest" responses by slowing down the heart rate, decreasing blood pressure, contracting pupils, and increases flow of saliva.

Several measures exist for the nervous system reactions. Among these are heart rate, heart rate variability, blood pressure, and galvanic skin response (Vedhara & Wetherell, 2005). On one hand, most of these measures require a medical practitioner and the use of expensive equipment. On the other hand, salivary alpha-amylase has recently been used as a measurement of sympathetic arousal in psychosocial research (Nater et al., 2005; Noto, Sato, Kudo, Kurata, & Hirota, 2005; Wetherell et al., 2006). The use of a saliva sample is also noninvasive and can be collected by the researchers with minimal training.

The Endocrine System

The endocrine system is another major participant in the body's response to stress. Two important pathways are of particular importance for the present research, namely, the sympathetic–adrenomedullary (SAM) system and the hypothalamic–pituitary–adrenal (HPA) axis (Wetherell et al., 2006). The SAM system is part of the sympathetic nervous system and the endocrine system. The adrenal gland is divided into two portions: the adrenal cortex and the adrenal medulla. The adrenal gland is a modified ganglion with neuron-like cells. The sympathetic nervous system innervates the adrenal medulla and causes it to release the catecholamine hormones, adrenaline and noradrenaline, into the bloodstream. These hormones, in turn, amplify sympathetic nervous system stress responses in, for example, the liver and the heart to mobilize endogenous energy stores and increase cardiac output.

The HPA axis, responsible for the longer-term effects of a stressful stimulus, reacts later: The resulting end product is produced 15–20 minutes after the initial stressor

(Maier, Watkins, & Fleshner, 1994; Miles & Gilbert, 2005; Wetherell et al., 2006). This slow response becomes important in the timing of saliva collection to measure cortisol. Corticocotropin-releasing hormone (CRH) is released from a part of the brain called the hypothalamus, which sits just above the roof of the mouth. It signals the release of adrenocorticatropic hormone (ACTH) from the pituitary gland. ACTH in turn signals the release of the glucocorticoid hormones into the bloodstream from the adrenal cortex. The principal glucocorticoid in people is cortisol, a stress hormone that suppresses the immune system, so that energy can be utilized by other systems to handle the stressor.

THE BIOPSYCHOSOCIAL MODEL

As interacting physiological systems, the immune system, ANS, and endocrine system play a role in adaptation to stressors. More than 30 years ago, Engel (1977) discussed the limitations of the biomedical model of treating disease. According to Engel, the biomedical model claimed that all illnesses, whether physical or psychological, have a basis in the physical body. Engel asserted that the biomedical model overlooked the social, psychological, and behavioral aspects of illness. Engel discussed two limitations of the biomedical model: reductionism and exclusionism. The "reductionist" viewpoint is that behavioral implications of disease must be proven by physiochemical principles; whereas, the "exclusionist" viewpoint excludes that which cannot be explained in physical terms. As a result, Engel proposed the biopsychosocial medical model that embraces both physical and psychosocial aspects of the disease process by leveraging the impact of modern psychology and systems theory. Systems theory supports the premise that all levels of organization are linked together, and that a change in one level effects a change in other levels.

PSYCHONEUROIMMUNOLOGY

The relatively new field of psychoneuroimmunology (PNI) is in alignment with Engel's proposed biopsychosocial model of medicine. PNI is the study of interactions that take place among the CNS, endocrine system, and the immune system (Fox, Shephard, & McCain, 1999). The immune system was once thought to be a closed system, depending solely on activity and processes of the immune system (Maier & Watkins, 1998). Early and ongoing research have revealed not only that the immune system interfaces with other systems, but also that the interface is bidirectional, implying that these body systems influence each other (Maier et al., 1994).

Although the term "psychoneuroimmunology" was not adopted until the late 1970s, the role of behavior's influence on the body was studied as early as 1914 by Cannon, who proposed the emergency reaction hypothesis, in which the body releases epinephrine in response to a threatening event (Mathews, Starkweather, & Witek-Janusek, 2005). Research in the field of PNI did not grow until the 1980s, after the monumental study by Ader and Cohen (Glaser et al., 1987). In their 1975 experiment with rats, Ader and Cohen incorporated techniques to determine whether immune response could be conditioned by behavior (Cohen, Ader, Green, & Bovbjerg, 1979). In this experiment, saccharine was paired with cyclophosphamide, an immunosuppressive agent. The results of this research indicated that behavior can impact immunity. As a result of this finding, the term "psychoneuroimmunology" was coined in 1977 by Robert Ader (Cohen et al., 1979). This finding gave impetus to numerous studies that have investigated a mind–body connection.

IMAGERY

The use of imagery or visualization as a complementary therapy has been explored in several studies (Bakke, Purtzer, & Newton, 2002; Donaldson, 2000; Giedt, 1997; Kolcaba & Fox, 1999; McKinney et al., 1997; Rider et al., 1990; Roffe, Schmidt, & Ernst, 2005; Spiegel & Moore, 1997; Van Kuiken, 2004). Van Kuiken's meta-analysis of guided imagery literature since 1996 reported that imagery has the potential to improve immunity and psychological resilience. Four different categories of imagery were identified: (1) pleasant imagery, (2) physiologically focused imagery, (3) mental rehearsing or reframing, and (4) receptive imagery. In pleasant imagery the participant imagines a calm place. By using active imagination, the person may visualize a location or even past memories that invoke a sense of calmness and well-being. In physiologically focused imagery, another form of active imagination, the participant imagines the body part or function that needs healing. This category may, in turn, require that the participant gain access to knowledge of physiological processes. In addition, this type of imagery may be of a symbolic nature used to symbolize bodily processes. Mental rehearsing or reframing imagery requires the participant to rehearse mentally a particular task. Research with positron emission tomography and functional magnetic resonance imaging has found that imagery engages the motor system and can impact the body in a manner similar to that in the actual experience (Kosslyn, Ganis, & Thompson, 2001). Last, receptive imagery is diagnostic and reflective, requiring the participant to be receptive to images that surface during the process. An example of this type of imagery is the body scan technique incorporated in the mindfulness-based stress reduction program, in which the participant scans his or her body mentally (Kabat-Zinn, 1990).

FEASIBILITY STUDY

In the process of designing our own study, we sought additional guidance (see the note at the end of this chapter) and consulted with Salimetrics, Inc., a laboratory resource for information regarding biomarkers and processing of the saliva samples. The Salimetrics staff assisted the research team in selection of biomarkers and the procedures for collection, codification, and shipment of the samples of saliva for analysis, providing extensive documentation on the procedures for collecting, storing, and transporting saliva.

We chose a homogeneous group, based on gender and cancer (men with prostate cancer), to limit the amount of variability in our results and allow for greater generalization. Our aim was to create a replicable, evidence-based study specific to stress reduction that incorporated both psychological and physiological measures. This multidisciplinary collaborative approach was integral to the hypothesis testing, randomization, and creation of an experimental and a control group. Because coloring a predesigned mandala had been used previously in art therapy research and was shown to reduce anxiety (Curry & Kasser, 2005) we decided to include it as the experimental task in our study. Members of the control group were given a simple maze puzzle to complete, so that they would be actively engaged in the same process, while the experimental group colored a predesigned mandala. Our pilot study examined the effects of coloring a predesigned mandala (the experimental group task) or working a maze puzzle (the control group task) on the levels of stress and anxiety in patients with prostate cancer in order to answer the research question: "Does coloring a mandala reduce levels of stress and anxiety in patients with prostate cancer?" In order to answer this research question, a biopsychosocial perspective was incorporated using the PNI framework of the HPA axis, SAM system, and immune system, resulting in the formulation of the following four hypotheses, involving physiological measurements comprising cortisol, SAM, immunoglobulin A (IgA), and the Adult State–Trait Anxiety Inventory for Adults, Form Y (STAI; Spielberger, 1983):

1. Coloring a predesigned mandala will lower stress, as indicated by a decrease in salivary cortisol (HPA axis).
2. Coloring a predesigned mandala will lower anxiety as indicated by a decrease in salivary alpha-amylase (SAM axis).
3. Coloring a predesigned mandala will enhance immunity, as indicated by an increase in salivary IgA (immune system).
4. Coloring a predesigned mandala will lower state anxiety, as indicated by a decrease in the State score of the STAI (STAI-S).

Because our research involved measuring the effects of a task—coloring a mandala (Figure 25.1) or completing a maze puzzle (Figure 25.2)—it was necessary to obtain pretest or baseline measurements prior to the task. Measurements were then taken after the task in order to have posttest measurement for comparison. Self-report measures of anxiety were obtained by administration of the STAI-S (Spielberger, 1983). We obtained physiological indicators of stress, anxiety, and immunity by collecting saliva to measure cortisol, alpha-amylase, and IgA.

In order to achieve randomization to either group, control or experimental, and to track the data throughout life cycle of the research, envelopes were prestuffed with all

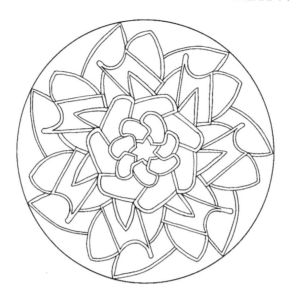

FIGURE 25.1. Experimental task.

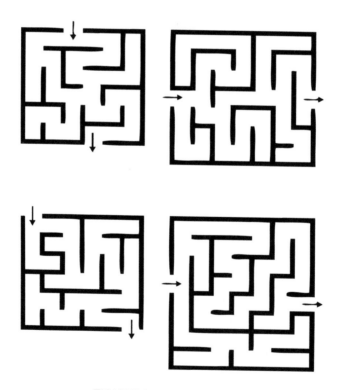

FIGURE 25.2. Control task.

necessary materials, including cryovials for saliva collection, and assigned a random-ized number. Assay results were formatted into spreadsheets at Salimetrics and sent to the co-investigator for statistical analysis. In addition, the STAI was scored by the co-investigator and entered into a spreadsheet.

Results

Because significance could not be achieved, the effect size of the mean change from baseline was calculated for each dependent variable within each task (mandala and puz-zle). Effect sizes were calculated using Cohen's *d*, which is obtained by dividing the mean differences by the pooled standard deviation (Cohen, 1988). Coloring the predesigned mandala resulted in decreased salivary alpha-amylase, a measurement of sympathetic arousal, and increased immunity, as indicated by an increase in salivary IgA. The study resulted in preliminary support for the hypothesis that coloring a predesigned mandala reduces levels of anxiety and has a beneficial effect on the immune system for prostate cancer survivors.

Discussion

It is noteworthy to discuss the two tasks used in this research when we consider the results of salivary cortisol. The maze puzzles, included as a control task, were not com-plicated, and their completion mimicked a simple line drawing in one shade of pencil. In contrast, the mandala was complex, requiring decisions regarding color usage for the many predesigned sections. In addition, more physical activity was required to color the mandala than to work the maze puzzle, which may have resulted in motor complications. The simplicity of the maze puzzle resulted in the participants completing more than one maze puzzle during the research, whereas neither participant coloring the predesigned mandala completed the coloring process during the 20 minutes. This may have resulted in a sense of urgency to complete the mandala coloring by the end of the 20 minutes, even though participants were informed prior to beginning that they did not have to finish the coloring. Moreover, coloring a mandala in itself may be a stressor for an older adult population, since commonly people do not make art or color past grade school. Consideration should also be given to the role of eustress, or "good stress," as it relates to the current research. Not all stress is considered bad, and a task such as coloring a man-dala or working a maze puzzle may in fact be a stressor, but one that is short-lived and has an end in sight. The body adapts to the stressor, then returns to a state of allostasis or balance.

Individual differences, situational factors, and specific characteristics of cancer patients contribute to the complications of cortisol measurement. There have been nota-ble differences in the diurnal cycle of cortisol for cancer participants compared to healthy participants in prior research (Turner-Cobb, Sephton, Koopman, Blake-Mortimer, & Spiegel, 2000). In addition, elevated levels of cortisol may be related to the chronic stress of those who have undergone cancer treatment; however, it is unknown whether this was true for these research participants. The stressor of driving to the research location from neighboring towns and finding a parking place, and the novelty effect of participating in research, not to mention the anticipation of driving home in busy traffic, may have contributed to an increase in cortisol. Elevated cortisol levels were related to anticipatory anxiety in a previous research study that examined cortisol levels in driving phobics (Alpers, Abelson, Wilhelm, & Roth, 2003). Therefore, the anticipation anxiety of driving home may have contributed to this unexpected increase of cortisol. Nonetheless, assessment of HPA activity is complicated, and accounting for individual and situational factors in addition to diurnal cycles is necessary (Wetherell et al., 2006).

Limitations

Even though we pioneered new territory in the field of art therapy research, this study was not without shortcomings. Limitations include the low number of participants ($n = 4$), lack of funding, lack of evidence-based art therapy research in the literature, and inexperience with saliva sampling. Given the low number of participants, only one of the hypotheses was supported by effect size results. Although the research protocol was modified to include smokers and any stage of prostate cancer, in order to attract a larger number of participants, only four participants were included in the research. This low participation rate is not uncommon for art therapy research, where sampled groups seem to be small by social science standards (Metzl, 2008).

We were new to the task of collecting saliva, which complicated our timing and measurement of saliva. Therefore, flow rate of saliva for measurement of salivary IgA was not included in the data analysis. Psychological variables that alter the rate of saliva flow can influence failure to account for flow rate of saliva (Miles & Gilbert, 2005). The results of cortisol analysis were not consistent with prior research, even though preventive measures were taken to account for the diurnal cycle of cortisol. A review of the literature indicated that most studies of cortisol included multiple samples of saliva throughout the day (Cruess, Antoni, Kumar, & Schneiderman, 2000; Schommer, Hellhammer, & Kirschbaum, 2003; Wetherell et al., 2006).

WHY BOTHER WITH BIOMARKERS?

Considering the small amount of information needed to measure biomarkers such as cortisol, one might ask why this is necessary. Why is it so important to measure physiological changes during the art making process? What can be gleaned from this type of research? As professionals we have made some strides in the design and implementation of evidenced-based research; however, there are no published art therapy studies demonstrating physiological change. This fact alone propelled us to conduct a controlled study examining biomarkers associated with stress and immunity through the collection of a simple, noninvasive saliva sample. In our opinion, research on "stress hormones" or cortisol is relevant to the work we do as art therapists. Prolonged stress can result in elevated cortisol levels, which then become depleted and contribute to further neurochemical changes in the brain. If we can biochemically prove that art-based interventions can decrease cortisol levels to a functional level, think about the implications for the field.

Replication is essential for advancing biomarker research in our field, which is why we include explicit procedures from our pilot study and discuss the limitations of the diurnal cycle. Because of the advancements of this type of research, it is important to stay current and to review similar protocols from different disciplines in developing the procedures for a design. We are currently replicating our own modified protocol, partnering with medical programs associated with George Washington University.

CONCLUSION

The result of our ongoing research has many implications for art therapy practice and research. Overall, the results of the feasibility study provide preliminary support for the hypothesis that coloring a predesigned mandala can reduce levels of anxiety and have a beneficial effect on the immune system for patients with prostate cancer. The use of a cost-effective, noninvasive task such as mandala coloring can be extended to other populations in which stress-reduction or deescalation is warranted. Incorporating the art task of coloring a mandala in an art therapy session can provide the element of relaxation necessary to enhance the therapeutic process. In our experience, conducting evidence-based research promotes the collaboration necessary to position art therapy as a viable option in the medical environment. This pilot study is important to the field of art therapy in that it provides initial evidence that an art task has a beneficial effect on the patient. The research design can be replicated for future studies that include a larger number of participants; the substitution of other art tasks in the research design can provide further information regarding the use of various processes and materials, which are unique to the field of art therapy.

NOTE

The 2006 study was conducted at Eastern Virginia Medical School, Norfolk, Virginia, in collaboration with Dr. Paul Aravich, Professor of Pathology and Anatomy at Eastern Virginia Medical School and an outside PNI specialist, Dr. John Rosecrans, Pharmacology Professor from Virginia Commonwealth University. Dr. Aravich was instrumental in assisting with the research design and provided the research team an understanding of the various physiological systems. Dr. Rosecrans taught a PNI course that John Lorance attended to assist with the review of the literature and to gain further understanding of PNI. Both Aravich and Rosecrans were research committee members. Elizabeth Warson was the primary researcher and John Lorance was the co-researcher. The research protocol was reviewed by Dr. Donald F. Lynch, Professor and Chairman of the Department of Urology of Eastern Virginia Medical School, and participants were recruited through the University of Virginia research department. Additionally, John Lorance met with Dr. Nancy McCain, a PNI researcher from Virginia Commonwealth University.

REFERENCES

Abbas, A. K., & Lichtman, A. H. (2005). *Cellular and molecular immunology* (5th ed.). Philadelphia: Saunders.

Alpers, G. W., Abelson, J. L., Wilhelm, F. H., & Roth, W. T. (2003). Salivary cortisol response during exposure treatment in driving phobics. *Psychosomatic Medicine, 65*(4), 679–687.

Bakke, A., Purtzer, M., & Newton, P. (2002). The effect of hypnotic-guided imagery on psychological well-being and immune function in patients with prior breast cancer. *Journal of Psychosomatic Research, 53*(6), 1131–1137.

Cannon, W. B. (1914). The interrelations of emotions as suggested by recent physiological researches. *American Journal of Psychology, 25*(2), 256–282.

Cohen, J. (1988). *Statistical power analysis for the behavioral sciences* (2nd ed.). Hillsdale, NJ: Erlbaum.

Cohen, N., Ader, R., Green, N., & Bovbjerg, D. (1979). Conditioned suppression of a thymus-independent antibody response. *Psychosomatic Medicine, 41*(6), 487–491.

Cruess, D. G., Antoni, M. H., Kumar, M., & Schneiderman, N. (2000). Reductions in salivary cortisol are associated with mood improvement during relaxation training among HIV-seropositive men. *Journal of Behavioral Medicine, 23*(2), 107–122.

Curry, N. A., & Kasser, T. (2005). Can coloring mandalas reduce anxiety? *Art Therapy: Journal of the American Art Therapy Association, 22*(2), 81–85.

Donaldson, V. (2000). A clinical study of visualization on depressed white blood cell count in medical patients. *Applied Psychophysiology and Biofeedback, 25*(2), 117–128.

Engel, G. (1977). The need for a new medical model: A challenge for biomedicine. *Science, 196*(4286), 129–136.

Fox, S., Shephard, T., & McCain, N. (1999). Neurologic mechanisms in psychoneuroimmunology. *Journal of Neuroscience Nursing, 31*(2), 87–96.

Giedt, J. (1997). Guided imagery: A psychoneuroimmunological intervention in holistic nursing practice. *Journal of Holistic Nursing, 15*(2), 112–127.

Glaser, R., Rice, J., Sheridan, J., Fertel, R., Stout, J., Speicher, C., et al. (1987). Stress-related immune suppression: Health implications. *Brain, Behavior and Immunity, 1*(1), 7–20.

Kabat-Zinn, J. (1990). *Full catastrophe living: Using the wisdom of your body and mind to face stress, pain, and illness.* New York: Delta.

Kolcaba, K., & Fox, C. (1999). The effects of guided imagery on comfort of women with early stage breast cancer undergoing radiation therapy. *Oncology Nursing Forum, 26*(1), 67–72.

Kosslyn, S. M., Ganis, G., & Thompson, W. L. (2001). Neural foundations of imagery. *Nature Reviews Neuroscience, 2*, 635–642.

Leardi, S., Pietroletti, R., Angeloni, G., Necozione, S., Ranalletta, G., & Del Guston, B. (2007). Randomized clinical trial examining the effect of music therapy in stress response to day surgery. *British Journal of Surgery, 94*(8), 943–947.

Maier, S., & Watkins, L. (1998). Cytokines for psychologists: Implications of bidirectional immune-to-brain communication for understanding behavior, mood, and cognition. *Psychological Review, 105*(1), 83–107.

Maier, S., Watkins, L., & Fleshner, M. (1994). Psychoneuroimmunology: The interface between behavior, brain, and immunity. *American Psychologist, 49*(12), 1004–1017.

Mathews, H. L., Starkweather, A., & Witek-Janusek, L. (2005). Applying the psychoneuroimmunology framework to nursing research. *Journal of Neuroscience Nursing, 37*(1), 56–62.

McEwen, B. S. (2004). *The end of stress as we know it*. Washington, DC: Joseph Henry Press.

McKinney, C., Antoni, M., Kumar, M., Tims, F., & McCabe, P. (1997). Effects of guided imagery and music (GIM) therapy on mood and cortisol in healthy adults. *Health Psychology, 16*(4), 390–400.

Metzl, E. S. (2008). Systematic analysis of art therapy research published in *Art Therapy: Journal of AATA* between 1987 and 2004. *The Arts in Psychotherapy, 35*(1), 60–73.

Miles, J., & Gilbert, P. (2005). *A handbook of research methods for clinical and health psychology*. New York: Oxford University Press.

Nater, U., Rohleder, N., Gaab, J., Berger, S., Jud, A., Kirschbaum, C., et al. (2005). Human salivary alpha-amylase reactivity in a psychosocial stress paradigm. *International Journal of Psychophysiology, 55*(3), 333–342.

National Cancer Institute. (n.d.). The prostate-specific antigen (PSA) test: Questions and answers. Retrieved May 3, 2008, from *www.cancer.gov/cancertopics/factsheet/detection/psa*.

Noto, Y., Sato, T., Kudo, M., Kurata, K., & Hirota, K. (2005). The relationship between salivary biomarkers and State–Trait Anxiety Inventory score under mental arithmetic stress: A pilot study. *Anesthesia and Analgesia, 101*(6), 1873–1876.

Rider, M., Achterberg, J., Lawlis, G., Goven, A., Toledo, R., & Butler, J. (1990). Effect of immune system imagery on secretory IgA. *Biofeedback and Self-Regulation, 15*(4), 317–333.

Roffe, L., Schmidt, K., & Ernst, E. (2005). A systematic review of guided imagery as an adjuvant cancer therapy. *Psycho-Oncology, 14*(8), 607–617.

Sapolsky, R. M. (2004). *Why zebras don't get ulcers* (3rd ed.). New York: Times Books.

Schommer, N. C., Hellhammer, D. H., & Kirschbaum, C. (2003). Dissociation between reactivity of the hypothalamus-pituitary-adrenal axis and the sympathetic–adrenal–medullary system to repeated psychosocial stress. *Psychosomatic Medicine, 65*(3), 450–460.

Segerstrom, S., & Miller, G. (2004). Psychological stress and the human immune system: A meta-analytic study of 30 years of inquiry. *Psychological Bulletin, 130*(4), 601–630.

Selye, H. (1956). *The stress of life*. New York: McGraw-Hill.

Sompayrac, L. (2003). *How the immune system works* (2nd ed.). Malden, MA: Blackwell.

Spiegel, D., & Moore, R. (1997). Imagery and hypnosis in the treatment of cancer patients. *Oncology (Williston Park), 11*(8), 1179–1189; discussion 1189–1195.

Spielberger, C. D. (1983). *State–Trait Anxiety Inventory: A comprehensive bibliography*. Palo Alto, CA: Consulting Psychologists Press.

Tortora, G. J., & Grabowski, S. R. (2000). *Principles of anatomy and physiology* (9th ed.). San Francisco: Benjamin Cummings.

Turner-Cobb, J. M., Sephton, S. E., Koopman, C., Blake-Mortimer, J., & Spiegel, D. (2000). Social support and salivary cortisol in women with metastatic breast cancer. *Psychosomatic Medicine, 62*(3), 337–345.

Van Kuiken, D. (2004). A meta-analysis of the effect of guided imagery practice on outcomes. *Journal of Holistic Nursing, 22*(2), 164–179.

Vedhara, K., & Wetherell, M. A. (2005). The measurement of physiological outcomes in health and clinical psychology. In J. Miles & P. Gilbert (Eds.), *A handbook of research methods for clinical and health psychology* (pp. 47–63). New York: Oxford University Press.

Wetherell, M. A., Crown, A. L., Lightman, S. L., Miles, J. N. V., Kaye, J., & Vedhara, K. (2006). The four-dimensional stress test: Psychological, sympathetic–adrenal–medullary, parasympathetic and hypothalamic–pituitary–adrenal responses following inhalation of 35% CO_2. *Psychoneuroendocrinology, 31*(6), 736–747.

Appendix

This final section of the book provides additional resources and information on art therapy and health care, including relevant organizations, ethical issues, cultural considerations, and art materials, safety, and infection control.

ETHICAL STANDARDS

Like other mental health professions, the field of art therapy has developed a specific set of ethical standards for practitioners. Art therapy codes of ethics generally reflect ethical areas common to counseling and psychology, such as patient welfare, confidentiality, research, and professional character and behavior. The role of art making in therapy poses unique ethical dilemmas and concerns for the therapist, and all therapists should be cognizant of these in introducing art to therapy. The most important of these include the following:

- *Confidentiality.* Art expressions must be recognized as confidential communications, just as verbal statements or videotapes are. Permission to display, exhibit, publish, or share art expressions must be obtained from either the client or, in the case of a child, the parent or guardian. If a client agrees to display of art expressions in any form, the therapist must be careful to consider if this is in the best interest of the client, based on the context and relevant factors in the client's treatment or status. Art therapists generally agree that the client's identity must be protected; this may include disguising any signatures or information found on the art product before displaying, publishing it, or sharing it in clinical or educational settings.

Art therapy in hospitals presents some unique challenges for confidentiality. While all art therapists and health care professionals follow rules set forth by their facilities and the Health Insurance and Portability and Accountability Act (HIPAA), they also provide services in settings that range from public waiting rooms and shared hospital rooms where complete confidentiality is often difficult at best. As described in Chapter 23, many patients want to show their artwork created while in a hospital, clinic, or other health care facility, so special attention to the ethical limitations of patient art exhibitions must be thoroughly considered before the artwork is shown. At the same time, art therapists are also cognizant of patients' needs and welfare and the important psychosocially curative factors inherent in sharing creative work with others.

- *Ownership.* Most art therapists believe that the client—the art maker—owns the art created in art therapy. In most cases, there is no question about this ownership. Art therapists generally keep cases notes on artwork created in therapy and only make photocopies, photographs, or digital images of client work solely for record-keeping purposes.

However, in cases in which there is an indication of suicide, harm to others, or possible physical or sexual abuse, for the patient's well-being, it is necessary for the therapist to retain art expressions. In work with various patient populations who are encountered in hospitals and clinics, art therapists often work with children and adults who may have experienced harm or express the intent to harm themselves or others. In these cases, art expressions are treated similarly to medical records that are retained in the patient's file for an extended period.

- *Digital Technology.* Like other mental health and health care professions, art therapists working in health care settings are concerned about the impact of digital technology on the confidentiality, storage, ownership, and electronic transmission of records and images. Currently, the field of art therapy has no definitive answers for these ethical dilemmas but is actively discussing issues inherent to emergent technologies, telemedicine, and healthcare laws for record keeping and electronic communications. Medical art therapists in particular are increasingly using digital technology as a platform for art making with patients, particularly children and adolescents (See Chapter 7 for more information). For example, when using hand-held technology, such as an iPad or digital camera, that is used by multiple patients for drawing, art therapists encounter unique situations involving confidentiality and secure storage of images.

The ethical standards mentioned in this section and others continue to be revised, and practitioners are advised to regularly consult professional ethical codes, HIPAA, and policies at their hospital or health care facility for more information. For a copy of the current *Code of Professional Practice* for art therapists, please contact:

Art Therapy Credentials Board, Inc.
www.atcb.org
3 Terrace Way
Greensboro, NC 27403-3660
Phone (Toll free): 877-213-2822
Phone: 336-482-2856
FAX: 336-482-2852
Email: *atcb@appnbcc.org*

CULTURAL CONSIDERATIONS FOR ART THERAPY IN HEALTH CARE SETTINGS

The topic of cultural sensitivity in art therapy includes not only attention to ethnicity but also degree of acculturation, environment, regionalization, family, extended family and peers, socioeconomic status, gender, disability, development, and religious or spiritual affiliations. Because it is such a broad topic, readers are referred to existing literature on art therapy and cultural issues for more information. Also art therapists who work in health care settings, like their professional counterparts in allied health and medicine, endeavor to provide service to others in a respectful, culturally sensitive manner and seek to increase their understanding of clients' worldviews through supervision, education, and self-evaluation of personal values and beliefs.

In regard to specific applications of art therapy with individuals who are coping with illness or disabilities, helping professionals using any creative methods in therapy consider how individuals appraise these methods, including biological, psychological, social, spiritual/religious, and cultural perspectives. They also include any developmental aspects and individuals' personal preferences for creative expression through art because diversity and worldview influence how adults and children perceive art materials and any associated props or toys offered. Helping professionals should have art media that are adaptable to various cultures, including clays and drawing materials in a range of tones that approximate different skin colors. Photo collage materials should reflect a variety of cross-cultural images, including ethnicity, families, lifestyles, and beliefs. Craft materials such as fabric, yarn, beads, and other objects may be helpful in stimulating individuals whose experience with art evolved around fabric decoration, jewelry making, or traditional arts.

In medical settings, art therapists are sensitive to cultural beliefs that influence patients' perceptions about illness and medical treatment. While all health care professionals involved in patients' welfare carefully consider their patients' values, art therapists specifically formulate psychosocial treatment plans with patients' cultural preferences and worldviews in mind. In the case of pediatric patients, this may also include the preferences and worldviews of parents, siblings, and extended family and community. Additionally, patients and families may have differing perceptions about how art therapy "works" or if it works. They may hold strong beliefs about art making that may or may not include its application as "healing" agent or may value specific practices that resonate with healing practices within their own culture or community.

Best practices for art therapy regarding cultural sensitivity in health care settings have yet to be sufficiently explored and defined. As art therapy with various patient populations continues to expand, practitioners are learning more about diversity, perceptions of how art therapy works, and personal as well as universal aspects of art expression for health and well-being (see the Resources section for more information on international art therapy organizations and arts in health care groups).

ART MATERIALS AND MEDICAL SETTINGS: SAFETY AND INFECTION CONTROL

Art therapy in medical settings presents some unique aspects regarding preparation and use of art materials with patients. For example, infection control is a high priority in hospitals. Art materials must meet standards for infection prevention when presented, for example, to children and adults whose immune systems are compromised. Organic materials such as many forms of clay and wooden brushes are contraindicated; in most cases, only new, unused art materials can be provided to patients in protective isolation and are left with the patient if they cannot be effectively sterilized after use. Sand for sand therapy or sand play may be autoclaved; certain tools and toys used in art therapy may also be sterilized with an autoclave.

Art therapists working with individuals in bone marrow transplant units, intensive care, burn units, or other settings that require patient isolation should consult with infection control specialists at the hospital or clinic in order to determine what materials are appropriate and safe for patients in restrictive environments. Additionally, there are a variety of helpful guides and standards for safety regarding art materials, including, but not limited to, the following resources:

Art and Craft Safety Guide, available from the U.S. Consumer Product Safety Commission, 4330 East West Highway, Bethesda, MD 20814, or at *www.cpsc.gov/cpscpub/pubs/art.html*.
Environmental Health and Toxicology Information Services, U.S. Department of Health and Human Service, Enviro-Health Links at *http://sis.nlm.nih.gov/enviro/arthazards.html*; free downloadable guides and information on arts and crafts materials.

RESOURCES

The following information is provided to help readers locate more information on art therapy, arts in health care, and art therapy organizations around the world. Because this information is time sensitive, updated information and links can be found at the International Art Therapy Organization at *www.internationalarttherapy.org*.

Art Therapy Networking

Art Therapy Alliance
www.arttherapyalliance.org

Art Therapy Without Borders
www.atwb.org

International Art Therapy Organization
www.internationalarttherapy.org

Arts in Health Care Organizations

Foundation for Art and Healing
77 Stearns Road
Brookline, MA 02446-6609
www.artandhealing.org

Society for the Arts in Healthcare
2647 Connecticut Avenue, NW
Suite 200
Washington, DC 20008
Phone: 202-299-9770
www.thesah.org/template/index.cfm

Foundation for Hospital Arts
4238 Highborne Drive
Marietta, GA 30066
Phone: 678-324-1705
www.hospitalart.com/about_us.html

Art Therapy Organizations

American Art Therapy Association
225 North Fairfax Street
Alexandria, VA 22314
Phone: 888-290-0878
www.arttherapy.org

Association des art-thérapeutes du Québec
57 Avenue Monkland
Montreal, Quebec H4A 1E9, Canada
www.aatq.org

Australian and New Zealand Art Therapy Association
www.anzata.org

British Association of Art Therapists
24-27 White Lion Street
London N1 9PD, United Kingdom
Phone: 020-7686-4216
www.baat.org

British Columbia Art Therapy Association
www.bcarttherapy.com

Canadian Art Therapy Association
www.catainfo.ca

Ontario Art Therapy Association
www.oata.ca

Chilean Art Therapy Association
www.arteterapiachile.cl/portal/index.php

Argentina Art Therapy Association
www.asoarteterapia.org.ar

Brazil Art Therapy Associations
Brazil: *www.arteeterapia.com.br*
Sao Paulo: *www.aatesp.com.br*
Rio Grande do Sul: *www.aatergs.com.br*

Art Therapy Italiana
www.arttherapyit.org/2009/art09_home.php

Association of Professional Art Therapists in Spain
www.arteterapia.org.es

Northern Ireland Group for Art as Therapy
www.nigat.org

German Art Therapy
www.dgkt.de/frameset.htm

Swedish National Association of Art Therapists
www.bildterapi.se/in-english.html

Israeli Association of Creative and Expressive Therapies
www.yahat.org

Hong Kong Association of Art Therapists
www.hk-hkaat.org

Taiwan Art Therapy Association
www.arttherapy.org.tw/about_en.php

Index